# Creative News Photography

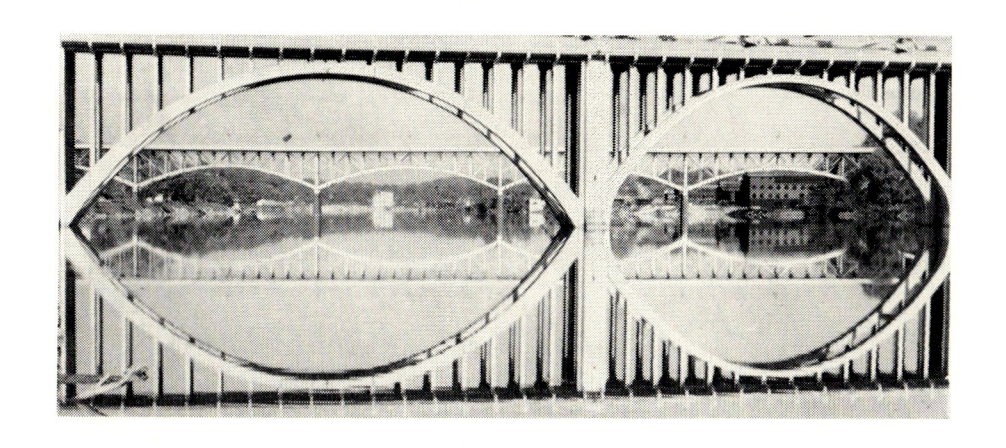

RODNEY FOX
ROBERT KERNS

© 1961 The Iowa State University Press
Ames, Iowa, U.S.A. All rights reserved

Composed and printed by
The Iowa State University Press

First edition, 1961
*Second printing, 1967*
*Third printing, 1969*

Standard Book Number: 8138-0370-5
Library of Congress Catalog Card Number: 61-10551

# The Authors

**RODNEY FOX** is co-author of **1000 Ideas for Better News Pictures** (Iowa State University Press, 1957) and author of **Agricultural and Technical Journalism** (Prentice-Hall, 1952). His photographs of Midwestern scenes appear frequently in the **Iowan** magazine. Professor of journalism at Iowa State University, he firmly believes that news photography not only can be, but should be creative. His classes are planned to instill this belief in his many students. Before devoting his talents to teaching and research, Fox was a working journalist on the staffs of the **Des Moines Register**, the **Mason City (Iowa) Globe-Gazette**, the **Iowa Falls (Iowa) Citizen**, and the **Sandy (Ore.) Post**.

**ROBERT KERNS** has been a consistent winner of state and national photo competitions, including NPPA, IPPA, and Inland Daily Press Association. He won the Don Christiansen Memorial Award for the best Iowa newsphoto of the year in 1959. Since his graduation in 1956 from the State University of Iowa, where he was a top flight campus photographer, he has chalked up an impressive record of creative news photography. He has worked on the pictorial staffs of the **Davenport (Iowa) Morning Democrat** and the **Cedar Rapids (Iowa) Gazette**, where he served as picture editor before becoming a photojournalist for the Goodyear Tire and Rubber Co.

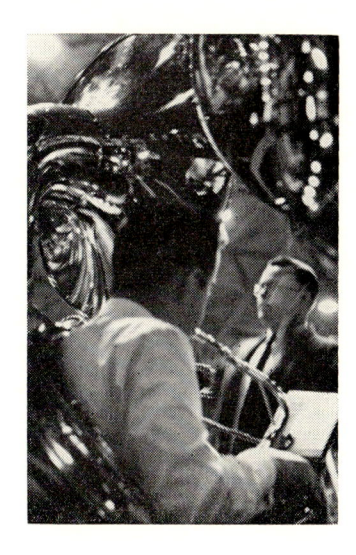

# This book is based on the belief...

... that photography can perform a vastly more important function than it now does in the communication of news, information and ideas.

Although in some publications photographs are used with magnificent effectiveness and in a great many papers play a vital and carefully planned part, pictures in newspapers and small magazines in general can be made to do much more than they do.

With today's communication increasingly in the form of television, radio, moving pictures and recorded words and sounds, it is essential that every available device be used to make the printed media as attractive and easily comprehended as their competitors. This is essential for their economic survival as well as for reasons of effectively discharging their responsibilities of providing information so basic to the continuance of a democratic society.

Pictorial presentations that range from comics to dignified and impressive books in such scholarly fields as history have demonstrated their abilities to attract readership and sales. Picture magazines have become enormously popular. Surveys consistently show the pulling power of news pictures, cartoons, comic strips. Advertising uses pictures lavishly. Promotional booklets, mailing pieces, funds solicitation appeals — all have turned increasingly to pictorial methods.

But in spite of all of these demonstrations of the worthiness of pictures in today's communication world, large segments of the press continue to be inadequately and ineffectively illustrated. Pictures are too few, too small and they tend to be of superficial subject matter while neglecting the magnificent materials that exist everywhere. Whether they depict shallow subjects or significant ones, photographs in much of the press tend to record objects and situations unimaginatively. Not many papers fully utilize opportunities to intensify feelings and meanings that can be conveyed by pictures through use of intelligent application of some knowledge of pictorial composition.

Even in some metropolitan newspapers and in some slick magazines and house organs, highly competent photographs follow a formula so closely that every issue looks as if it had exactly the same pictures as the preceding one, leaving readers with the feeling that they have seen all this before.

It makes little difference whether the

blame for this lag on the part of many publications to use fully the miracle of pictures should be placed against publishers not yet converted enough to provide sufficient funds for photography, against editors too stubborn to break away from tradition and habit, against unimaginative photographers or against the inadequacy of schools of journalism charged with training newsmen. The important thing now is that as full and effective as possible use of pictures be made in the greater part of the printed media.

These chapters are intended to help editors and photographers in their efforts to improve the pictorial contents of their publications, especially those without art departments or trained pictorial experts.

Main contentions in this book are that:

1. With Americans steadily demonstrating their delight in television and other forms of pictorial presentation, newspapers and other printed publications will do well to use more and better photographs;
2. Opportunities exist in almost every news situation for taking something better than routine record pictures;
3. Digging deeply into a news situation can reveal wonderful opportunities for interpretative reporting in depth *in pictures*;
4. Pictures possess the potential for delivering a considerable emotional impact *in addition to* that provided by subject matter, an impact available through good planning and organization of the elements within the pictures.

Achievement of increasingly effective results with photography has been made easier because of the magnificent improvements in cameras and photographic materials, advances that resulted from research. Use of research also has contributed much to what is known about pictorial composition, has demonstrated the popularity of pictures and has helped in the understanding of some problems of news values. But as yet, researchers are struggling to find answers to myriads of questions that perplex editors and photographers. This suggests the need for continuing research in this difficult field. It also indicates that here is an area in which effective results must depend on good sense and intuition combined with use of the fragments of solid information produced by scientific studies.

Obviously, much of the content of this book is not made up of facts revealed by research and so, it is hoped, will be considered only as stimulating suggestion. Certain ideas advanced are sure to be rejected by some editors and photographers, in some cases with a degree of violence. But even the process involved in considering an idea and refusing it can be stimulating.

The authors wish to thank the many individuals and publications who have contributed pictures, information and help. Special thanks are due to J. Winton Lemen, manager, Photo-Press Sales Division of Eastman Kodak Company, for his help with the chapter on ROP Color; to David E. Archie, publisher and editor of *The Iowan* and to the *Rochester* (N.Y.) *Times-Union* who provided use of the color plates; and the *Davenport* (Iowa) *Democrat* and the *Cedar Rapids* (Iowa) *Gazette* for permission to publish many pictures from those newspapers. All pictures in this book used without credit lines were taken by Robert Kerns, and most of them have appeared in the *Gazette* or *Democrat*.

RODNEY FOX
ROBERT KERNS

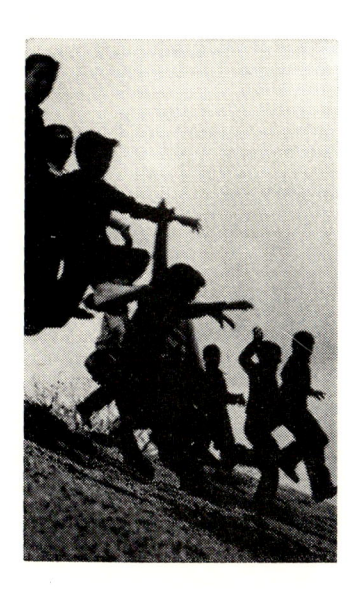

# Contents

**Part 1**
*MORE PICTURES... MORE CIRCULATION... MORE PRESTIGE*
1. Pictures – the Key to Reader Attention, 11
2. Subject Matter Is Most Important Factor, 17
3. Depth Reporting With Pictures, 31
4. Picture Stories, Essays and Layouts, 35
5. Agricultural Revolution Deserves Intensive Photo Coverage, 41
6. Women's Page Pictures Attract Readers, Delight Advertisers, 48
7. Winning Readers With Pictures of Leisure-Time Fun, 55
8. Pictures To Lure Young Readers, 64

**Part II**
*HOW PICTORIAL ORGANIZATION INCREASES APPEAL*
9. The "Organized" Picture, Does It Really Pay? 77
10. Balance Makes Pictures Look Comfortable, 80
11. Shapes, Lines and Curves As Picture Elements, 89
12. Repetition, Rhythm and Pattern Give Pleasure, 99
13. Texture Brings Fun of Touch to Pictures, 105
14. Tone Values and the Magic of Light, 111

**Part III**
*PRACTICAL PHOTO PROBLEMS REQUIRE PRACTICAL SOLUTIONS*
15. ROP Brightens America's Newspapers, 121
16. How To Load Pictures With Action, 131
17. Good Portraits Tell a Story, 140
18. Variety Is the Spice of Group Pictures, 148
19. Cutlines Help Pictures Tell Their Stories, 156
20. Don't Be Niggardly About Picture Size, 163
21. Retouching Can Save Many Pictures, 167
22. Creative Imagination, 172

Other Books You Might Want To Read, 188

Index, 189

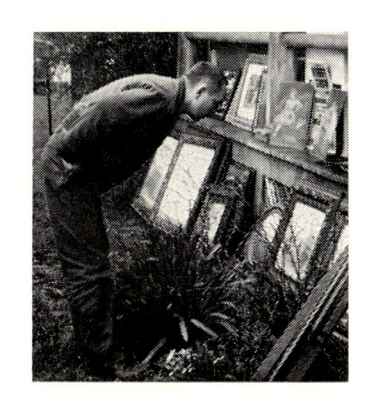

PART 1

More Pictures...More Circulation...More Prestige

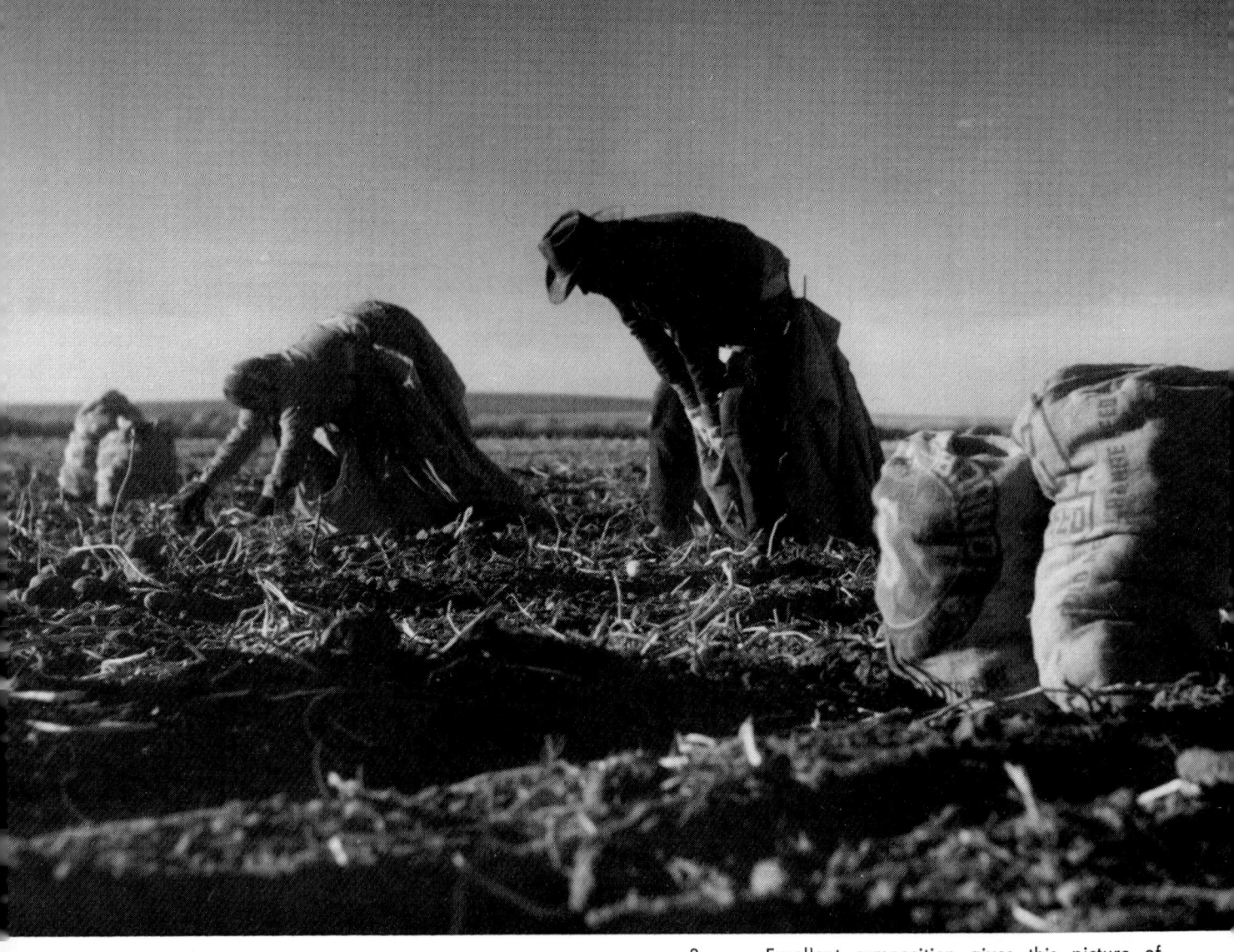

2   Excellent composition gives this picture of field workers some of the qualities of a masterpiece painting. Notice repetition with variation in figures and sacks. (See Chapter 11)

*Bob Woody in Burley (Idaho)* Herald — Bulletin

CHAPTER 1

# Pictures—the Key To Reader Attention

EXCELLENT LOCAL PHOTOGRAPHIC COVERAGE unquestionably is one of the big answers to the intense need of printed news media to maintain circulation, readership and prestige in an era characterized by fierce competition for the time and attention of readers.

Americans have demonstrated their delight in pictures by going to quantities of movies for a half century, by buying vast numbers of picture magazines for over 25 years and by attaching themselves by the millions to television sets for more than a decade.

Now seems the time for more newspapers, house organs and magazines to realize that if they can't lick this mounting tide of pictorial communication, they had better join it. Publications already using pictures extensively and competently are well aware that they constantly must seek means to increase photographic effectiveness. They recognize that they are involved in a bitter and never-ending war.

That pictures today are an essential method for presenting information and ideas to people is largely accepted by those who produce brochures, annual reports and promotional literature for industry and institutions. Presentations of that sort have turned to extensive use of pictures to "sell" ideas, as advertising has long done in its effective efforts to sell both commodities and ideas.

All publications striving to improve their picture coverage today enjoy simplified production problems because of the enormously improved cameras, photographic materials and engraving processes available. With the mechanics of photography becoming constantly simpler and better, photographers can more easily and quickly become technically competent and then apply their energies to planning pictures and solving the problems of what to take and how to do so.

### Help Available for Improvements

These problems of what pictures to take and how most effectively to plan them must be worked out by each publication against the background of its special needs and situations. But, for help, editors and photographers can investigate the successful achievement of others and turn to the results of research when available. Active imaginations

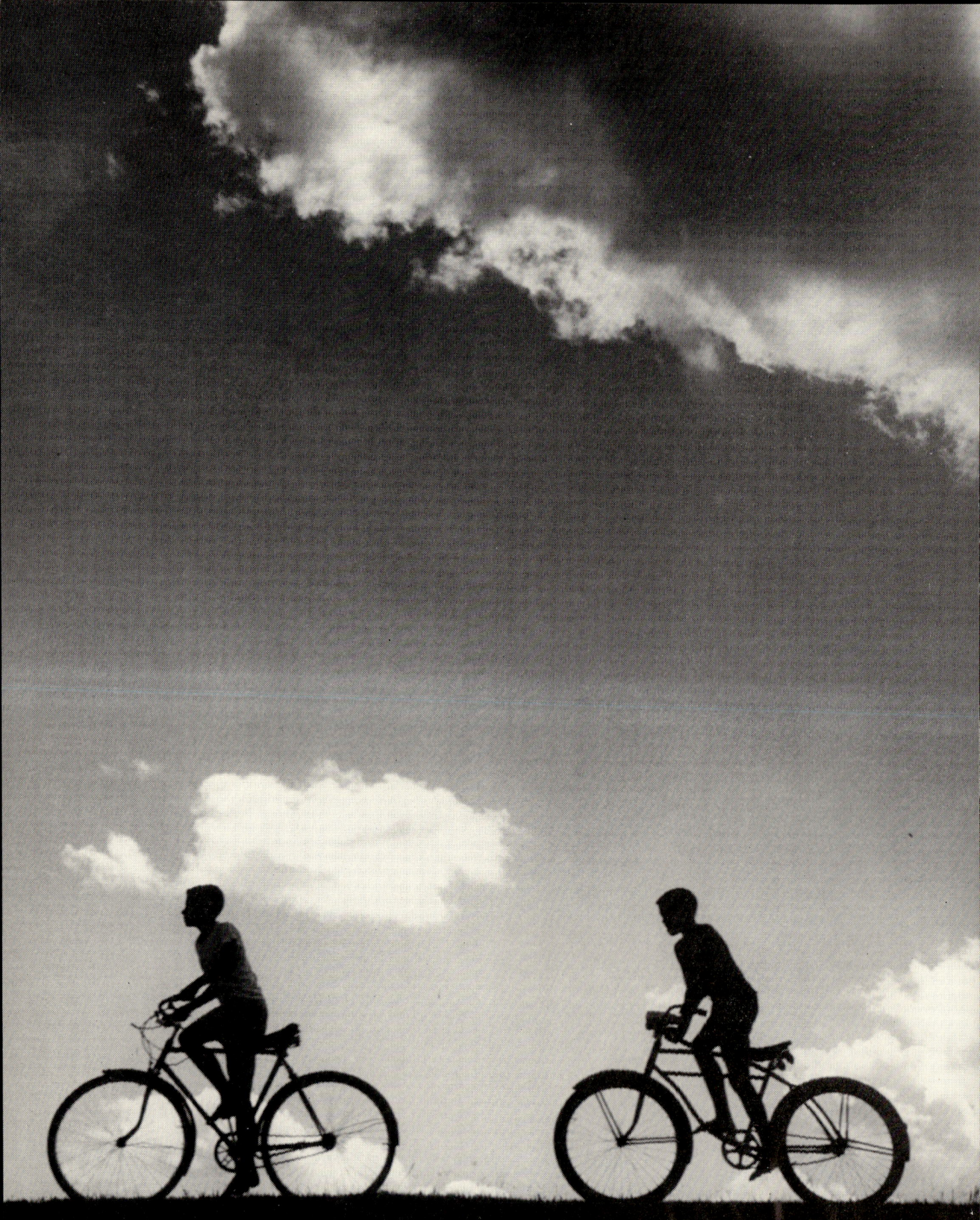

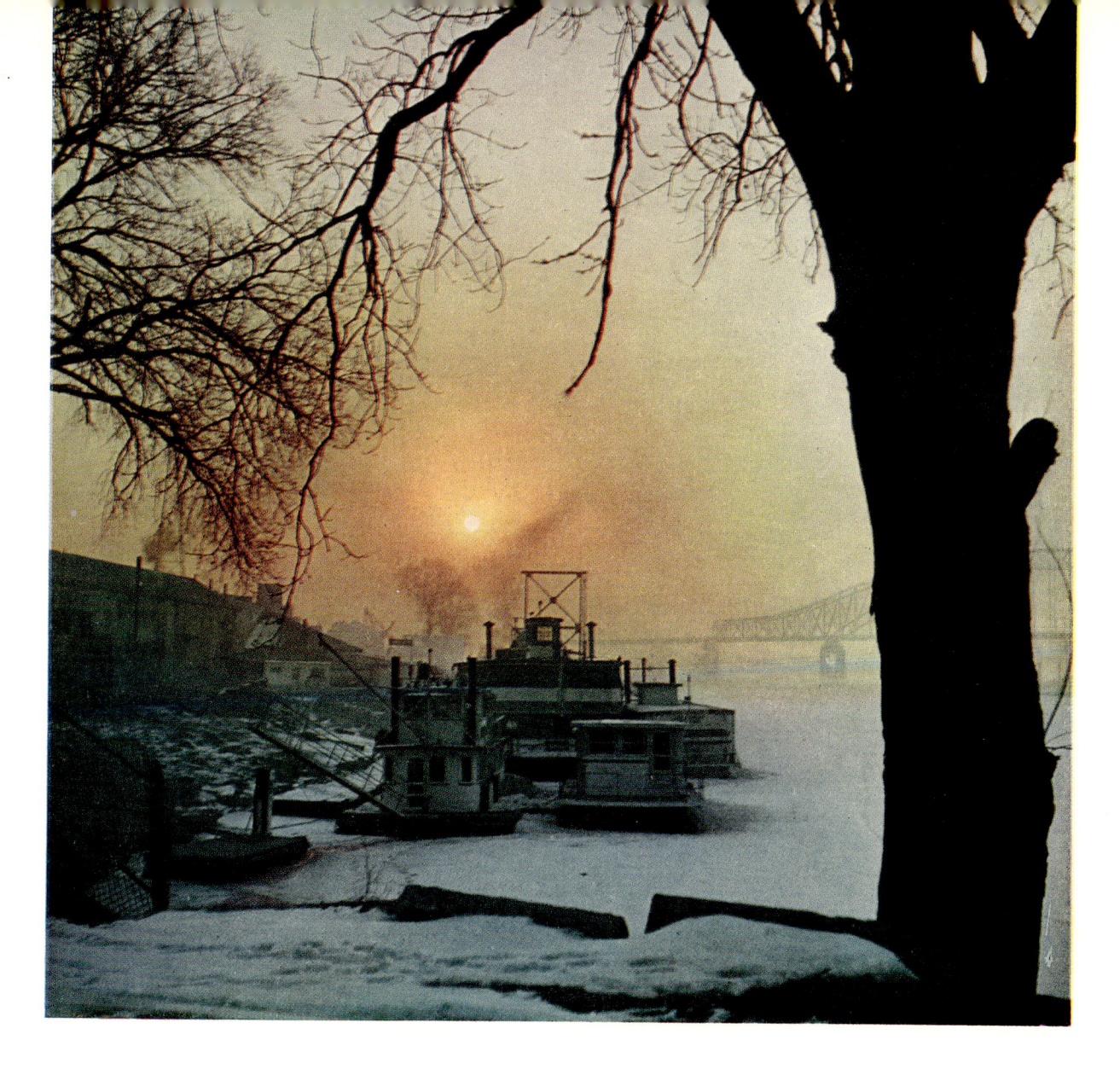

4   Many people enjoy scenes reminiscent of the past. *Bert Vogel in* The Iowan

working with such information can see ways to apply the experience of others, find different applications of current practices, discover combinations and modifications of ideas already in use and, in the process, sometimes hit on new ideas.

Achievement of this better and more extensive pictorial coverage not only should provide a strong asset in building up readership and popularity, but also should help publications discharge their obligations of providing information to readers in a form they will look at, understand, and appreciate.

**Pictures Called Challenge of Decade**

"One of the greatest challenges to the newspapers in the sixties will be in the field of pictorial journalism," declared John J. Colburn, managing editor of the Richmond, Virginia, *Times-Dispatch*.

"Editors will have to do a better job of graphically illustrating the news. That means a better understanding of pictures, maps,

When a picture tells a story of carefree youth on a [su]nny summer day, it's sure to appeal to many readers. [Br]uce Roberts, *staff photographer,* Charlotte *Observer*

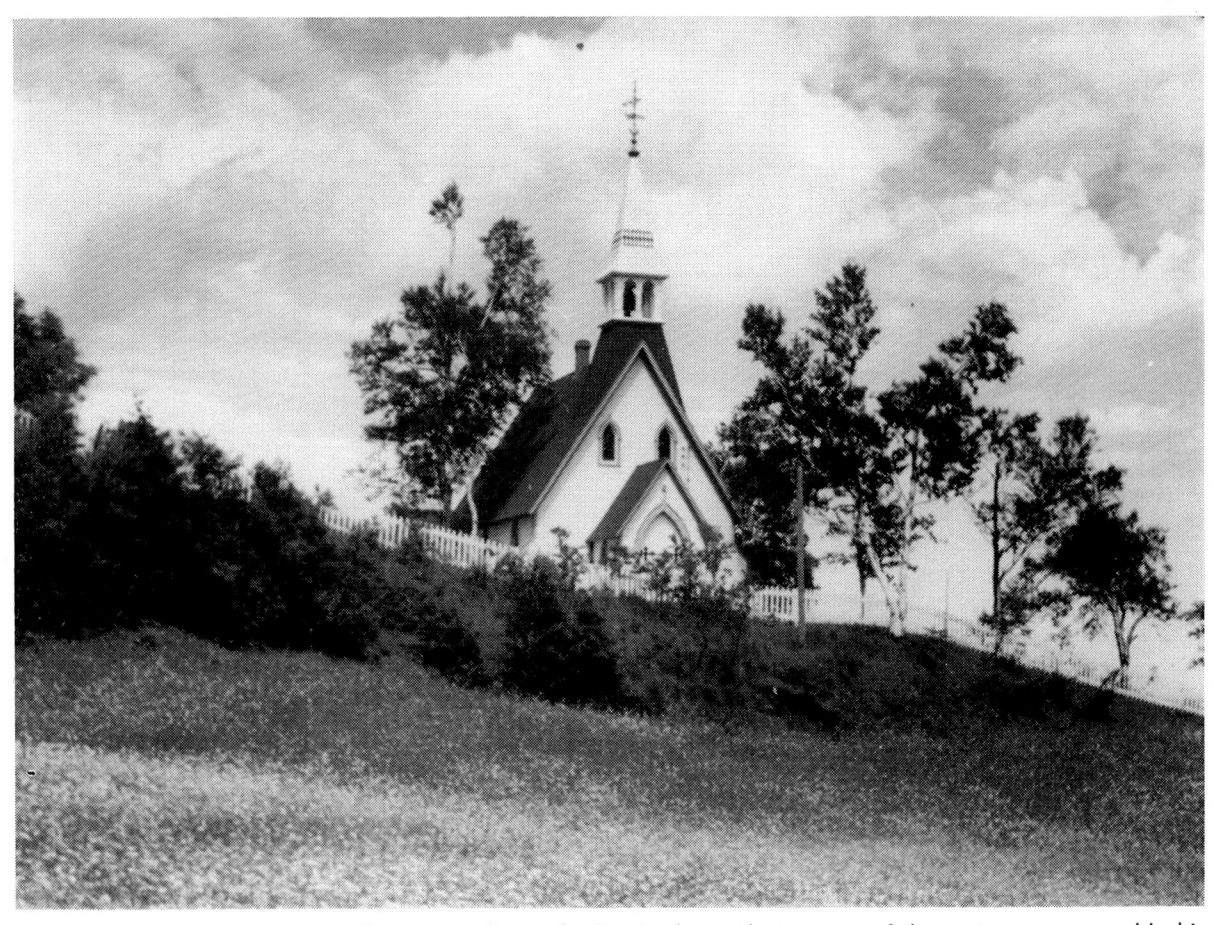

5    To those who live in the strident uproar of the contemporary world, this photograph of peaceful quiet offers escape. To rural residents, it dramatizes the familiar.

*Photo by Tom Merryman*

charts and pictodiagrams. Photographers must become more than mere technicians."[1]

**Pictures Credited for Bigger Circulation**

One publisher of a weekly newspaper has credited roughly half of his circulation to the favorable reception of pictures in his paper. That publisher, Mel H. Ruder of the *Hungry Horse News*, Columbia Falls, Montana, a paper with an ABC circulation of 3,292, wrote, "We are not a county seat town, and I believe if we weren't a picture paper, we'd have about 1,500 circulation. Pictures aren't the whole answer. Our mail brings comments about editorials, country columns, but most of the comment is about pictures."

Another weekly newspaperman calls photographic equipment tools of the profession like typewriters and words. That man, R. O. Burrows, Jr., of the Burrows Publishing Company, which produces good papers in two Iowa towns, declared, "Today's newspapers, whether they are the smallest weeklies or the largest of dailies, are dull listless masses of words without pictures to give them life. The thousands of engraver's dots that form the pictures in modern-day newspapers

---

[1] Colburn, John H., "Pictorial Journalism Is Big Challenge of '60s." *The Quill*, April, 1960.

prompt people to read not only the captions, but the adjoining news stories at a rate unprecedented since Gutenberg invented movable type."

**Pictures Called Cheaper To Run Than Words**

Evidence that extensive picture coverage, with all its advantages, doesn't need to increase costs is contained in the statement that pictures are cheaper to run than words, made by Dick Beecroft of the Bridgeton, New Jersey, *News,* a suburban paper.

"Inch for inch pictures are cheaper than type," Beecroft declared. "It costs less to run them than anything else put in the same space. Not only that, they are good salesmen for your paper. This is especially true on small-town dailies which I've been on for 25 years." [2]

**Pictures Help Sell Advertising**

In addition to building up news, local pictures sell advertising better than anything else, Edmund C. Arnold wrote in *Publishers' Auxiliary.* Arnold said that photographs not only helped sell advertising, but also helped the advertisers sell their merchandise.[3]

**A Quiz To Take**

To test whether your publication is achieving the ultimate benefits from really modern

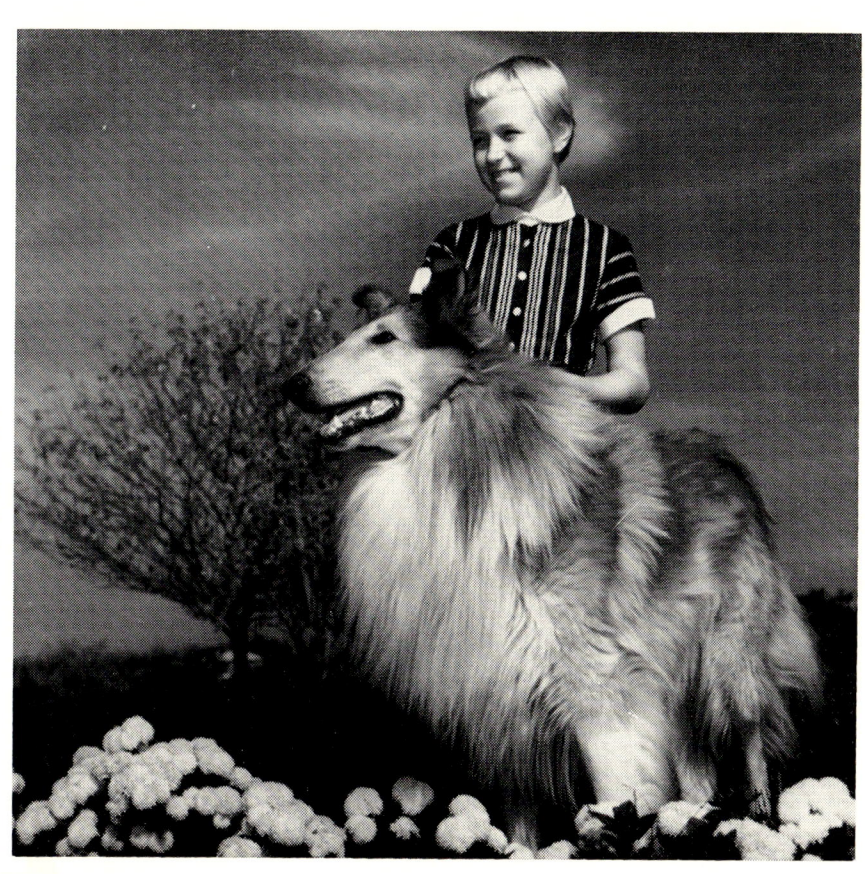

[2] Collings, James L., "Pix Cheaper to Run Than Words: Beecroft," *Editor and Publisher,* Oct. 24, 1959.

[3] Arnold, Edmund G., "*Nothing Sells Like Local Photos,*" *Publishers' Auxiliary,* Nov. 8, 1958.

6  Without such excellent composition and technical quality, this picture of happiness itself might have been just another photograph of a child and a dog.

*A. Martin Herrmann,
The Pittsburgh* Press

— 15

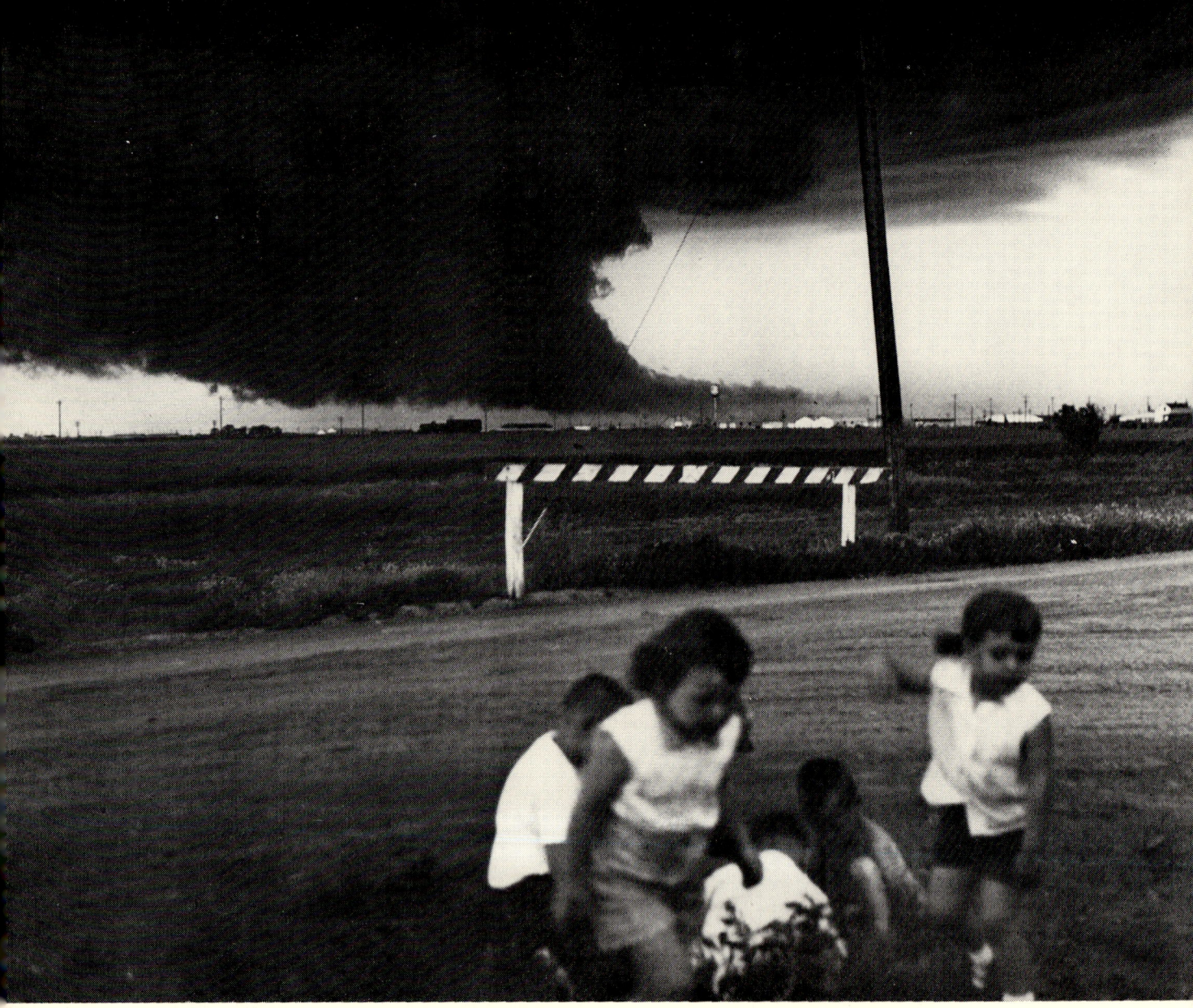

7   Threat of impending death for children gives this picture enormous power.   *Fargo (N. Dak.) Forum by Alf T. Olsen*

photographic coverage, you might ask yourself:

1. Do we use enough pictures?
2. Is the proportion of pictures to word material right for our publication?
3. Do our pictures really add to the story, or do they just fill space?
4. Do we use pictures large enough to be effective?
5. Are we selecting the best possible available subject matter for our readers?
6. Are our pictures planned, cropped and organized to make them as effective as possible?
7. What ideas and practices should we add to what we already are doing to improve the quality of our photographic presentations?
8. How can we escape the monotony that results from a too close adherence to a formula without becoming slaves to another one?

It is hoped the following chapters will provide ideas and information you can use as you work toward answers to these questions. But since no two publications are exactly alike or have the same problems, the answers you reach must be unique.

CHAPTER **2**

# Subject Matter Is Most Important Factor

NOTHING IS SO INTERESTING to most people as people. For the best possible subject matter for news pictures, photograph people.

Human beings are fascinated by themselves, by their mates and children, their neighbors, members of their community, their countrymen, people in faraway places — even by their enemies.

Bigtown newspapers can photograph the people in the day's news, many of them famed or at least prominent, some of them heretofore obscure souls suddenly transformed into newsworthiness by a sudden stroke of luck, trouble or tragedy. Readers welcome pictures of the familiar faces of the famed as though they were of acquaintances, even though that acquaintance is through news pictures only. Toward the obscure person suddenly tossed into the news, the thousands of other obscure ones react with the feeling, "Golly, that might have been me."

In smaller towns where every man — even the least consequential — still is of comparative importance, pictures of local people have enormous punch. In smalltown papers, pictures make news.

The publisher who credits pictures with gaining about half of his circulation, Mel Ruder of the *Hungry Horse News,* said he doubted if a youngster could grow up in his

8   This crowd contains the raw material for the best news photographs in the world, because nothing is so interesting to people as people.

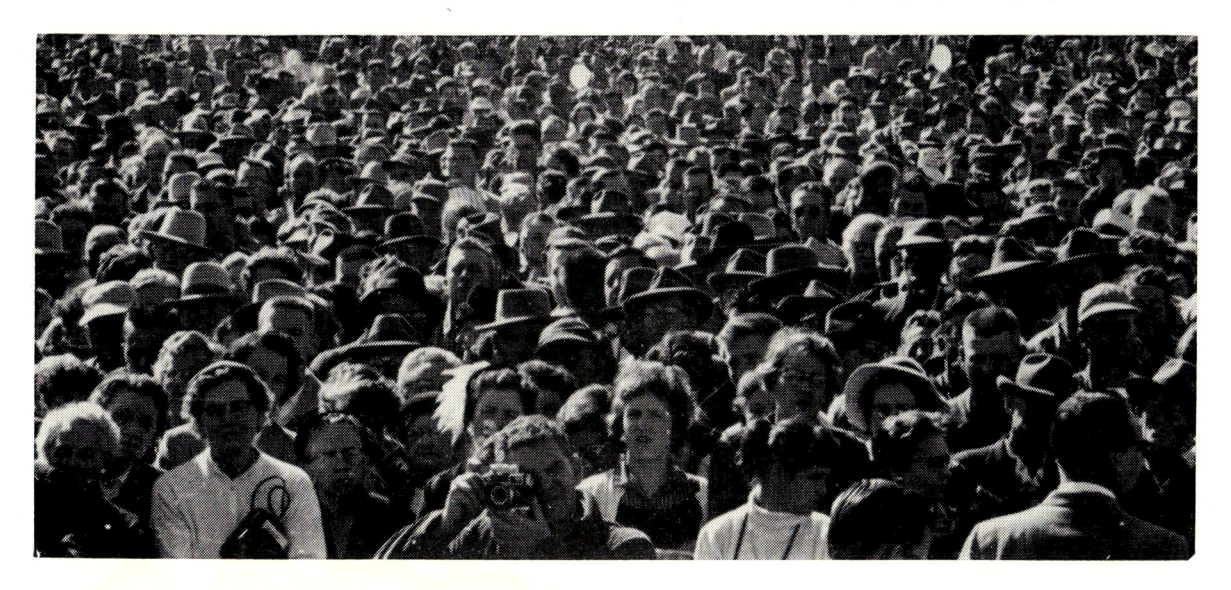

— 17

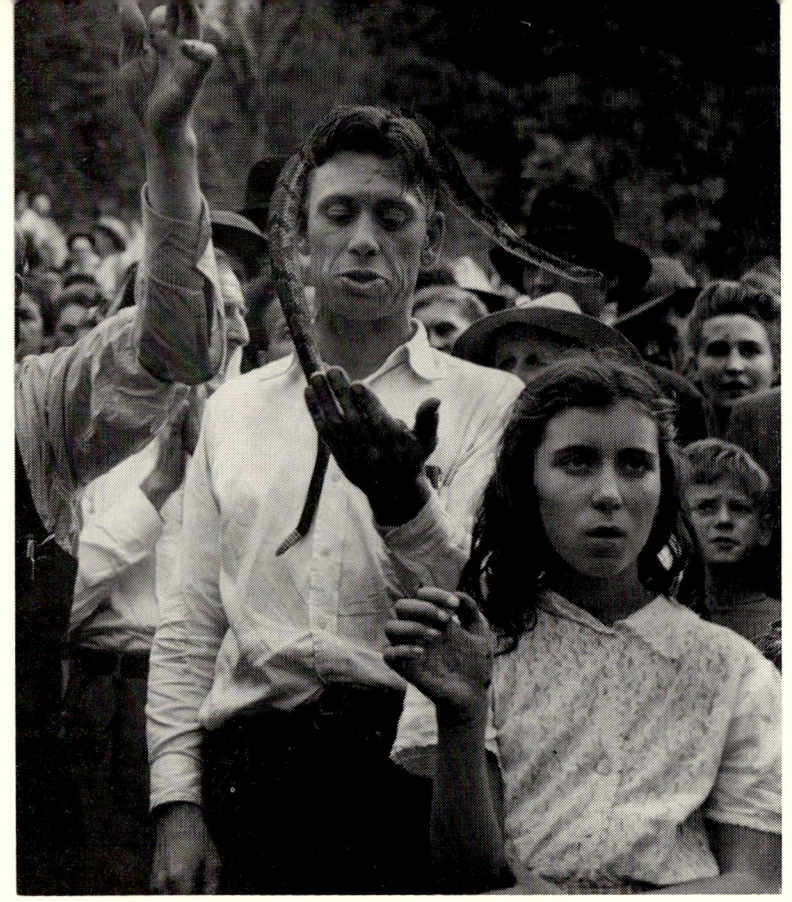

9   People — all people — are intensely interesting.
*The* Courier-Journal *(Louisville, Ky.),*
*Thomas V. Miller, Jr.*

town without having his picture in the local paper at least three or four times. While taking a picture in the seventh grade room, the publisher asked for a show of hands of how many had been pictured in his paper previously. Something like 75 per cent had, as tots with Santa Claus, while getting polio shots, at Cub Scout award nights, at junior bowling banquets or for some other reason.

10   But a pretty young woman is the most charming kind of person to picture.
*L. W. Ward*

**Why Are Some Pictures Superior?**

Just as obvious as the interest of people in people is the fact that some pictures of people have much greater newsworthiness than do others. What situations involving people make the best news pictures? Research has provided some answers to this question, but much still remains to be proved. Until full scientific proof is available, editors and photographers will have to continue to rely on accumulated lore, good sense and such evidence as research has provided.

Potentially most powerful news situations, probably, are those that have to do with hu-

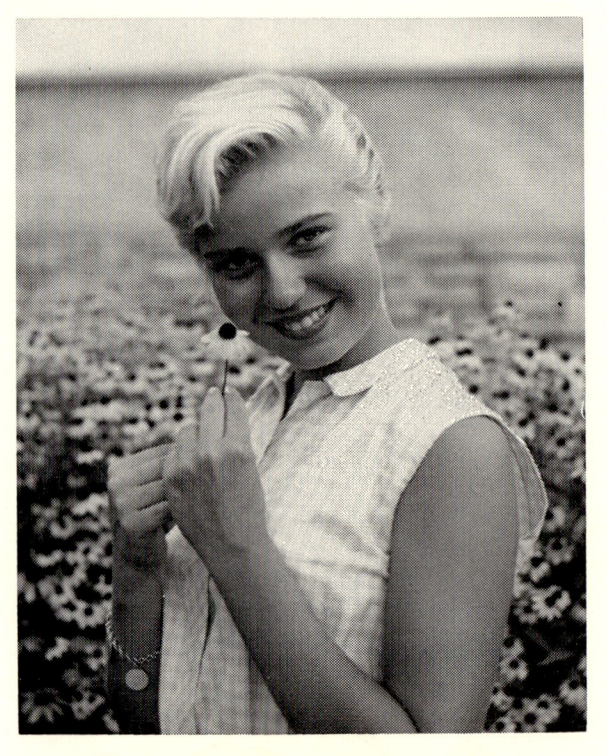

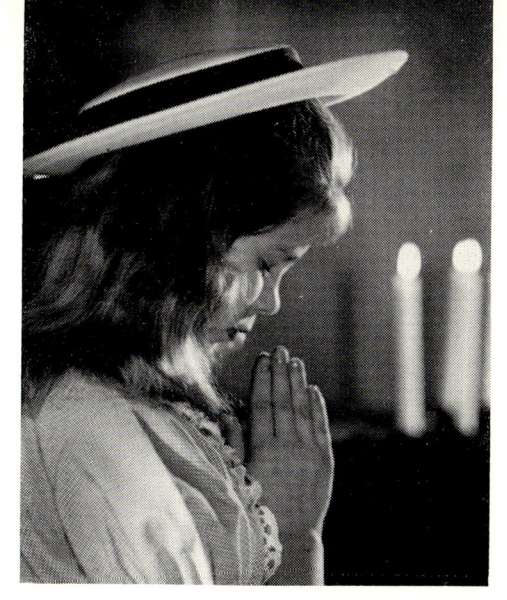

11 Except, perhaps, a good and pretty little girl.

Frontier Enterprise, *Lake Zurich, Ill., Joyce L. Klug, publisher, (Photo by Safranek)*

man survival, with life and death. So violent are the reactions inspired by pictures of this sort that often they must be handled with restraint or left out. Too vivid a portrayal of death with its attendant horrors can easily be overwhelming and revolting. But pictures that have to do with rescues and escapes and dangerous situations and with health contain this strong appeal, attached to the desire of men, in common with all living things, to survive.[1]

[1] The idea that news value of pictures is based on four elemental human themes of survival, sex, ambition and escape was advanced by Laura Vitray, John Mills, Jr., and Roscoe Ellard in *Pictorial Journalism*, McGraw-Hill, New York, 1939.

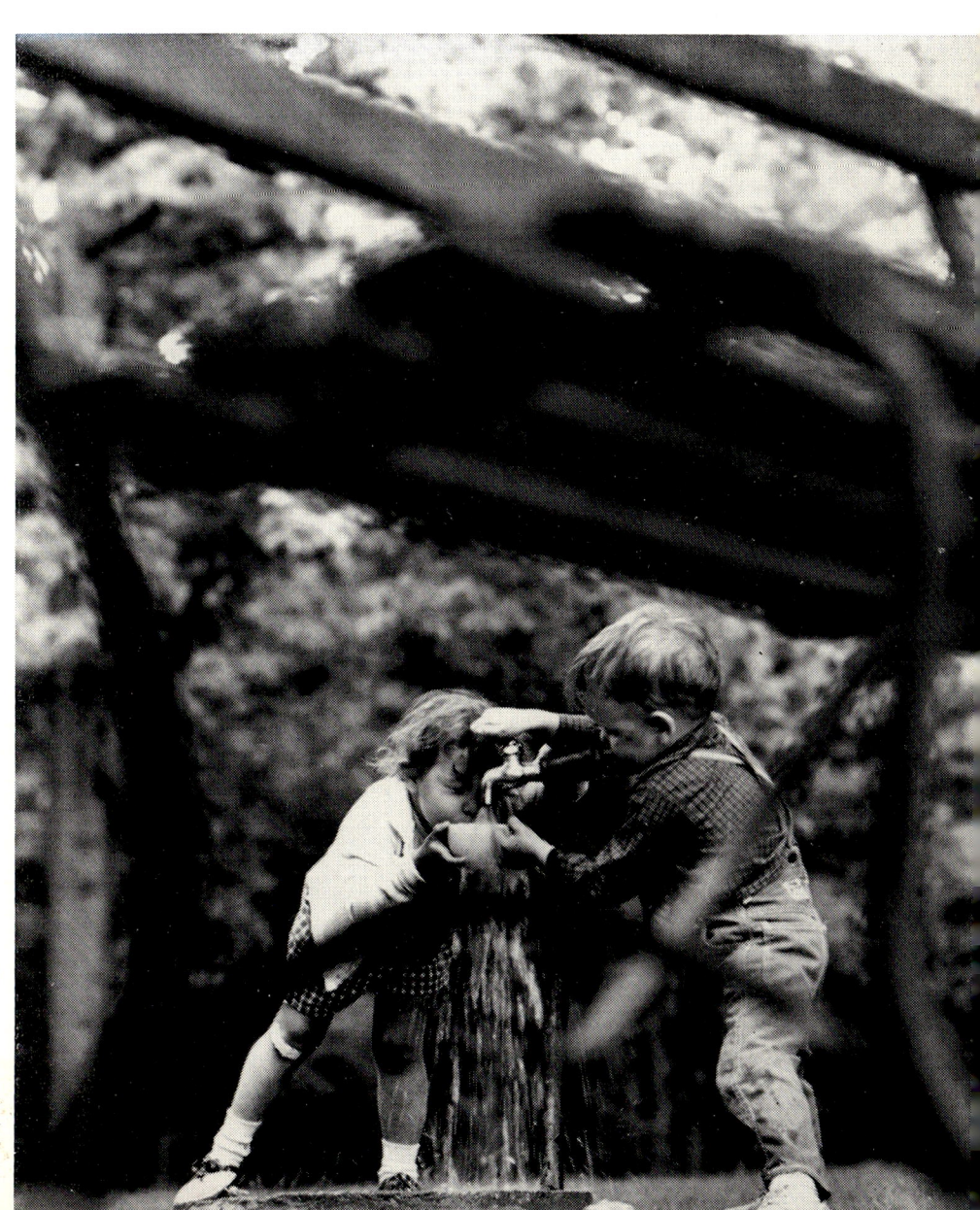

12 Or maybe a little boy and girl can be twice as charming as one child.

*Dale Stierman, chief photographer, Dubuque (Iowa)* Telegraph-Herald

### Sex and News Pictures

Obviously and without question, one of the great basic urges that results in the interest of people is sex. It can be argued, of course, that sex is only an aspect of the urge for survival, an expression of the long-range desire of all species for continuance.

Although a part of the newspaper and magazine press has exploited lurid aspects of sex until much criticism of journalism has resulted, the fact remains that its powerful appeal can be utilized tellingly within the confines of what is generally accepted as good taste in conservative, family-style publications.

After all, sex can't be ignored in a paper that makes any pretense of picturing life realistically. For in its broadest aspects, sex explains most of human affections, including the tenderness most people feel toward children and toward gray-haired elderly people who stand as parent images, even the love of pets who serve as child substitutes. Sex has vastly broader implications than these, and although much of the field at present is taboo for general publications, some sound knowledge of the findings of science about sex can be of great help to editors and photographers who want to do an intelligent and compassionate job of covering many stories.

Because of the intensity of interest in sex and because it is entangled in laws, mores and religious beliefs, obviously pictures that involve it to any considerable degree must be handled with the greatest discretion and understanding.

Since to ban all pictures with at least some sex implications would mean eliminating almost all news pictures, each publication must find its own answers to the problems set up by the intense appeal of sex versus the restrictions and taboos placed around it. Answers to these problems reached by a conservative rural weekly and by a metropolitan tabloid obviously will be quite different. The pictures that sell a "girlie" magazine would wreck a family newspaper.

When a strong social conscience rather than business exigencies determines how materials strongly involving sex shall be edited, two seemingly opposed results probably follow: Greater restraint is applied to some matters; and some materials now generally considered taboo are published.

### Photographers Can Exploit Ambition

Human beings find satisfaction of deep urges in pictures of other human beings because such pictures help the individual establish for himself his position in society. Most everyone is eager to know where he stands in his group and in society in general, is desirous of feeling that he is at least equal to and preferably superior to others.

Pictures can provide a temporary satisfaction of ambition for a viewer by permitting him to enjoy vicariously the prestige of the successful character pictured. Photographs of presidents and movie actors and heroes on parade provide this momentary fulfillment for millions. The picture of a high school football player may do the same thing for a younger boy; or the society page picture of a hostess pouring tea may do it for a socially ambitious woman; or the picture of a newly elected company president may do it for a business man.

If an individual can find satisfaction of his ambitions by imagining for a moment that he is the successful person pictured, certainly his delight must be vastly deeper when he sees himself or a member of his family, or even a member of his social group, pictured in a success role. Such pictures not only help measure prestige but also help build it.

Opportunities for news photographers to utilize successfully at the local level the normal, almost universal surge of human ambition are limitless.

### Conflict Always Exciting

Pictures of conflict, whether in war or sports or local politics, interest men end lessly. Conflict involves survival in many cases; conflict has to do with the ambitions of men to win, whether in a Parent Teachers Association election or a gang fight; conflict and sex often are entangled.

**Pictures As Means of Escape**

Pictures offer to most men a way to escape, for a moment at least, the seemingly dreary here and now of their routine lives. As men seek this escape through sports and the theater and hobbies, they can learn to find it, too, in news pictures. And news cameramen can attempt to provide in their pictures this much-sought escape.

The pictures that best do this job, probably, are those that offer the viewer a chance to live for a time the life of somebody else, to participate in some problem not his own, to get away from this moment and this place. To best provide this release, a picture should

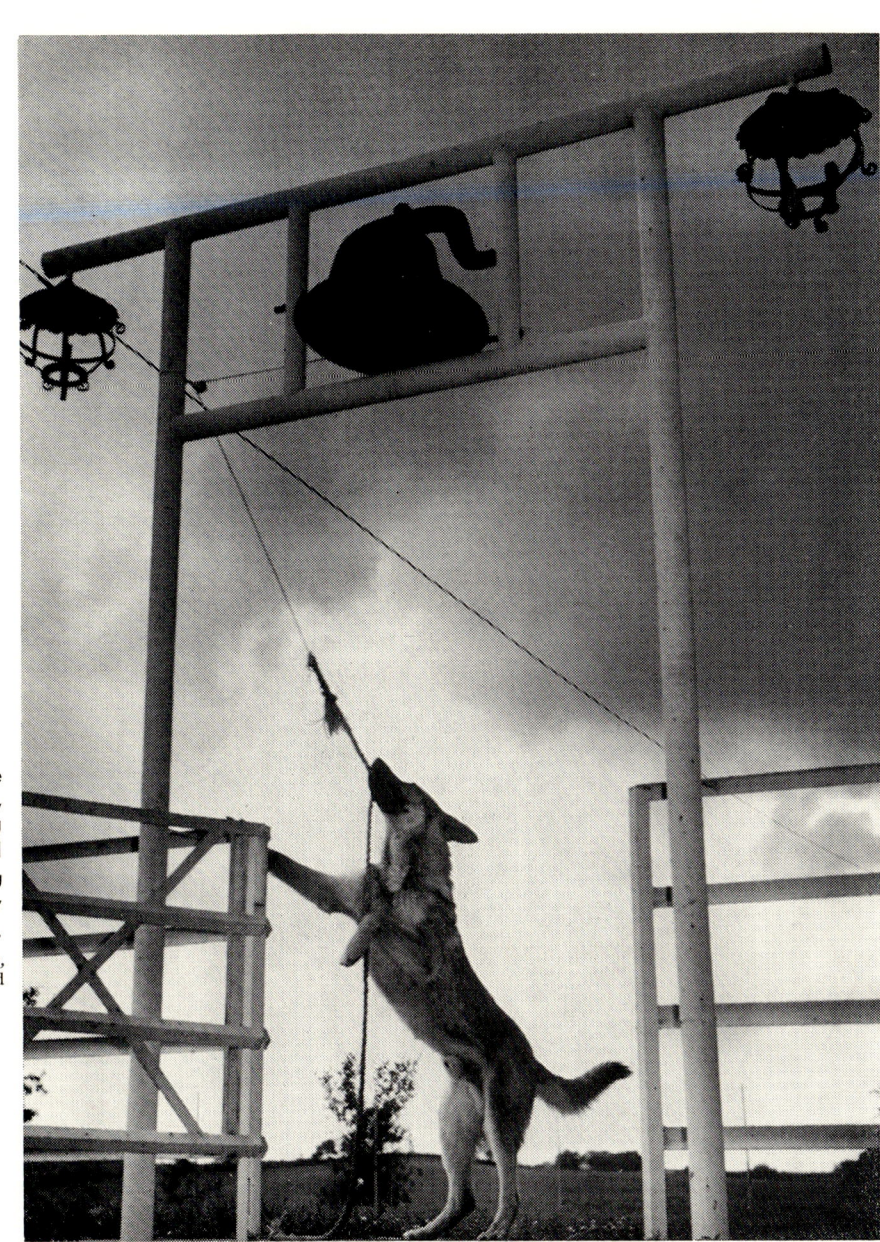

13 Animals provide wonderful subject matter, too. This dog rings a bell instead of barking when somebody approaches his home.
*Dale Stierman, chief photographer, Dubuque (Iowa)* Telegraph-Herald

14   Two animals can be even more delightful than one, as are this mother and kitten.
*Bruce Roberts, staff photographer, Charlotte* Observer

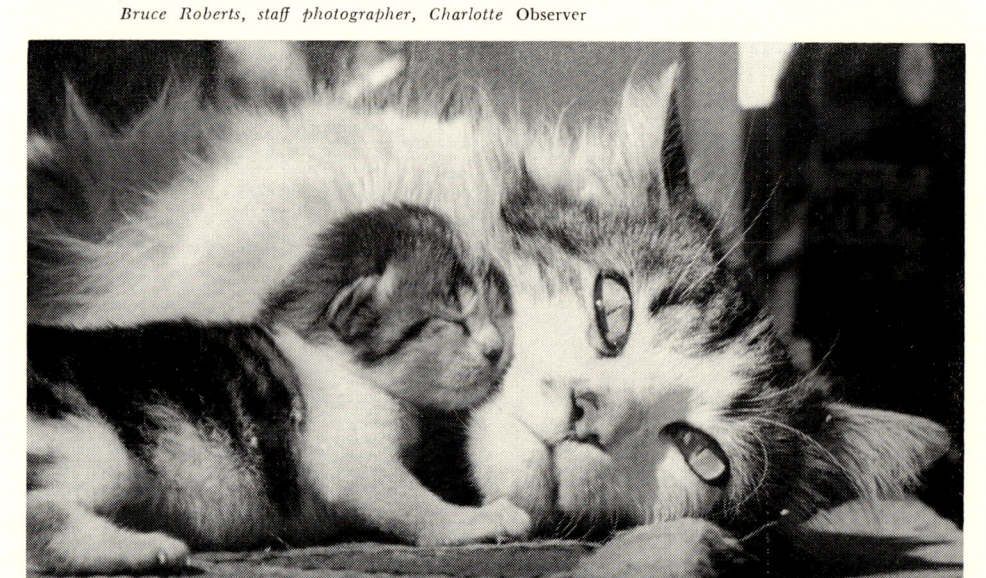

15   See what fun it is when you picture a man and an animal together.
*Bruce Roberts, staff photographer, Charlotte* Observer

16   And notice how newsworthy a small boy and his injured puppy can be.
*Davenport (Iowa)* Morning Democrat

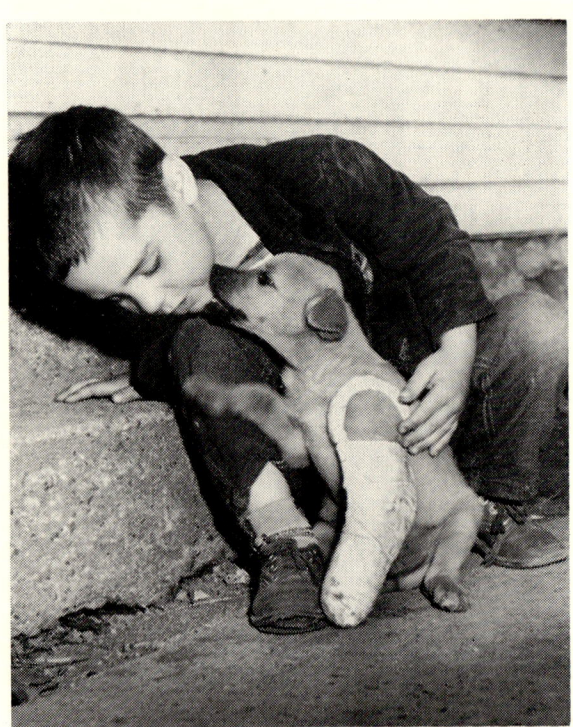

present a story-telling situation colorfully and clearly, especially with a deep touch of emotion whether it be humor, pathos, anger or some other sentiment.

### Animal Pictures Appeal

Next to the interest by human beings in others of their kind, perhaps, is their interest in animals. Some of this interest can be explained, probably, because some people think of pets, especially young ones, as child substitutes. But there seems to be a deeper reason than that for the fascination animals hold for men. Men seemingly always have struggled to understand their relationship to the animal world, for animals have been dangerous enemies as well as a food supply, and animals obviously are fellow living creatures. Some of man's earliest pictures represented animals.

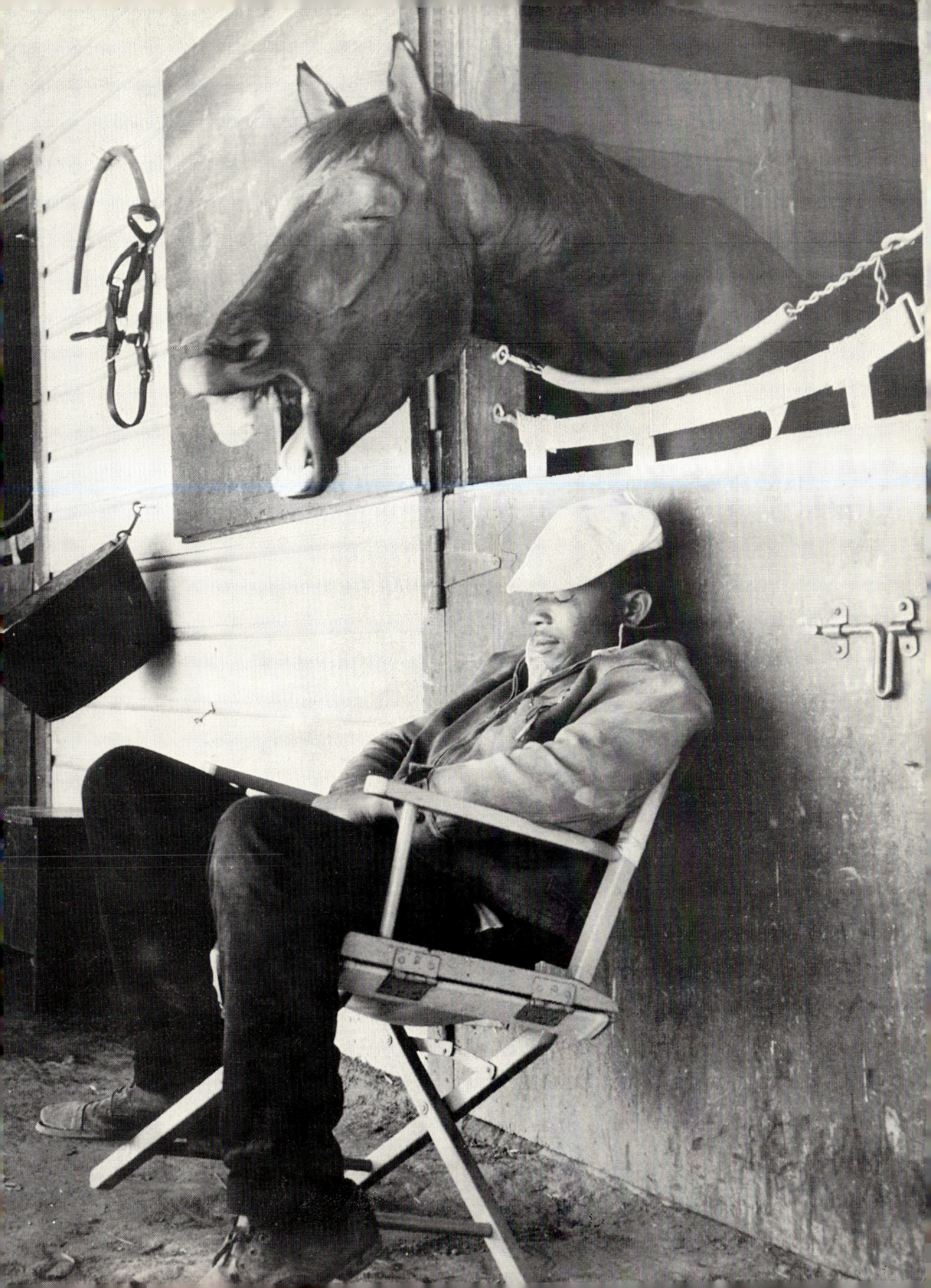

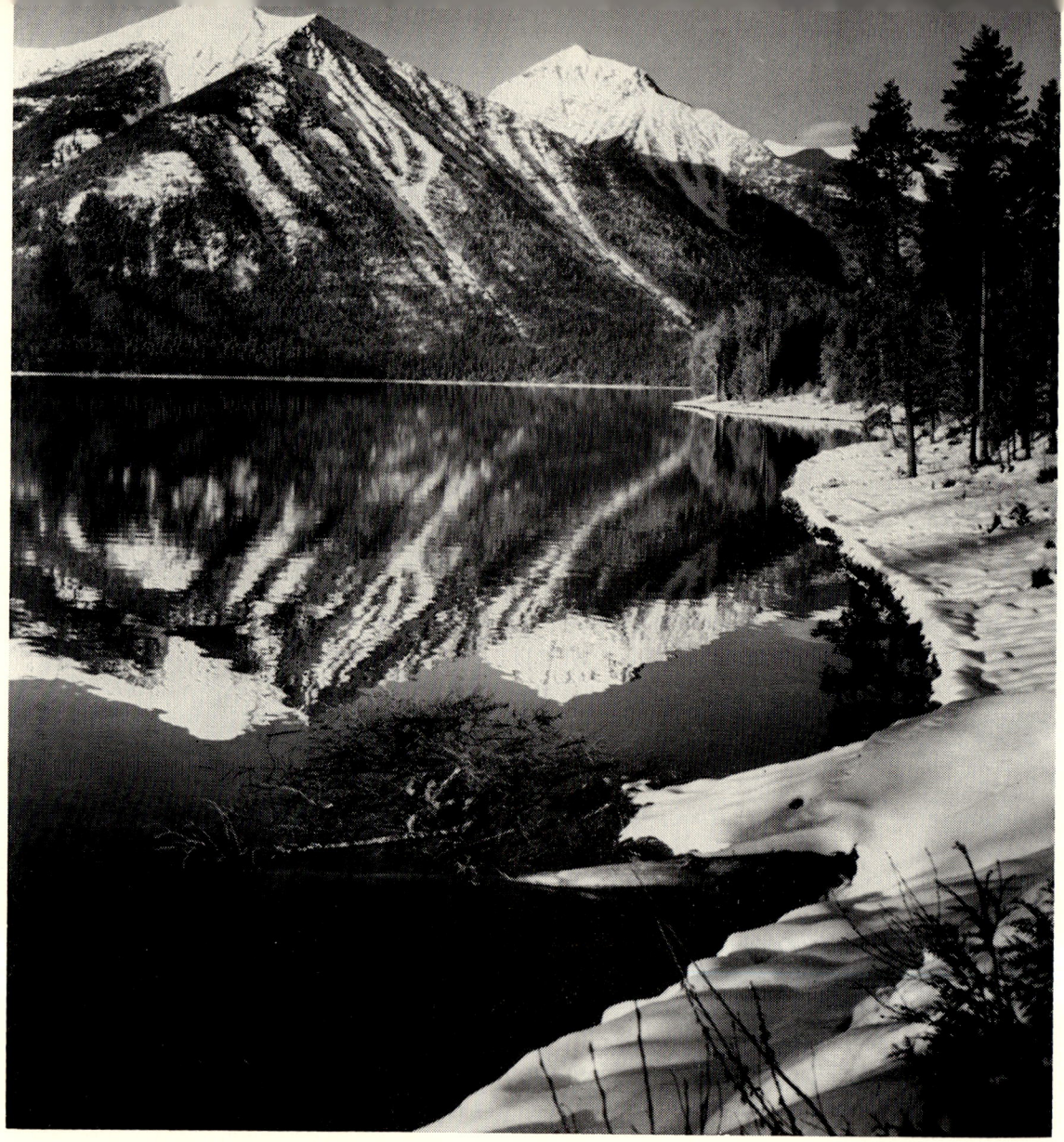

### Environment Needs Picturing Too

Not only is man greatly interested in his own kind and in his fellow creatures, the animals, but also he is fascinated and often deeply moved by the environment that surrounds and sustains all life — the earth and the universe. This background for living all too often seems neglected by news photographers in their preoccupation with picturing humankind.

After suggesting that the use of the small camera by news photographers has resulted in such a minute dissection of the human personality that in some respects pictures of people have become "monotonous repetition of behavior, mannerisms, gestures, relationships, situations," Jacob Deschin, camera editor of *The New York Times,* wrote:

"The world offers far more opportunity for the photojournalist and for all photographers affected by his inspired and searching response to life, than human visage, grimace and bodily gyration alone.

"What of man's environment, so generally neglected in these days of photojournalism's greatest triumph? What has happened to landscape photography, to the 'character' delineation of a street, a city square, or a

17   Man often is deeply moved by pictures of his environment, whether they be of mountain majesty. . . .

*Mel Ruder Photos for* Hungry Horse News, *(Columbia Falls, Mont.)*

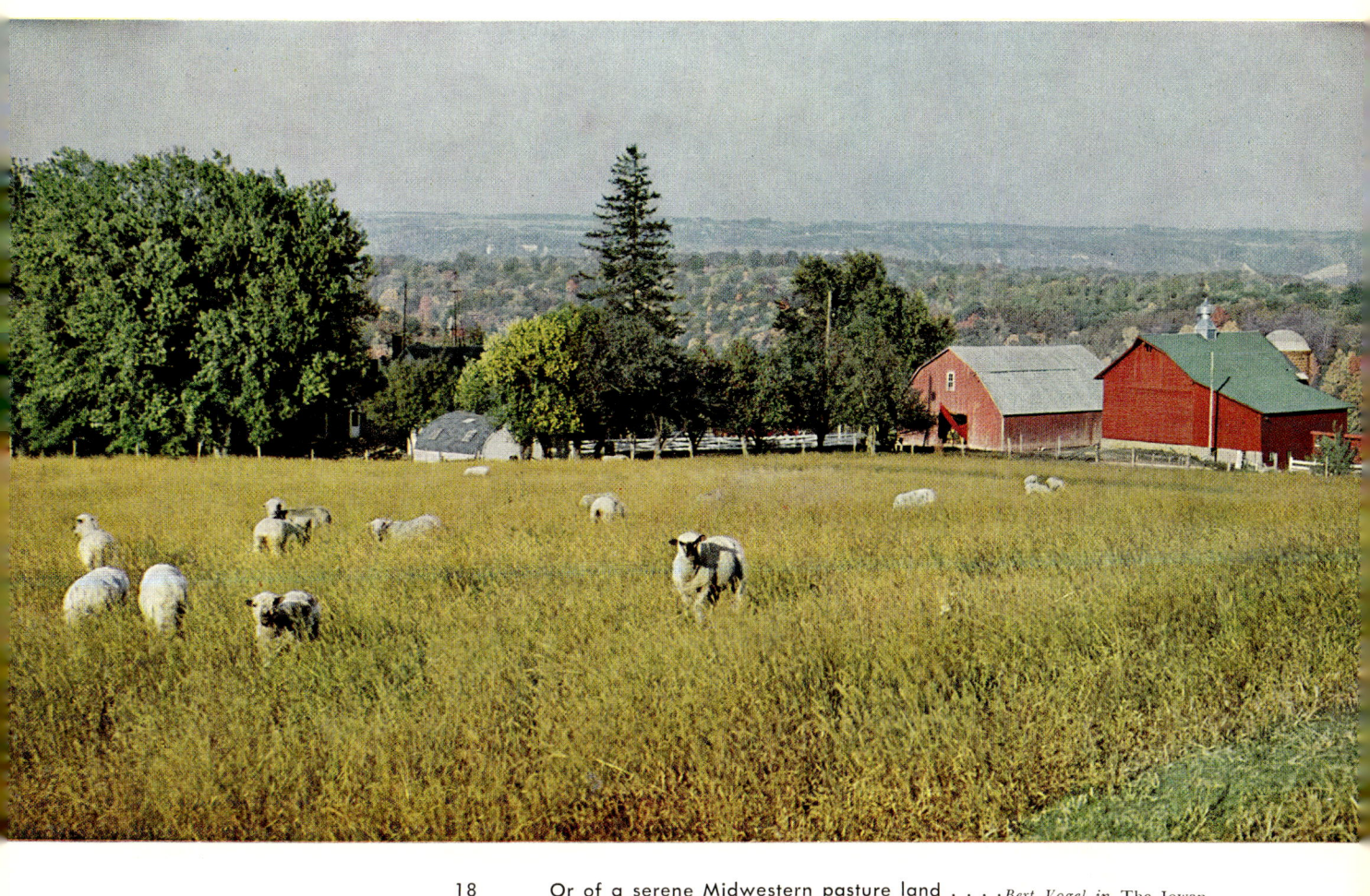

18   Or of a serene Midwestern pasture land . . . . *Bert Vogel in* The Iowan

country lane, and to the intimate nature scene?

"What of the qualities of texture, surface, and shape in objects, places and scenes; of the descriptive and mood-suggesting properties of light itself? Would not photography be better served by such diversification of material and treatment than by imitating photojournalism's preoccupation with human behavior?"[2]

Mankind is greatly excited now by the infinite spaces that surround the earth. But most individuals are much more warmly interested in the familiar, nearby landscape, in city streets, in the land, the sky, the waters — all those elements that sustain, comfort or

[2] Deschin, Jacob, "Photojournalism Too Much With Us?" *Popular Photography*, June, 1960. Page 38.

19   Or of the promises or threats of the overhanging sky. . . .
*Bob Beasley* The Cooperative Consumer

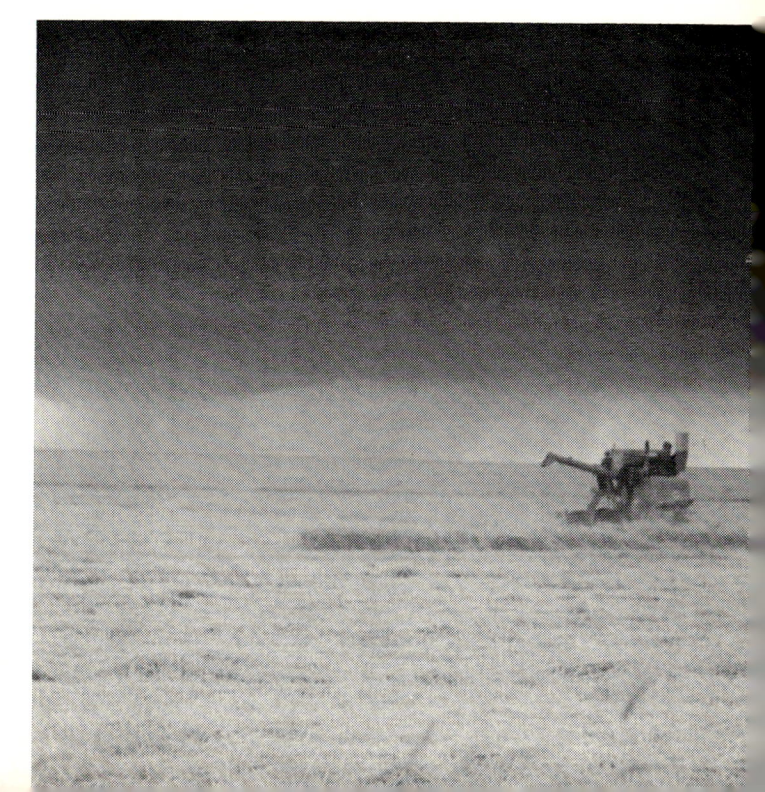

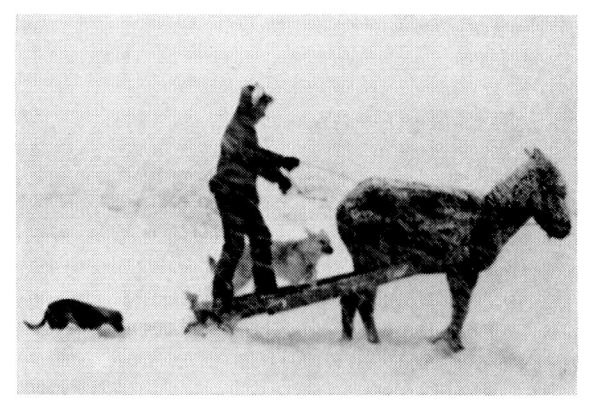

20     Or of winter's blinding storms. . . .
*James Forrest in Albuquerque* Journal

21     That create extra chores. . . .

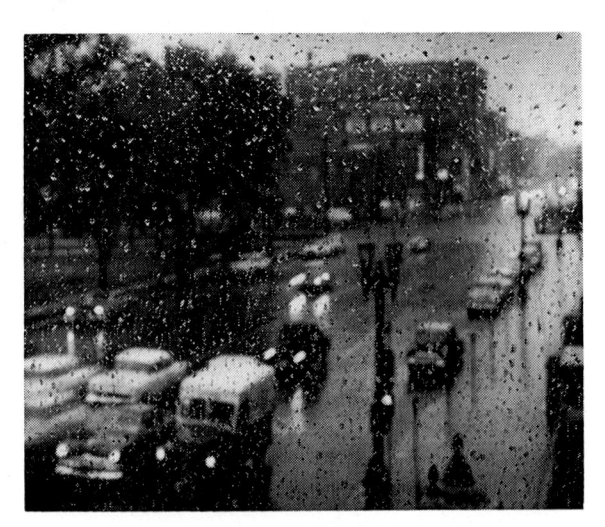

22     Or of an unexpected summer thunder shower. . . .

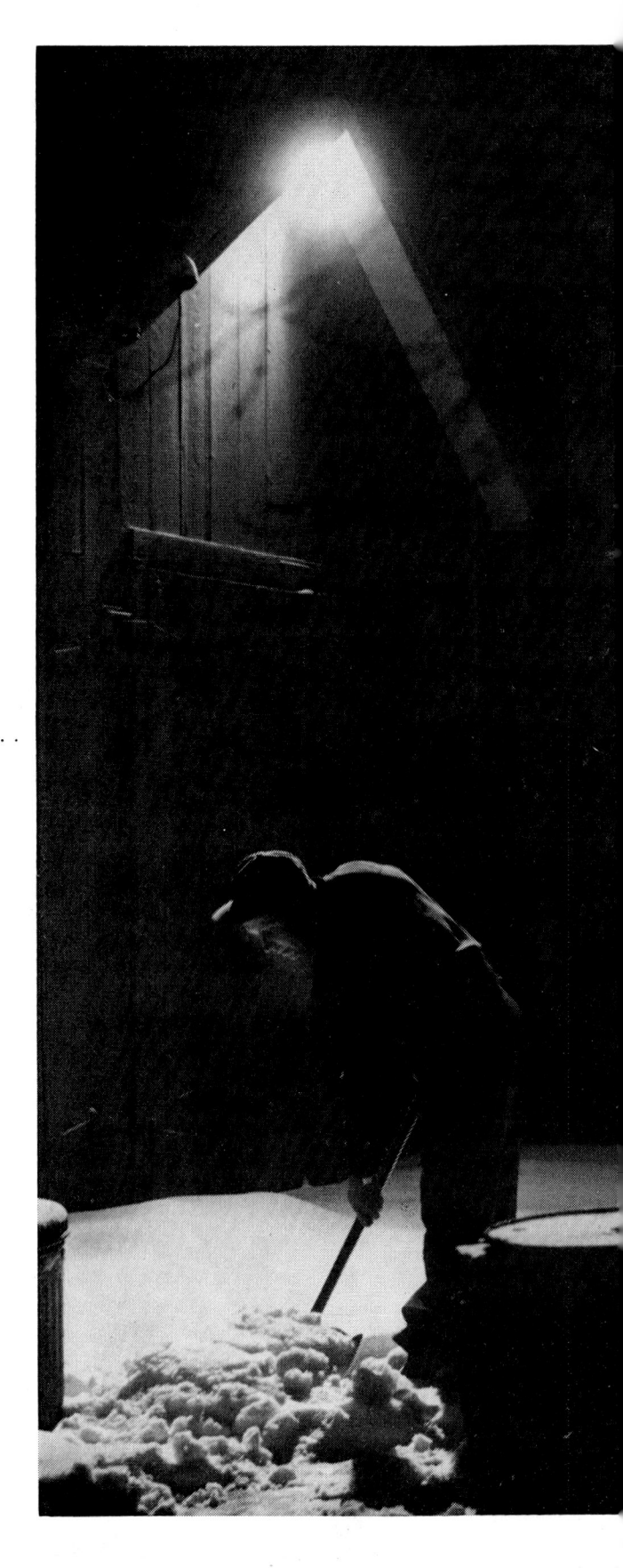

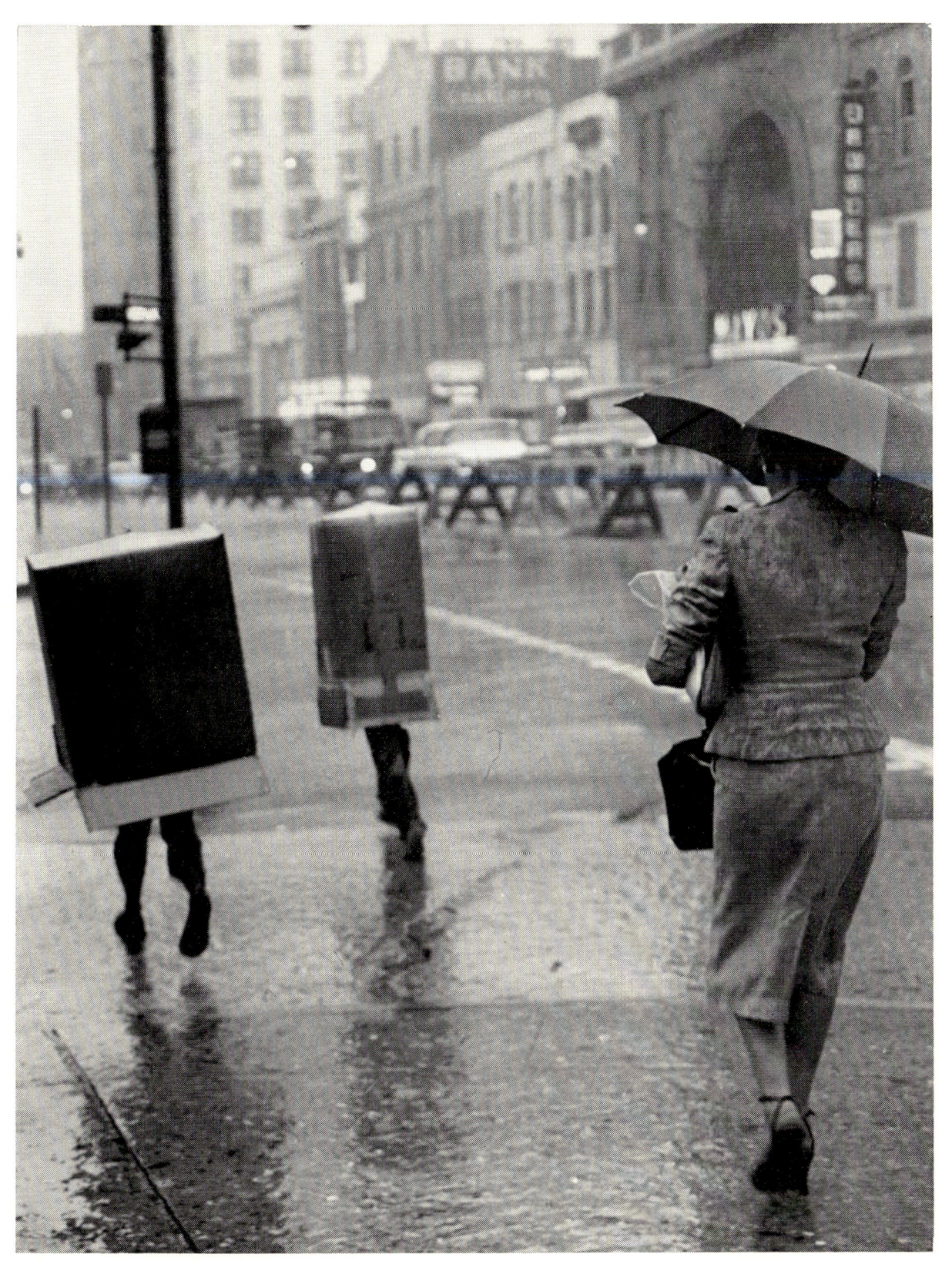

23   That calls for desperate measures.
*Bruce Roberts, staff photographer, Charlotte* Observer

threaten mankind. The weather still is the most talked about news, and it and the pageant of the changing seasons offer photographers unlimited subject matter.

Because men treasure their memories and recollections, they sometimes like pictures of the old and familiar, of locally historical places, of scenes that arouse nostalgia. A familiar place seen through the camera of an imaginative photographer is dramatized and enhanced. The local environment offers endless opportunities to such cameramen.

**Uses of Symbolism**

The complex but fascinating problems involved in the use of symbolism and in symbols are of great importance to news photographers and editors. The ability to use symbols is basic not only to almost all human communication but to most thought as well.[3]

From the practical standpoint, a photographer can make many uses of his understanding of symbols and the symbolization process. He can use such obvious symbols as the cross, the flag, the hammer and sickle within his pictures where they convey in simple terms their often enormously complex meanings. KKK and an arrow scrawled on a wall may be, for some, only a sign pointing to the meeting place of an organization, but to others the sign becomes a symbol of great emotional intensity. Incorporated in a picture, that KKK may provide, because of its symbolic nature, meaning and feeling far different and more intense than would mere lines of chalk on a brick wall.

The tricky thing about symbols is that the meanings and feelings they arouse will not be exactly the same for any two persons and will be violently opposite for some. The significance of the cross will be vastly different for a devout Christian and for someone taught to hate and condemn Christianity.

At another level, almost any representation may assume intense symbolic meaning. The picture of a bejeweled woman at the opera opening, of a dirty child on the steps of a slum dwelling or of a union picket are factual representations of those persons, and at the same time they are almost certain to take on additional meanings because they also become symbols in the eyes of those who look at them. The picture of the picket will become a symbol with intense meaning both to devoted union members and corporation executives, but the symbolic meaning read into the picture by them obviously will be very different.

Some knowledge of symbols and how they operate can be intelligently utilized to enhance the meaning and the emotional content of pictures. Some such knowledge is necessary to avoid permitting pictures to say things they aren't intended to communicate. A picture that is strictly objective when considered only as a photographic representation of the objects shown can become a violent comment when a viewer interprets certain objects or combinations of objects and situations in the picture as symbols. A picture that is absolutely accurate as a representation of the objects shown may be considered inaccurate by a viewer because of the meanings he has drawn from the picture as a result of certain symbolisms he has found in it.

---

[3] Interesting discussions about symbols are contained in *An Essay on Man* by Ernst Cassirer, Doubleday & Co., New York, 1953, and in *Symbolism* by Alfred North Whitehead, Capricorn Books, New York, 1959.

24   News photographers often can use symbols and a knowledge of symbolism to produce emotional contrasts.

*Lowell Georgia, Green Bay (Wis.) Press-Gazette, staff photographer*

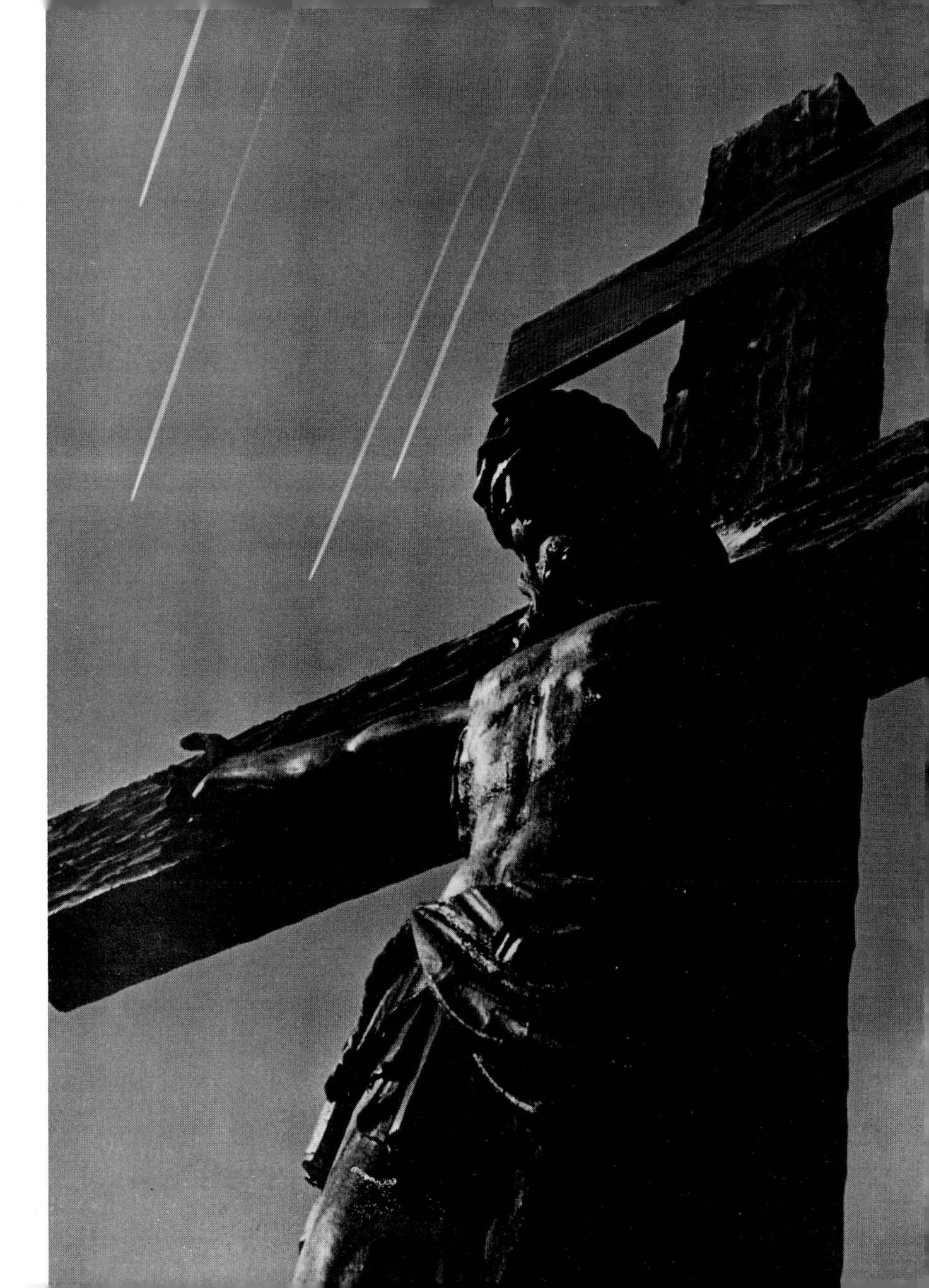

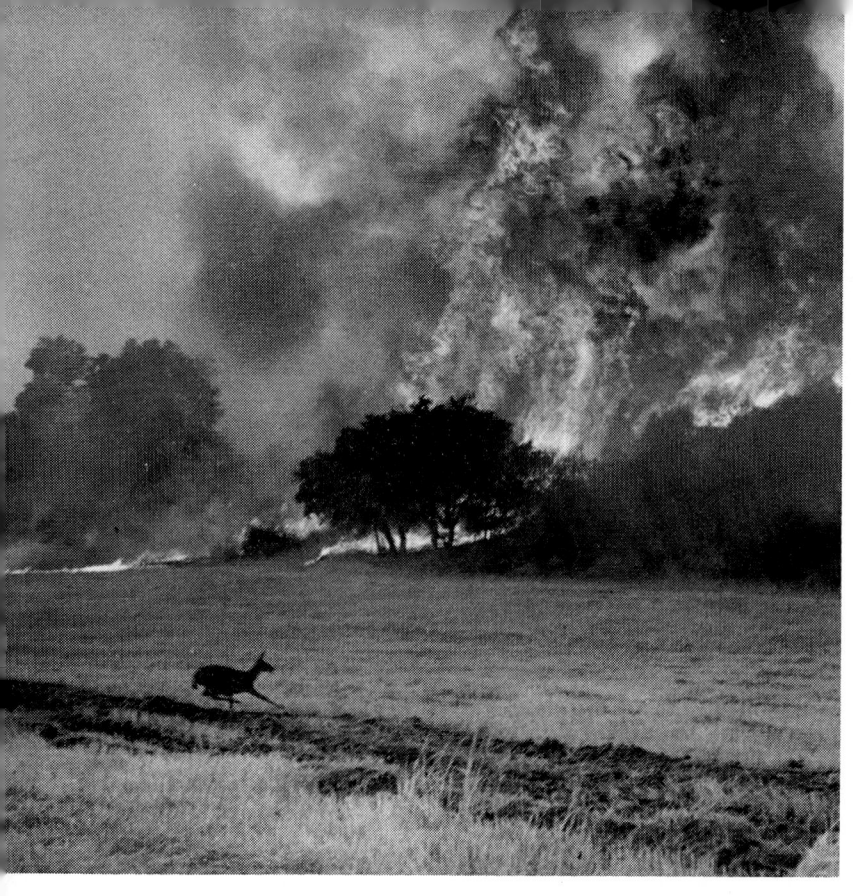

25   Perhaps no photographs have deeper emotional impact than those illustrating the desire to survive, like this one of the fleeing deer. . . .

*Photo by Phil Glickman, Los Angeles Examiner*

**News Pictures Must Be News**

News pictures, which are pictorial stories, must have the same qualities as written news articles. They need to be rich in such qualities as recency, nearness, importance, human interest. In addition they must bring added understanding to the story by visualizing information which cannot be adequately described in words alone.

Too, it's necessary that news photographs be of high technical quality. Poor photography shows itself in poor reproductions. Exposure, development and printing all must be properly done. Good print quality will be rewarded by better reproduction.

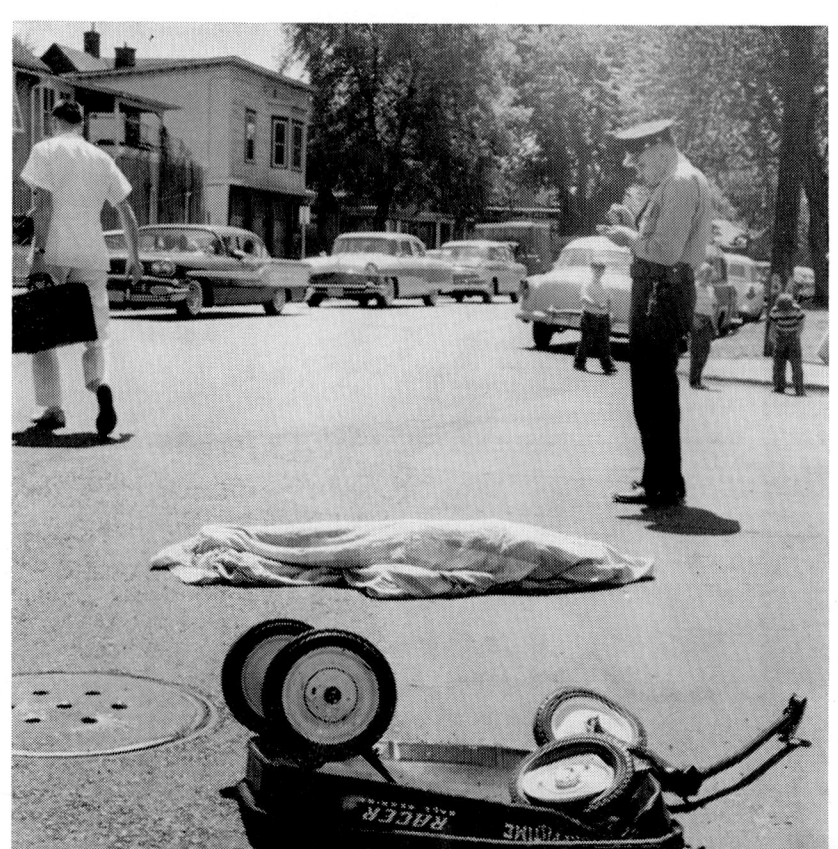

26   And this photograph by William Seaman that tells so vividly the story of a child who did not survive.

*Photo courtesy of Minneapolis Star*

CHAPTER 3

# Depth Reporting With Pictures

SOME NEWSMEN of late years have been talking a great deal about the need for reporting in depth. It's not enough, they say, to cover a significant story with the who, what, when and where questions answered lightly and with perhaps a flippant and superficial touch of answers to the how and why questions.

If news stories are to be meaningful, if they are to be more than superficially interesting, if news is to function as an integral part of the democratic process, stories must be covered much more fully, it is argued. It's not enough just to tell that something happened. If the story is to do its job fully, it must thoroughly explain why the incident occurred, probe deeply the historical backgrounds, develop the personalities of the principal characters involved, perhaps explain what the incident probably means.

**Depth Needed in Picture Coverage**

If such arguments for the verbal coverage of stories are sound, then isn't it logical that the men who report with their cameras should work in depth, too, at least with the more than routine stories?

Pictorial coverage of local news generally seems much more shallow than do verbal reports. If in many American cities and towns a century from now a historian turned to a newspaper file as a source for a picture history of a city, readers of his book would be convinced that events of the mid-1900's consisted only of accidents, fires, crimes, queens and drum majorettes in parades, men shaking hands, sports events and the emergence from boots of cute kittens or puppies. Even the crime, fire and sports pictures would reveal only glimpses of disconnected actions.

**Lens Can Cover in Depth**

There seems to be no unanswerable reason why photographers can't probe as deeply with their lenses as reporters do with their pencils. Whether a photographer is "illustrating" a story being done principally in words or is working out a picture story or essay, his camera can turn up penetrating information. Some answers can better be made in pictures than in words. Many photographers have demonstrated this magnificently.

Here is an example of local picture reporting in depth . . .

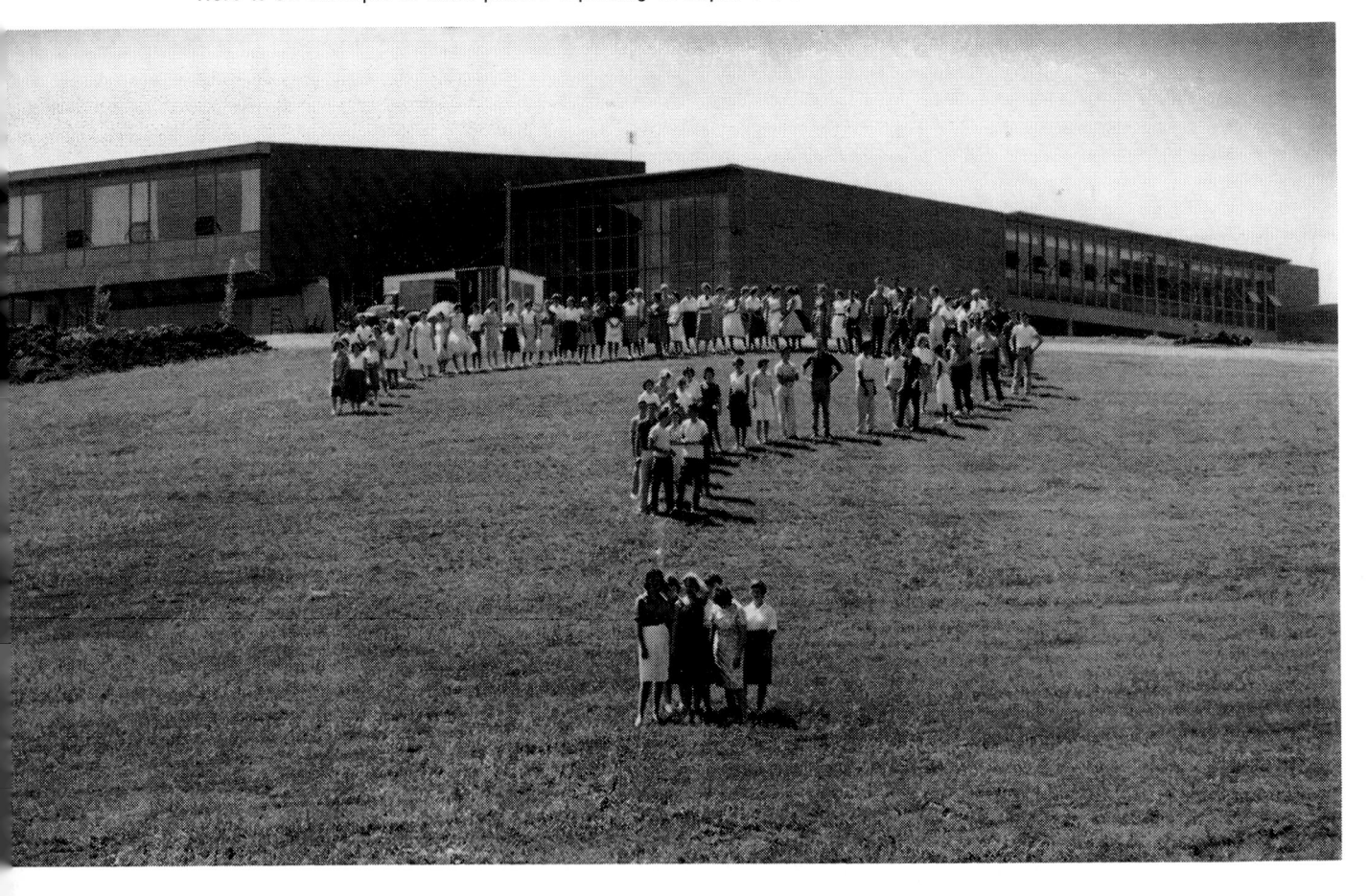

## Our Increasing School Problem

This high school building is only 3 years old and has no room this year for the enrollment of the students forming the question mark.

## The Cause . . .

The main cause of our increasing school problem is the almost unbelievable population rise over the past few years. The Chamber of Commerce estimates 5 new families a week are moving into town. Five new residential areas have been developed within city limits in the last 2 years.

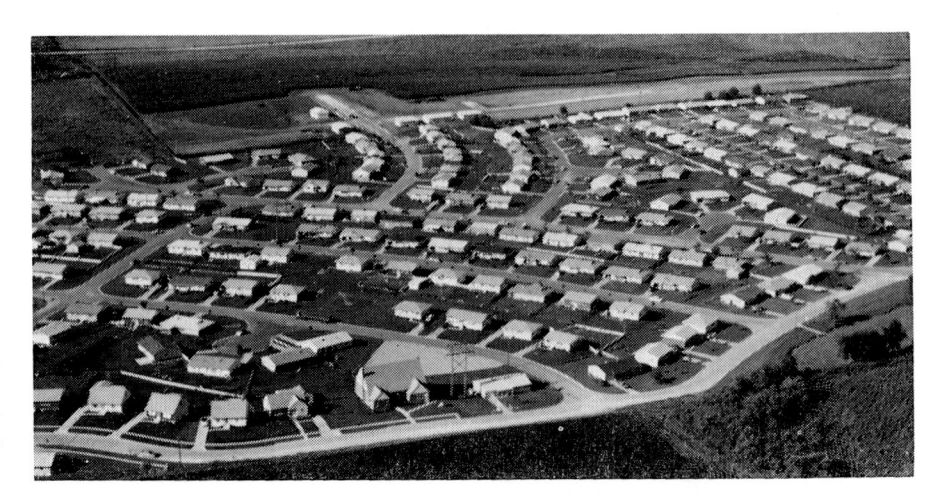

# Problems . . .

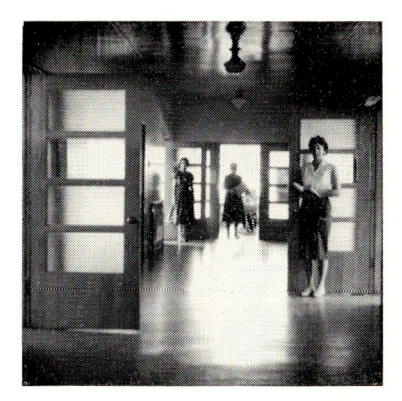

**NEED QUALIFIED TEACHERS**
We have an increasing need for qualified teachers. Who will stand in this empty doorway next year?

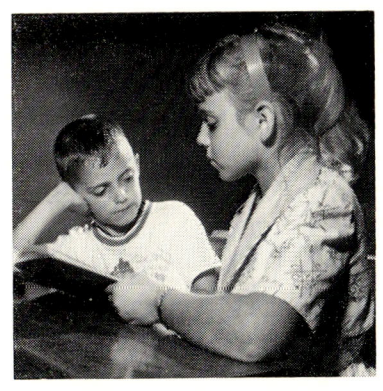

**ANTIQUATED METHODS**
Here, two children must read from the same text. Boredom and disinterest all too often result.

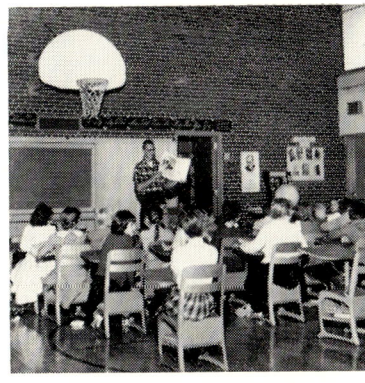

**CROWDED CLASSROOMS**
Many of our new schools have already run out of class space and are forced to use gyms and stages.

# Some Solutions . . .

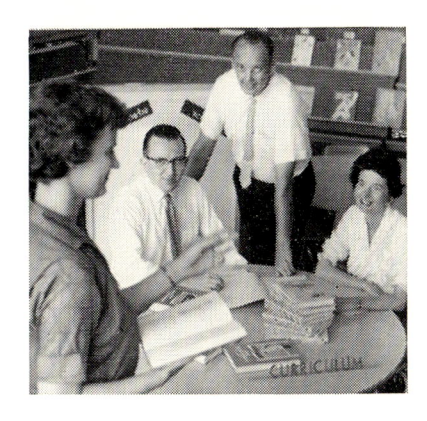

**CURRICULUM PROGRAMS**
A curriculum committee headed by a salaried expert would help plan and guide children's education.

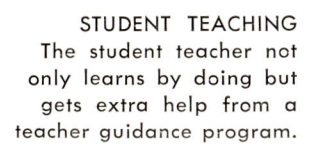

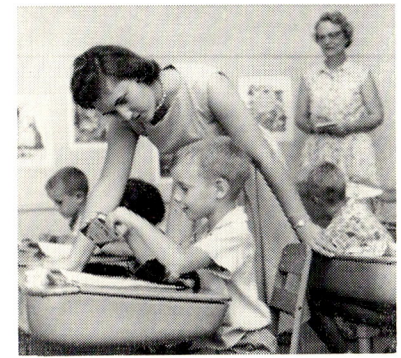

**STUDENT TEACHING**
The student teacher not only learns by doing but gets extra help from a teacher guidance program.

**NEW FACILITIES**
The cost of improving our educational system is very little compared to the price of delinquency and prison programs.

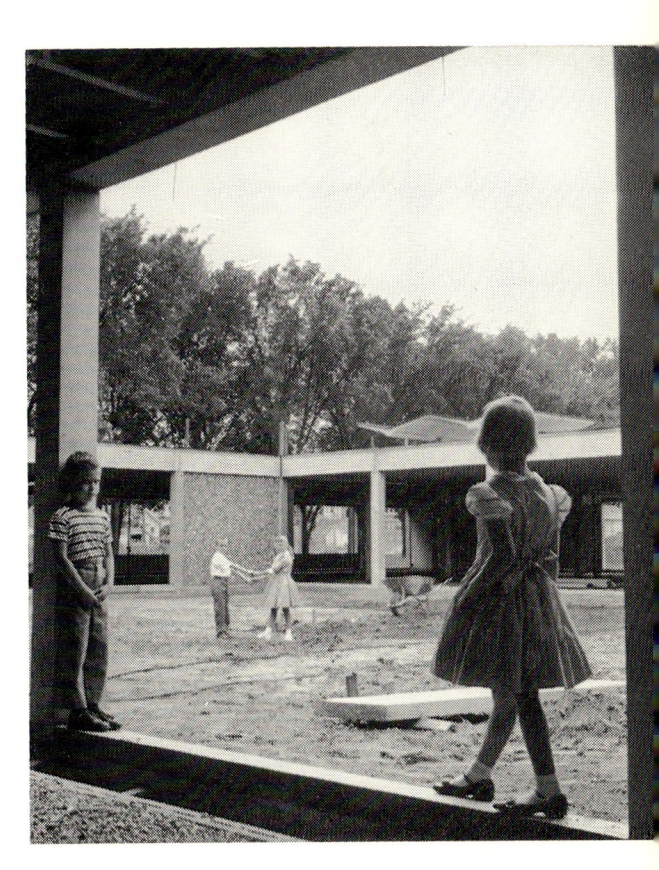

**How To Cover a Story**

How can a significant and important story be covered in depth through a lens? Make that lens find answers to the questions of why this incident happened — not just quick, superficial answers but the deeper answers that explain. Make the lens satisfy questions as to what this incident signifies. Make the lens probe deeply into how the incident happened. To do this takes thinking, always hard work. And several pictures probably will be required, and that takes time and effort. But the job can be done and done magnificently in pictures.

Suppose that a country correspondent reported that the century-old Maple Hill church, a landmark 10 miles east of your city, will close forever after next Sunday's service. Obviously this event offers a chance for a sentimental story with pictures of the pastor locking the weathered doors, of gray-haired women looking sadly at the sun-flecked markers on graves of the church founders beneath the great maples.

But such pictures, effective as they might be, are only answers to the what. The church is closing because the rural population has dwindled until not enough farm families remain in the neighborhood to support the institution. The rural population has dwindled because efficient new machines and improved crops have resulted in the combination of many small farms into a few big ones and the elimination of most hired farm help.

The photographer can use the pictures of the closing of the church as the news peg for a much larger story. He can photograph abandoned farm homes near the church, big, tractor-drawn machines, towering hybrid corn, the empty store building that, with the now abandoned church, is the only remnant of a once busy farm town. That series of pictures might explain to many readers the cause of the great agricultural adjustment that is now shaking rural America and its social and economic life so deeply. The story of that adjustment needs to be more widely known than it is.

**Method Has Many Uses**

This method could be used to investigate and report in depth many local public affairs. What is the situation of the local schools? What is the local juvenile delinquency situation and what efforts are being made concerning it? What are the arguments for and against annexation of great new areas to the city?

**Will Depth Coverage Pay?**

But will enough people read socially significant stories reported in depth to justify the time and expense required to obtain them? It would be interesting to try some depth reporting — either picture stories or copiously illustrated verbal stories — and then take a readership survey.

The amount of expense and space justified in providing better coverage in photographs is a matter each publisher has to decide against a background of his operation. Some of the factors he might consider include not only direct profits and loss, but also his responsibility to provide significant information in effectively readable form in fulfillment of the obligations of a free press in a democracy.

CHAPTER 4

# Picture Stories, Essays and Layouts

PICTURE STORIES and essays can be used to report in depth events and public affairs of the greatest importance.

Or they can be used to present delightful features that amuse, beguile and delight through skillful use of whimsey, humor, pathos.

They seem to have been developed so far to their highest form in magazines, but they can be used in many ways in newspapers to report general news or on sports, society or farm pages. There seems to be no special reason why they can't be used more often even on editorial pages which, in general, have largely resisted extensive use of pictures even though photographs sometimes can be enormously persuasive.

**The Picture Story**

A true picture story must have a plot, which implies that it must have a beginning, a middle and an ending. It needs to start with an attention attracting picture that functions as a lead does for a story told in words. After the lead the story development follows, evolving finally into a climax, or ending. Good picture stories have been as brief as four photographs. Some good books are only long picture stories.

The Picture Essay

A photo essay is simply a collection of pictures around a central theme. Although it doesn't have a plot, it may discuss, philosophize about, scrutinize and even argue a point about the material of its central theme.

Although a plot isn't involved, a photo essay should be tightly constructed. Every picture in it should contribute definitely and not repetitiously to what is to be said.

As with a picture story, a picture essay needs a "lead," a picture that can be splashed to draw attention.

A layout is just a collection of pictures about a common subject, but it can be effective and requires less planning than does a close-knit essay or story. As with stories and essays, the layout is more attractive if one "lead" picture is splashed and variety provided.

**Stories, Essays, Layouts Have Much in Common**

Certain procedures and requirements, in addition to "lead" pictures, make both picture stories and essays more effective.

1. At least one picture should show an over-all view to help orient the viewer.

Effective picture stories carry you with them . . .

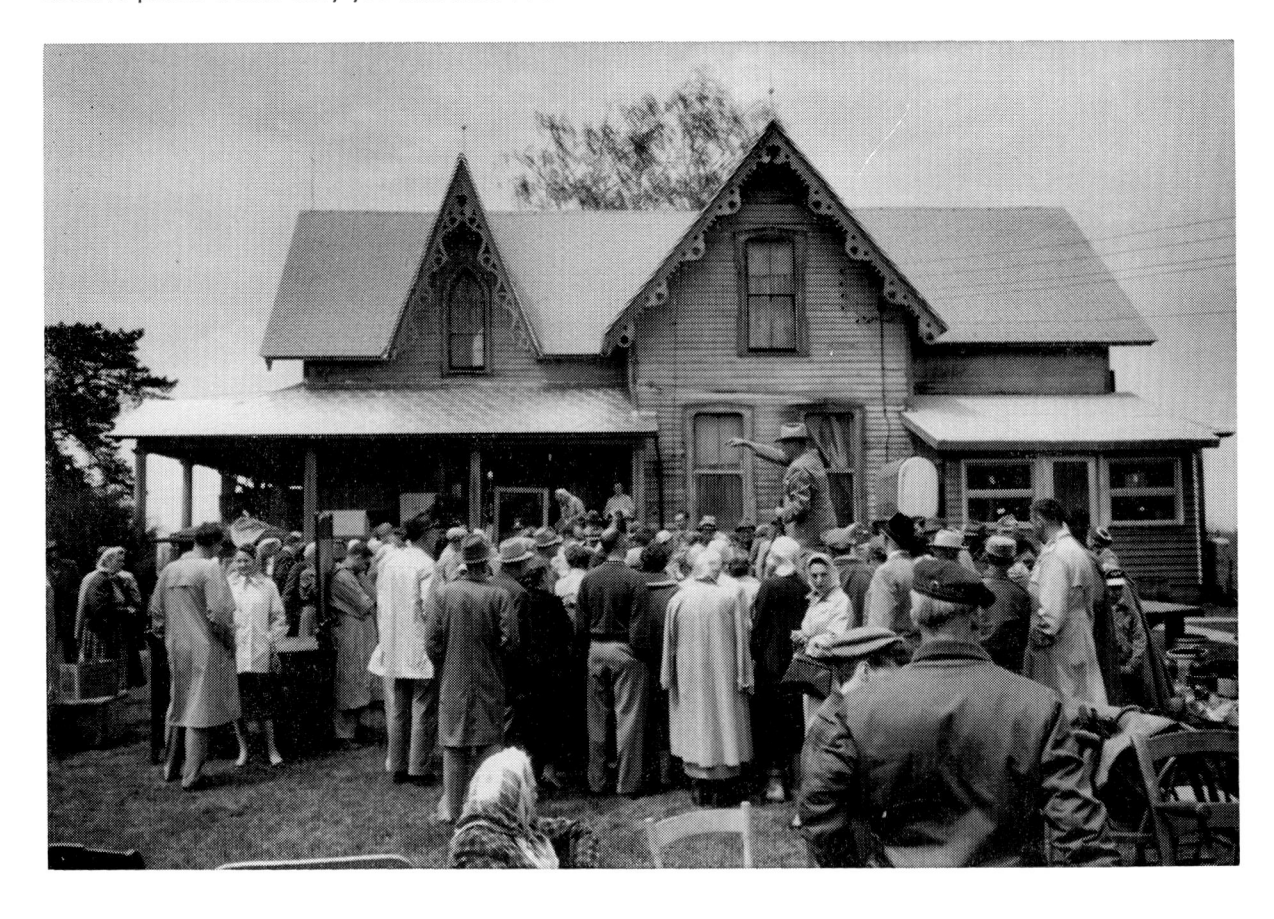

# Auction Today

**Photographs by NILS LINDQUIST**
from MINUTES, magazine of Nationwide Insurance

*" . . . 11, I got 11, 11, 11, I got 12, 12, 12, I got*

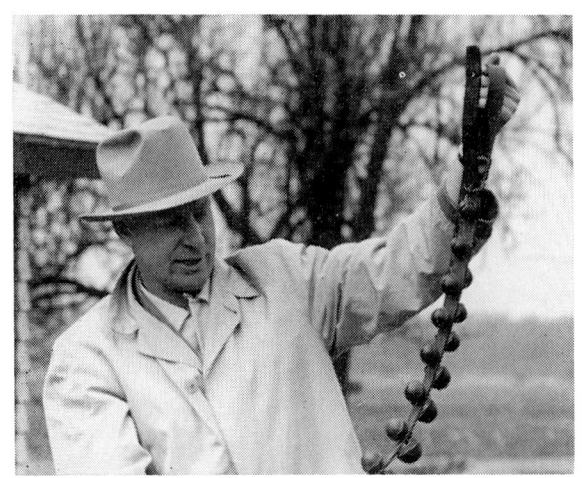

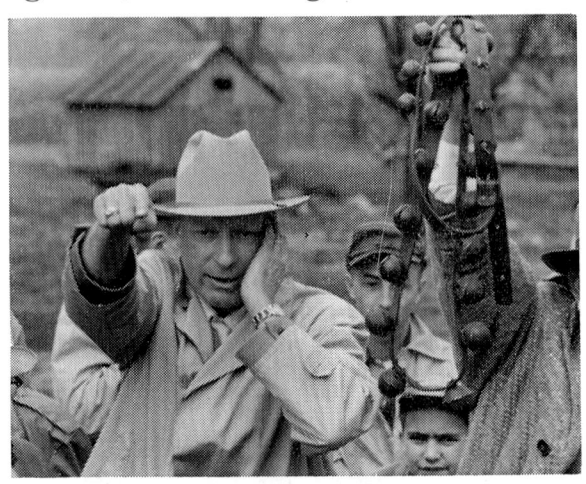

36 —

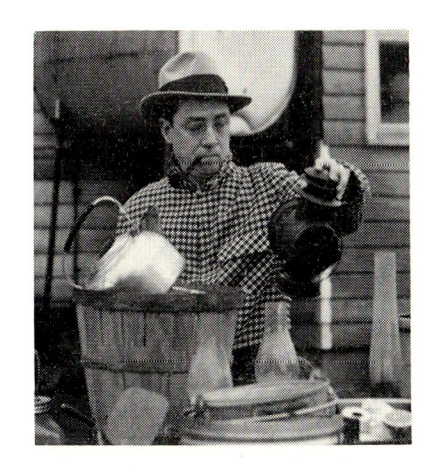

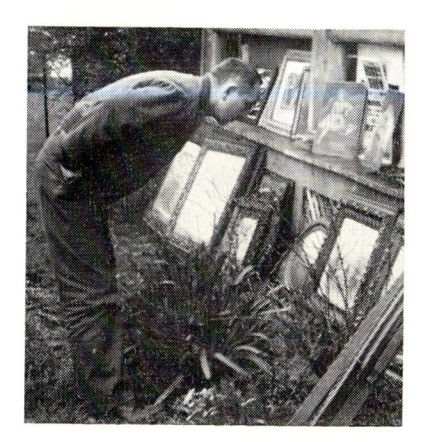

*Appraisal*

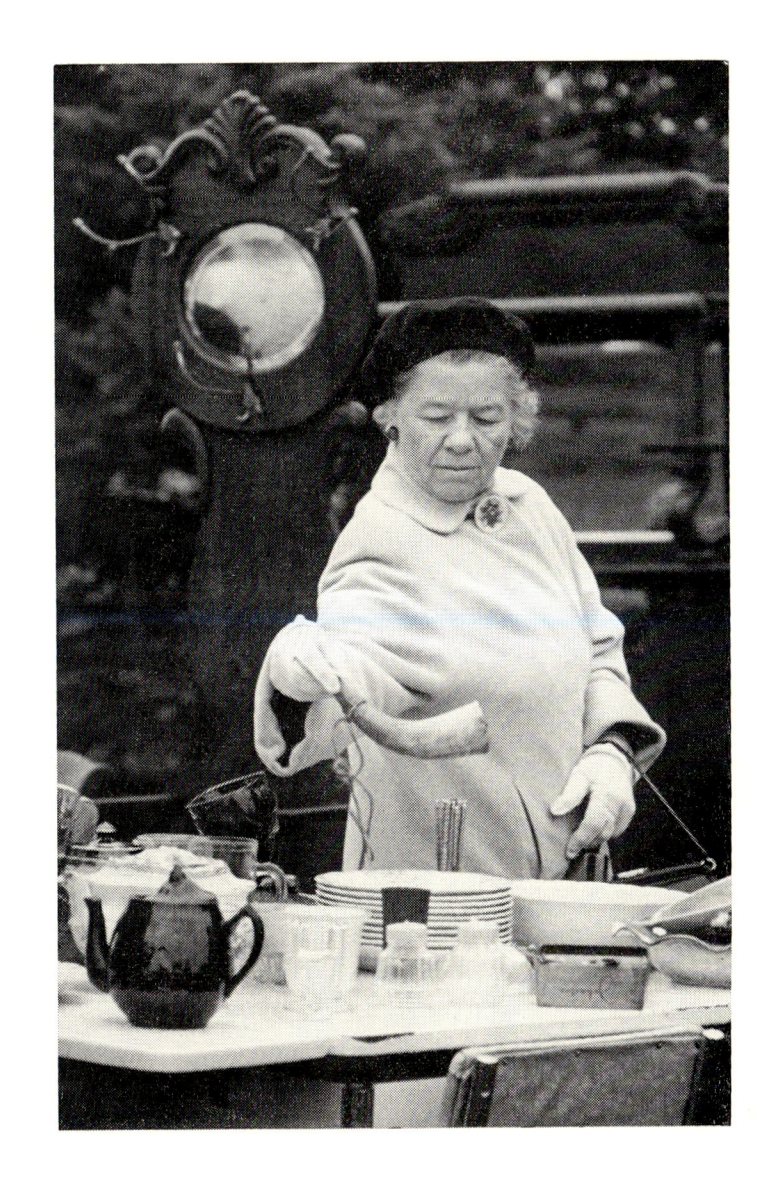

13, 13. All done? Sold, 13! Now look, I got . . ."

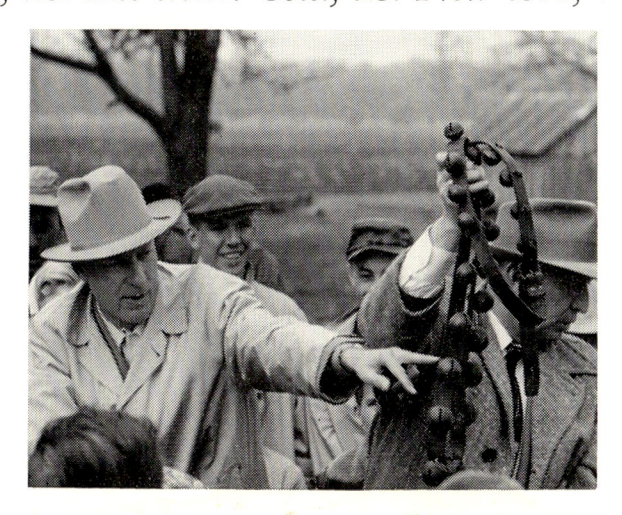

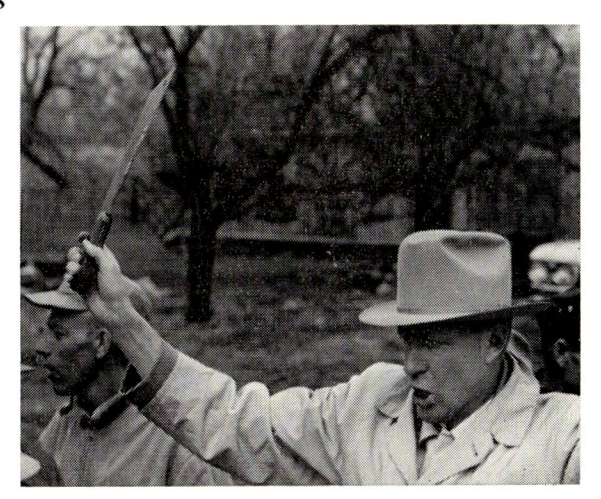

— 37

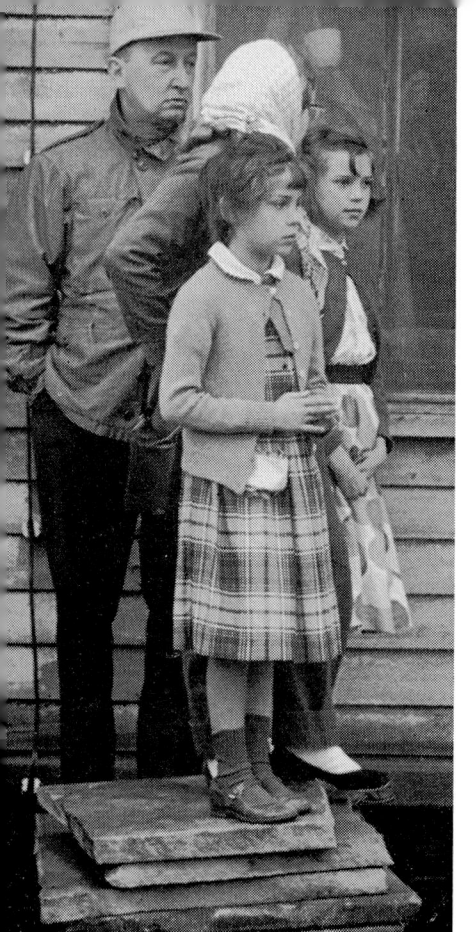

*Vantage Point*

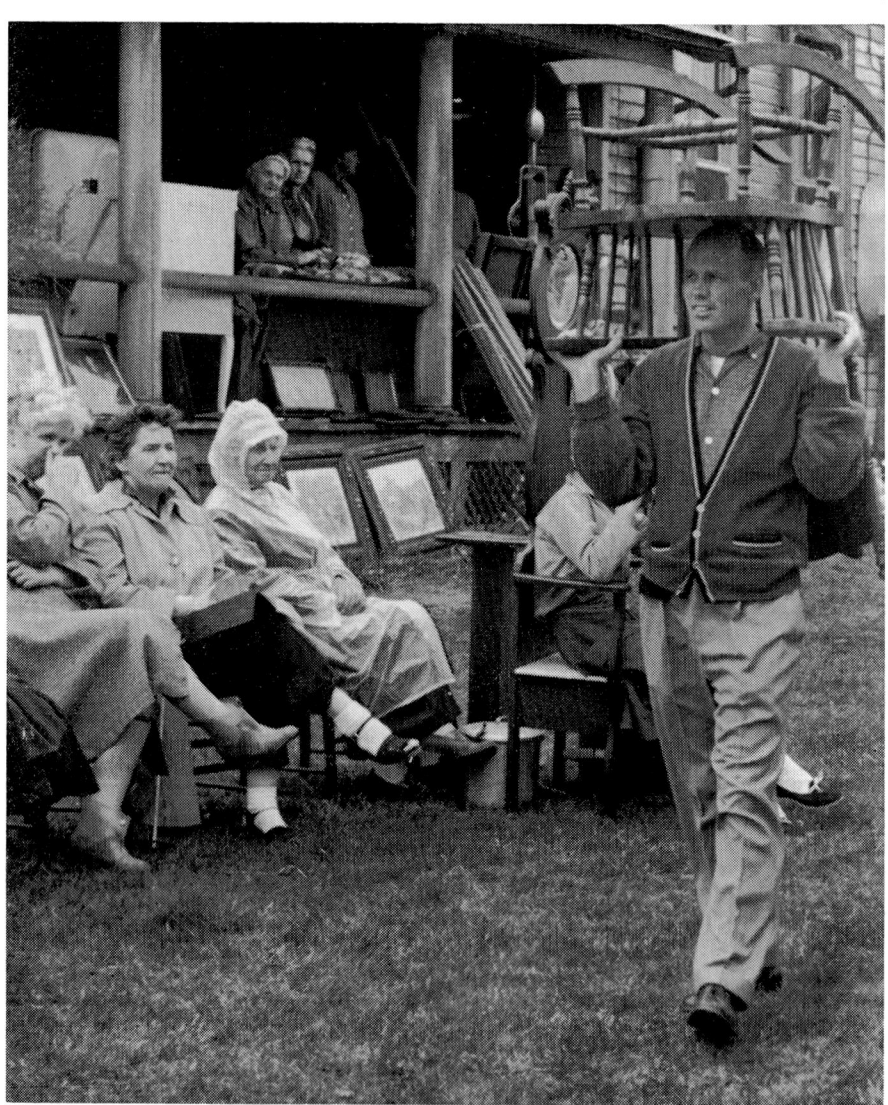

*Victor*

2. Some pictures need to be closeups that show detail.
3. Some pictures need to be taken from middle distance.
4. Photographs should be varied in other ways to combat monotony. Low, high and normal angle shots, night shots and day shots, perhaps, as well as other means can be used.

Pictures should be used in different sizes and shapes.

5. Pictures that contribute mood or feeling perform a valuable function.
6. Pictures should fit together into a unified whole with no unbridged gaps that the reader's understanding cannot cross.

7. Pictures that don't contribute significantly to the central plot or theme should be cut mercilessly. Don't use pictures just because they are pretty or of good quality. Each picture should do a job that no other picture in the series does.

In taking single news pictures, most photographers strive to gather all elements into the single unit. In a series it would be nice if each picture could stand as an individual unit, but there seems to be a tendency for pictures in a story or essay to lean on each other. This is all right if together they create a complete and satisfying whole.

The more pictures used, the greater the opportunity for subtlety; a story told with fewer pictures sometimes is more direct and forceful.

**Careful Planning Needed**

Because picture stories and essays require considerable effort, time, expense and space, they should be carefully planned to avoid waste.

A script should be prepared and worked on until it is decided how many pictures are needed, what they are, how they should be distributed to produce the right proportion of various kinds of shots needed. Unless careful plans are worked out and written down in advance, a photographer deeply involved in shooting a story easily can forget to obtain some pictures vital to the proper telling of a story.

Because so much time and effort are involved, it would be well for the photographer and his editor to go over the script together until they reach agreement. Things don't always work out exactly as planned, but preparation goes far in cutting down waste.

Planning a picture series doesn't mean that the event needs to be staged. Best results usually are obtained when the pictures are of a real event. Some pictures may have to be taken before or after an event, such as backgrounds, closeups and subjects not obtainable at the time of the event.

Generally, it is better to photograph persons involved rather than bringing in a model or somebody to pose. For instance, if you are showing how a product is made in a local factory, picture one of the regular machine operators rather than bringing in some cutie from the front office. Her long fingernails might get caught in the machine, and your pictures probably would reveal her inability to operate it.

47     A nice sports page sequence capturing the actual "splintering" of a broken bat hit, and showing the player's automatic "follow-through."
*Carl Franks, Cedar Rapids (Iowa)* Gazette

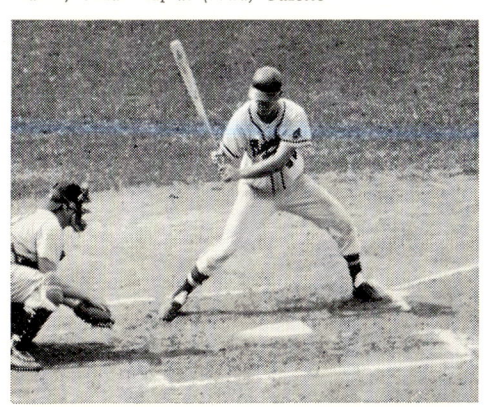

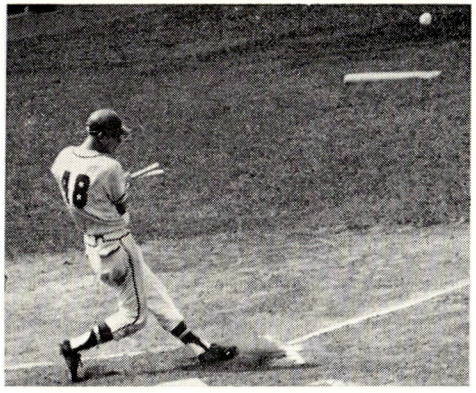

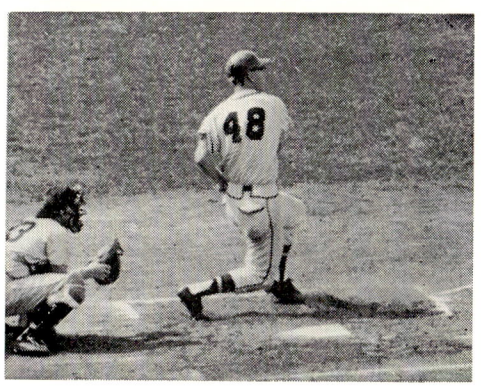

— 39

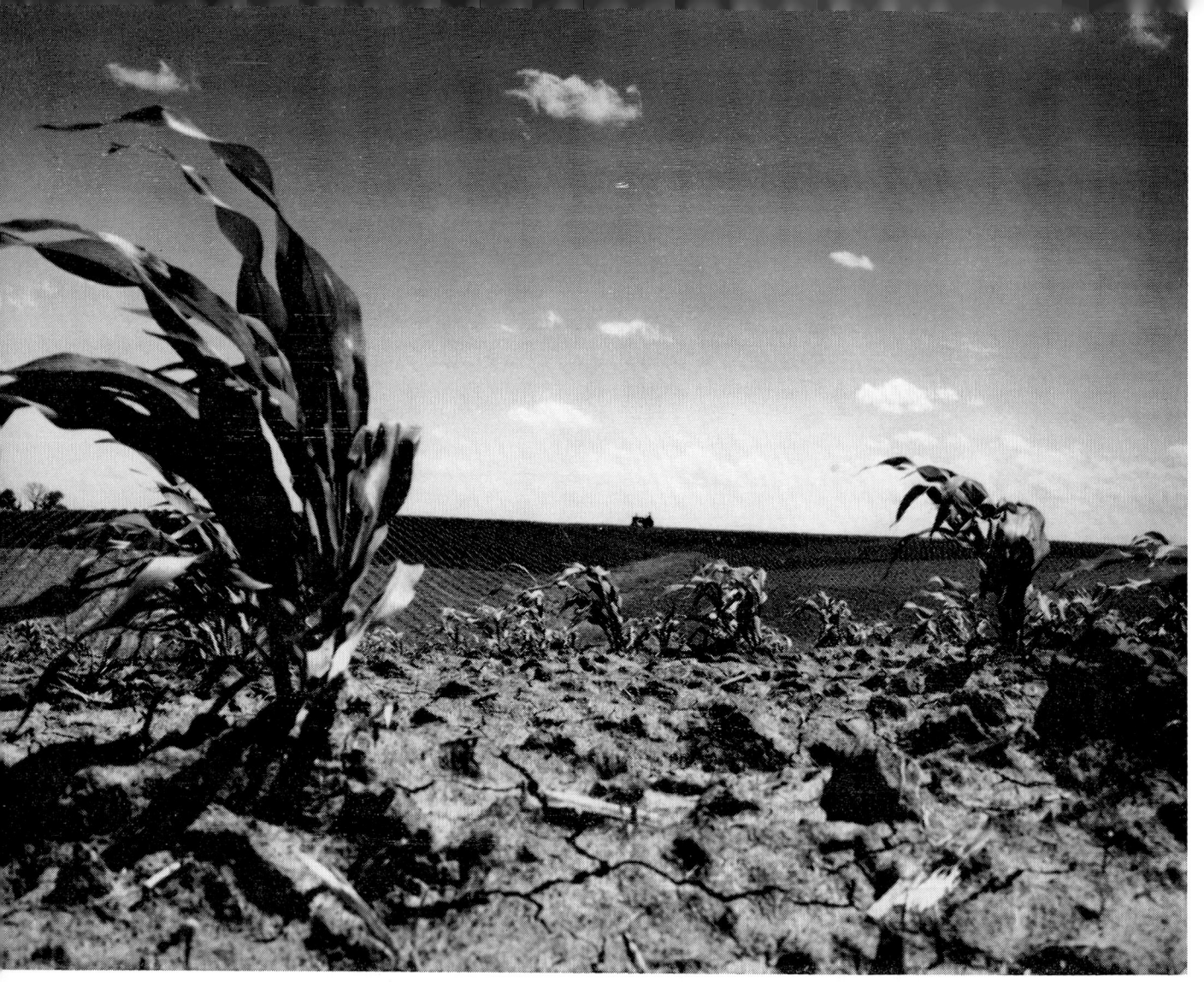

48     During this time of adjustment, agricultural reporting must concern itself more with explaining the industry to all citizens and the changes in agriculture to farmers and ranchers.
*Jack Brinton, Des Moines* Register *photo*

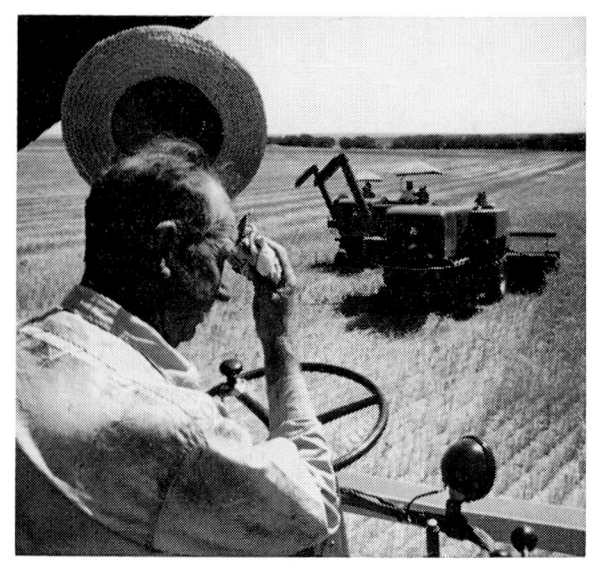

49     The great summer effort of agriculture to feed mankind is typified by this picture of a Colorado farmer in the heat of harvest.
*Dave Mathias, Denver* Post

CHAPTER 5

# Agricultural Revolution Deserves Intensive Photo Coverage

PROFOUND CHANGES in the pictorial and verbal coverage of farm news are needed to match the revolutionary adjustments in agriculture now in progress. These needed changes include greatly increased and intensified coverage of agricultural news as the vast industry — the one that furnishes the food and most of the fabric for the nation — gropes its way toward a new stability.

Because most of this stepped-up coverage of agricultural news needs to be directed toward the general public rather than toward farmers alone, pictures can play an especially important function in catching the attention and interest of urban people who may not be fully aware of the enormous importance of agriculture to themselves.

**Farm News Needed in Urban Press**

Pictures and stories that explain to non-farmers the fundamental economic, social, political and international importance of the current agricultural situation are probably the most urgently needed. And perhaps such information is most needed in metropolitan papers where interest of publishers and editors about such matters is low, partly because they think agricultural news is of little interest to their readers.

But small city daily papers, even in agricultural areas, and the country press often also slight coverage of agricultural news, and especially fail to provide information that helps explain the enormous changes and problems wracking agriculture today. Such information is badly needed because even farmers and small town people most concerned with the upheaval in agriculture often have little understanding of it.

Photographs should be especially effective in arousing public interest in agriculture because farm pictures can be loaded with fundamental, ready-made appeals to the general reader, appeals that concern many of the vital interests of mankind. For farm pictures have to do with the creation of food and clothing — the basis of survival for all men. Farm pictures have to do with the weather, still the most important news item in the world, and with the dramatic changing of the seasons. Farm pictures have to do with animals and plants, and with the great relationships of nature. Agricultural pictures have to do with forests and woodlands and streams. And agricultural pictures, too, deal

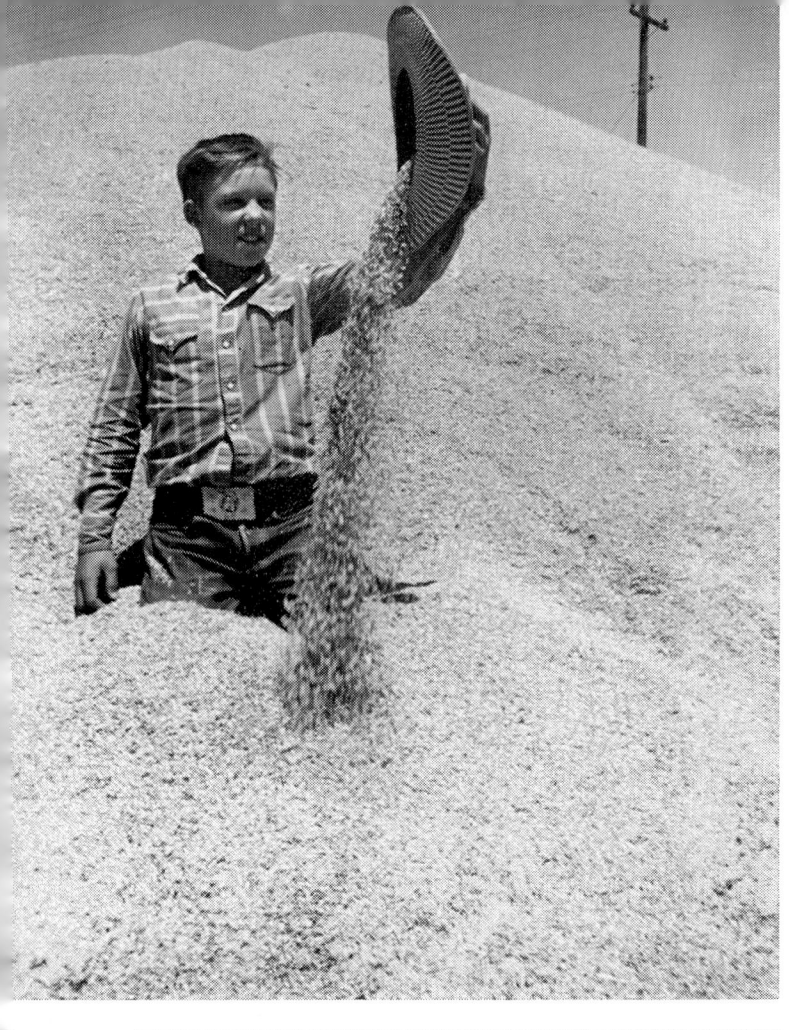

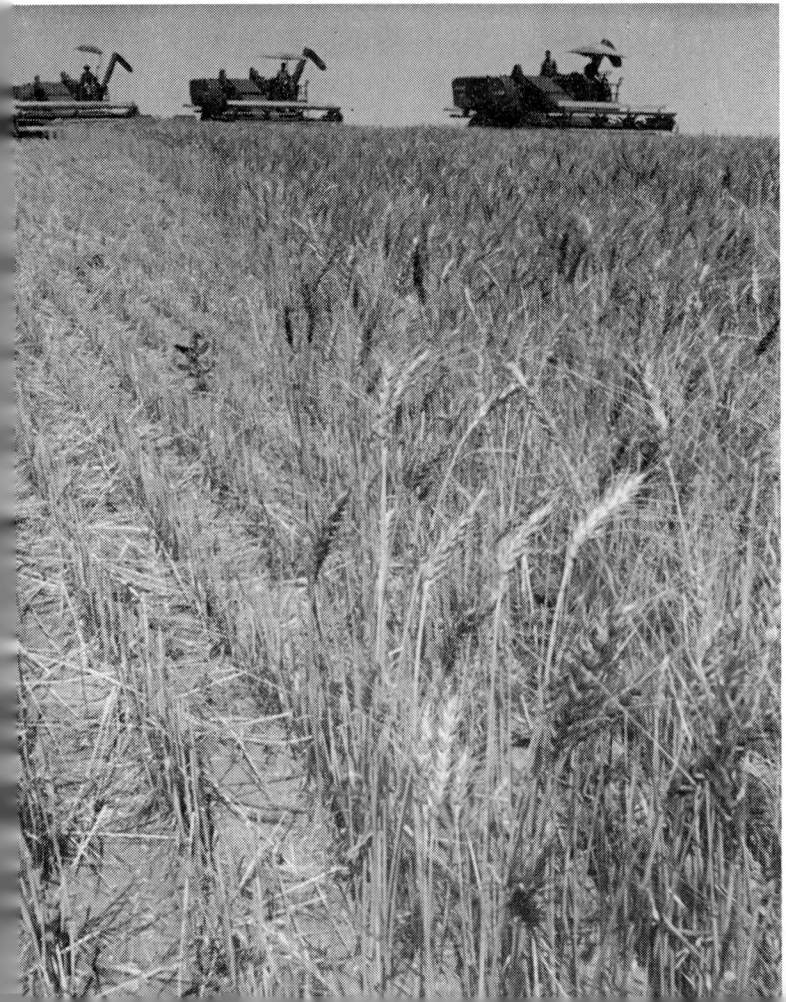

50   Mountains of grain symbolize the triumph of farmers over nature, but paradoxically create enormous problems.
*Dave Mathias, Denver Post*

with men and women and youths, with social life and rural customs and with the traditions of our nation.

Many a city dweller, tired of the noise and frantic struggles of urban living and surfeited with television and newspaper accounts of murder, mayhem and sadism, might be expected to turn with relaxation and relief to pictures of the rural scene.

**Pictures Can Help Explain Changes**

In human terms, pictures can reveal the pain that accompanies the displacement of a considerable proportion of the farm population, the difficulty of adjustment to new ways of life faced by thousands, the dismay caused by the decay of hundreds of recently prosperous small towns whose jobs were to supply the farmers. For pictures of closing-out farm sales, of abandoned farm homes, empty schools, Main Streets with half of their stores closed, of farmers and their wives commuting to industrial jobs to supplement their incomes and hold their farms a little longer, all bring home the human element in the situation.

**Pictures Reveal Reasons**

Photographs, too, can picture the underlying reasons for this basic revolution in agriculture with its repercussions in the general economic, social and political life of the nation. Pictures show dramatically the huge and complex machines planting, cultivating and harvesting the amazingly big and productive crops that have sprung from agricul-

51   Ever more effective machines help farmers feed the world — and are an important factor in creating agricultural problems that demand adjustment.
*Dave Mathias, Denver* Post

tural research. Looking at such pictures, urban readers readily can understand that the 125 acre farm with its old-fashioned plows, mowers and binders can no more stand up in competition with the fantastic new machines and crops and livestock than the hoe, spade and scythe could compete with horse-drawn binders and cultivators. Such pictures explain why farms must be larger units, why the number of people needed for farming is decreasing.

**Photographs Make Statistics Live**

Statistical aspects can be explained by simple graphs, decorated with and accompanied by photographs. Pictures of great heaps of corn beside overflowing cribs can dramatize

52  The appeal of rural landscapes that show farming operations in progress makes it comparatively easy for pictures to attract the attention of the general public to agriculture.
*Bob Beasley*, The Cooperative Consumer

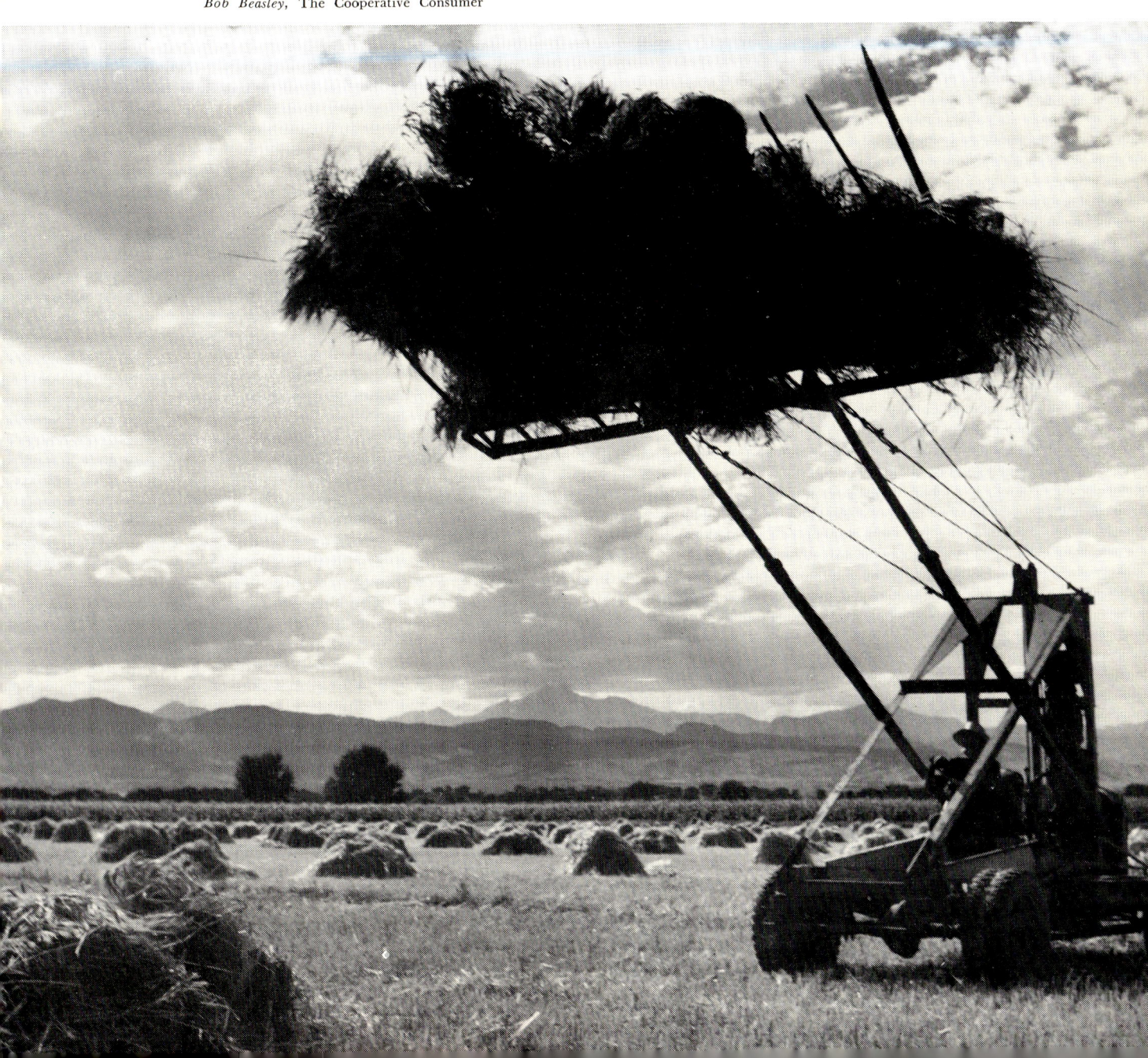

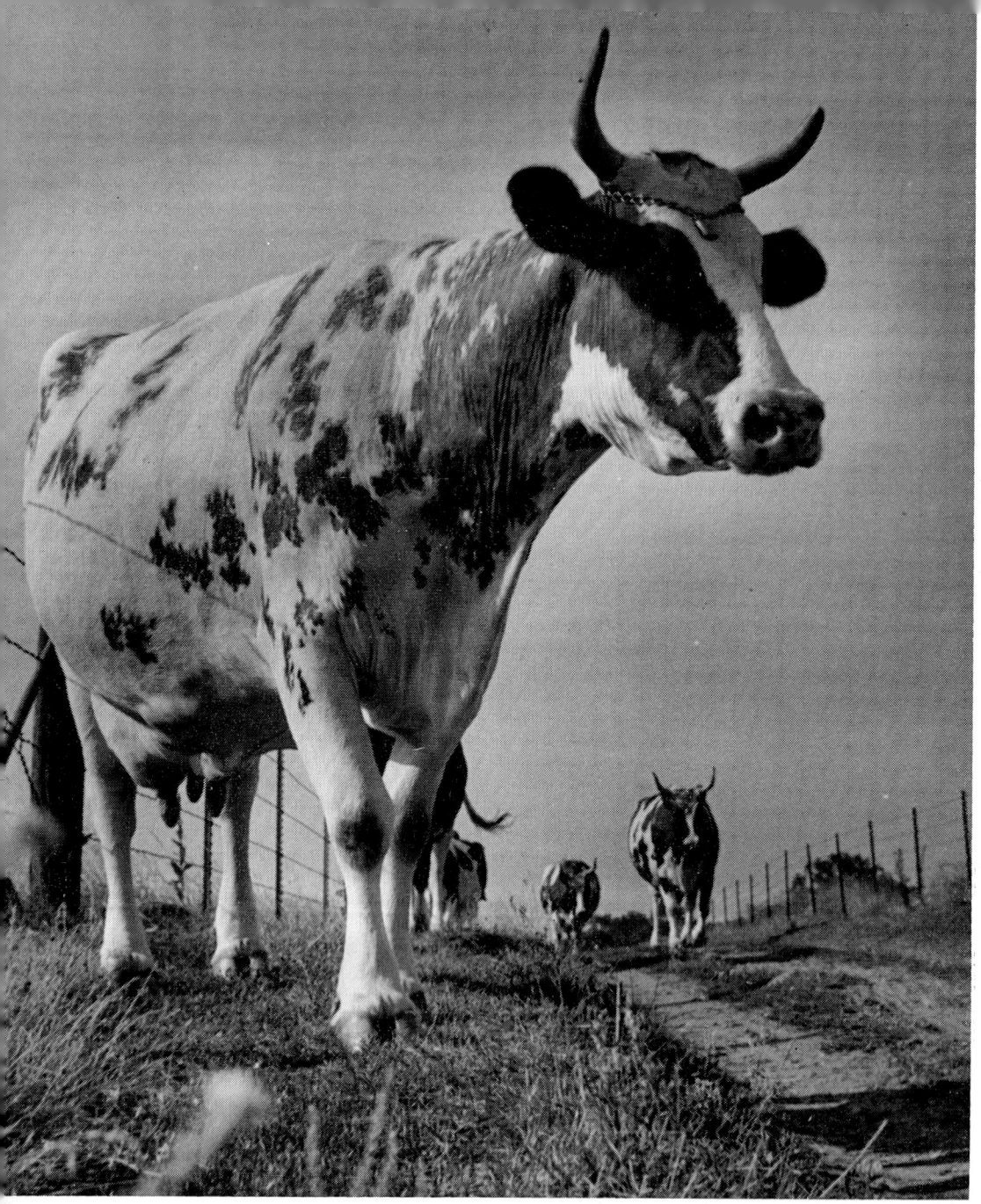

53 The photogenic qualities of a cow make her good picture material for newspapers, whether rural or urban.
*George P. Miller in Harvester World. International Harvester Company*

the enormous problems of chronic overproduction that contribute to low incomes for farmers and to the general farm problem. Pictures of hillsides eroding under crops that shouldn't have been planted on them, of the last trees being cut from streamsides to provide more cropland will point up the desperation of farmers for more cash even when their efforts only add to the burden of overproduction. And such pictures will point to the desperate need to relieve the situation. Airviews can vivify the concepts of acres in ways figures can't. Photographs can make statistics come alive.

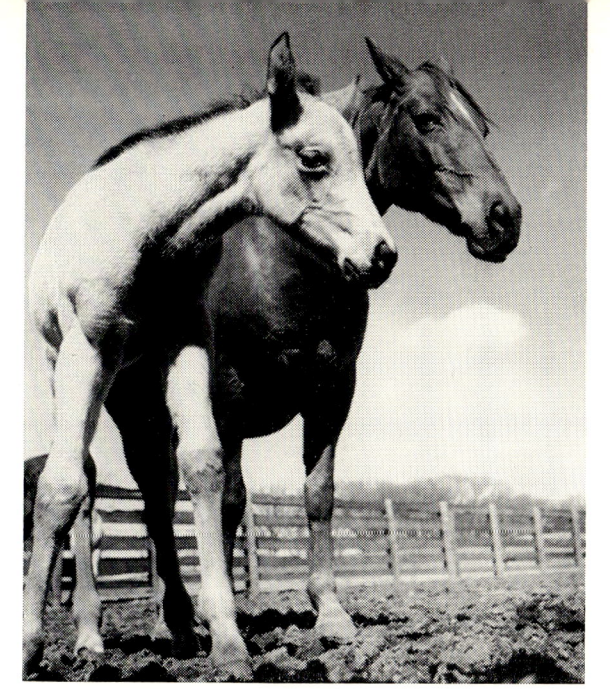

**54** This picture of a mare and colt should attract attention almost anywhere.
*Bob Johnson in Ames (Iowa)* Daily Tribune

**55** There is real drama in this picture of a hog collapsed from heat being revived with use of spray from a fireman's hose. The animal survived.
*Photo by Bob Bartley, Herald-Register Grinnell (Iowa)*

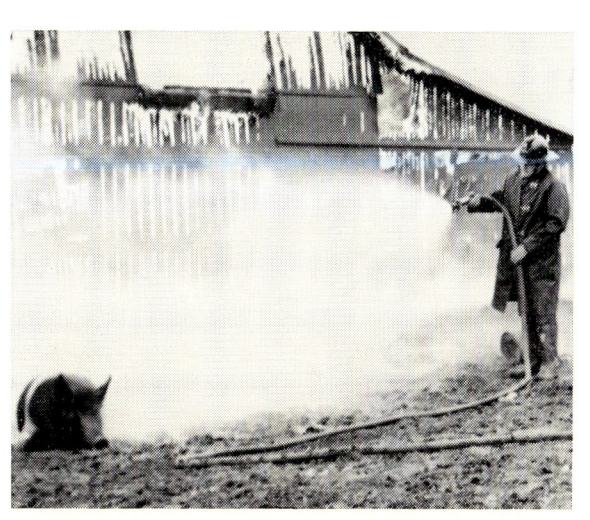

**56** Although agriculture is changing fast, many good old ways of doing things persist, like this "God's Acre" project to aid a rural church.

## Farmers Need Picture News Too

But while the great responsibility of today's agricultural reporting, especially in pictures, may well need to be directed toward the general public, the specific news needs of farmers must not be neglected by newspapers. Especially is this true in areas in which agriculture is of great importance.

Although the farm population is decreasing rapidly, many families continue to operate farms, many of them greatly enlarged.

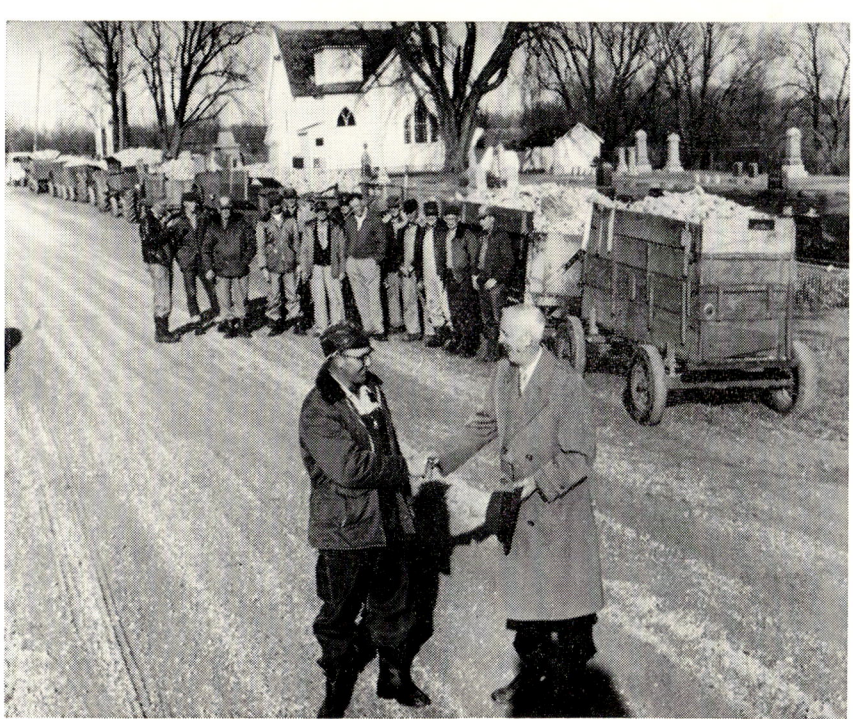

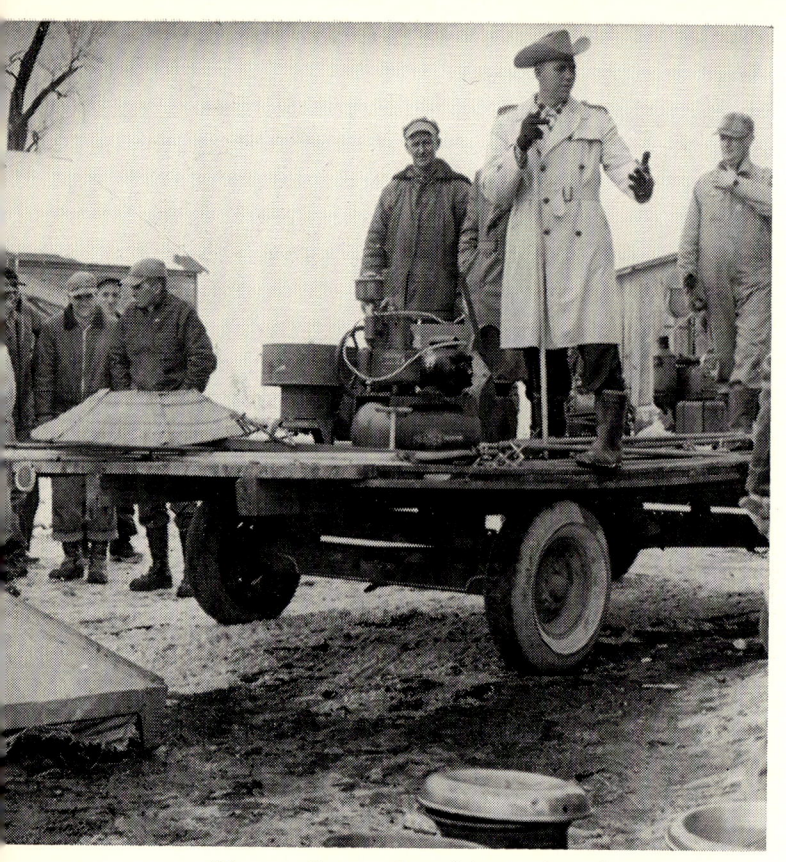

**57** Farm sales of livestock and equipment remain important and newsworthy events although to some they seem sinister because today they symbolize the diminishing number of farms.
*Paul Andre, Cedar Rapids (Iowa) Gazette*

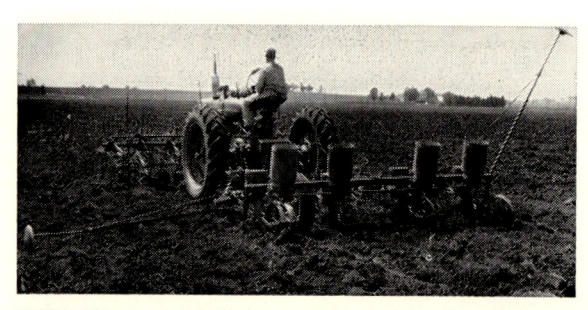

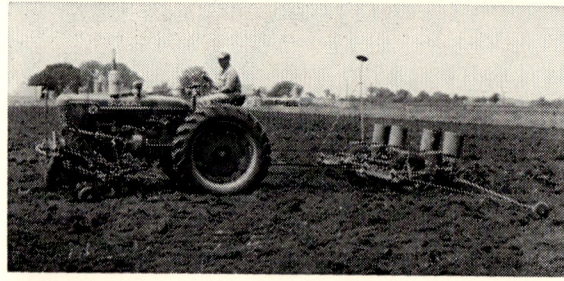

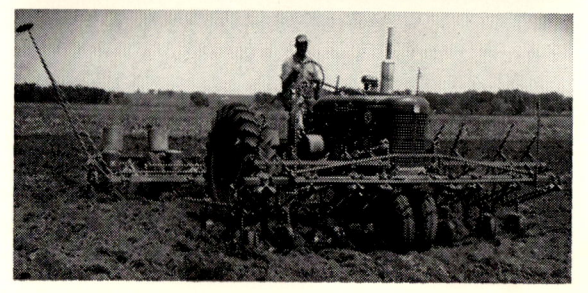

Their buying power continues great, and in agricultural areas their political importance remains large. Newspapers need these farmers as subscribers and as friends.

As with agricultural news intended for general readers, special news for farmers can be carried to an important extent in pictures. The new kind of farmer, with his huge acreages and enormous investments in machinery and land, needs to keep abreast of the rapidly developing advances in agricultural technology and needs quick and ready access to much news if he is to survive in this highly competitive business operation.

Local picture stories can bring this type of farmer reports concerning research in production, processing and marketing. Competing farm journals are doing an excellent job in this field, largely in pictures. But with their greater space and frequency of publication, local newspapers often can supplement and do a more intensive job than can the journals. Even though a farm magazine exploits a story first, the newspaper farm editor can publish picture stories about the experiences of local farmers who try new practices, can obtain information from local authorities who might suggest specific methods to apply locally.

Even though the radio with its immediacy can do a discouragingly good job of bringing current market reports to farmers, the printed publications can outdo radio in backgrounding market situations by using maps, graphs, photographs as well as printed words.

**Government Picture Coverage Helpful**

With their large operations, farmers must keep well informed about federal, state and local government. Here, too, pictures can help keep farmers informed about current and proposed farm programs, legislation, policies and reforms.

**60** For newspapers in farm areas, bread and butter farm photos reporting continues to consist largely of pictures of ingenious ideas farmers like to know about — such as these showing how a disc and planter operate when attached to the same tractor.
*Paul Andre, Cedar Rapids (Iowa) Gazette*

Likewise, with some quite militantly political farm organizations exerting pressures, coverage of their affairs at least partly in pictures is important as a portion of the presentation by newspapers of political matters of special interest to farmers.

**What Topics Most Interesting?**

What topics about agriculture most need to be spread before readers of American newspapers? A group of editors representing all major areas of the United States checked what they considered the most important agricultural subjects for newspaper use.[1]

In the order of importance assigned by the editors, here are the 25 topics considered of greatest interest:

1. Surplus, how much, why
2. Causes of farm troubles
3. Farmers' cost-price squeeze
4. Long-range prospect for agriculture
5. Significance of agriculture in our economy
6. Free prices (government out of farming)
7. Ownership trends, family farm
8. Effects of population increase
9. Is farming a way of life or a business?
10. Farm income level now and what society wants it to be
11. Numbers, especially decreasing farm population
12. Conservation's effect on current and future output
13. American society's obligation to agriculture; why shouldn't government help agriculture adjust?
14. Basic maladjustments
15. County, township and town government problems
16. Soil bank or some other voluntary land adjustment
17. Inelastic resources, demand, prices
18. New uses for farm products
19. Co-operatives
20. Farm organizations
21. Consumer food prices, now and outlook for future
22. Increasing technology and its effect
23. Processing efficiency
24. Advertising to increase consumption
25. Insufficient amounts, when and why?

Ingenious photographers and editors can devise ways of using photographs, maps and graphs to present pictorially such topics as these to a democratic society that needs such information if it is to make intelligent decisions about an important segment of its national life.

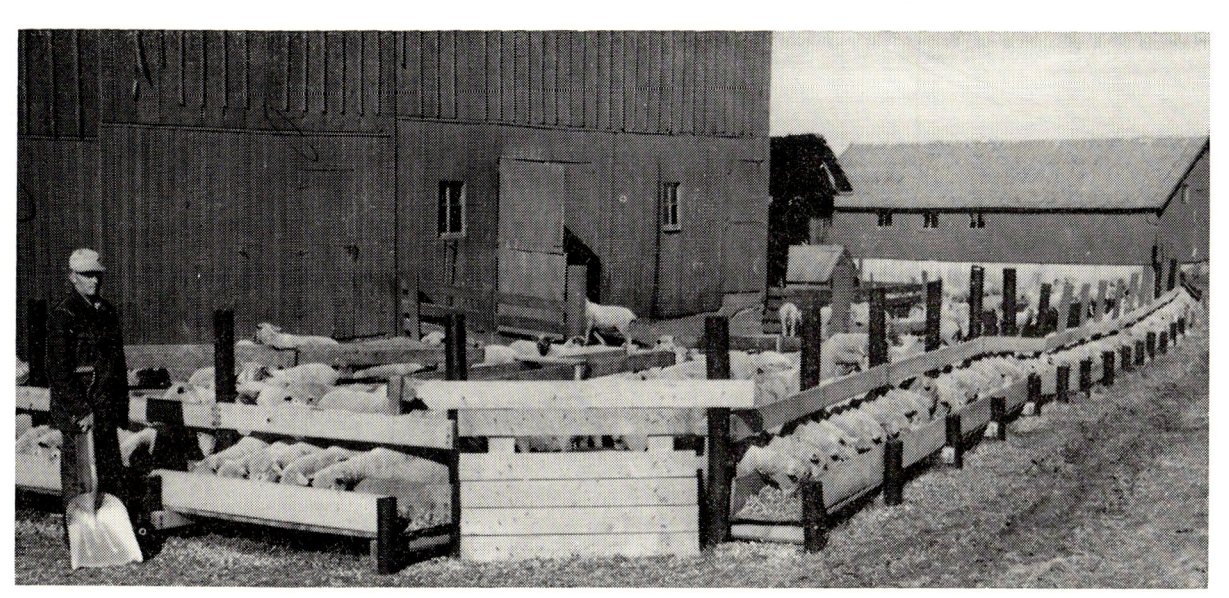

[1] Carlson, Jerry, *Editors' Judgements Concerning Appropriate Content for an Agricultural Adjustment Handbook.* Unpublished, Iowa State University graduate seminar report, 1960.

61  This picture of a method of feeding sheep is the practical kind farmers like to see on their farm pages.

*Paul Andre, Cedar Rapids (Iowa) Gazette*

CHAPTER **6**

# Women's Page Pictures Attract Readers, Delight Advertisers

BECAUSE WOMEN'S PAGES and society sections deal with some of the most basic matters of life, women's page editors have a chance to use some of the most exciting and emotion evoking pictures in a paper.

After all, what subjects are more important than marriage and babies, food and the decoration of homes, the social strivings of a community expressed in parties, receptions, gatherings? Not infrequently love — or lack of it — is discussed in stories and columns on women's pages.

Yet in spite of these wonderful potentials, women's and society pages in the non-metropolitan papers tend to be as little pictorial as any section with the exception, perhaps, of classified advertising. And the pictures used incline toward the highly conventional, routine and unimaginative.

**Society Pictures Can Be Alive**

It's true that many society pages publish quite a few pictures of weddings, wedding

62   One of the happiest moments in a woman's life can be illustrated in many ways more delightful than the usual formal head-and-shoulders picture.
*Davenport (Iowa)* Morning Democrat

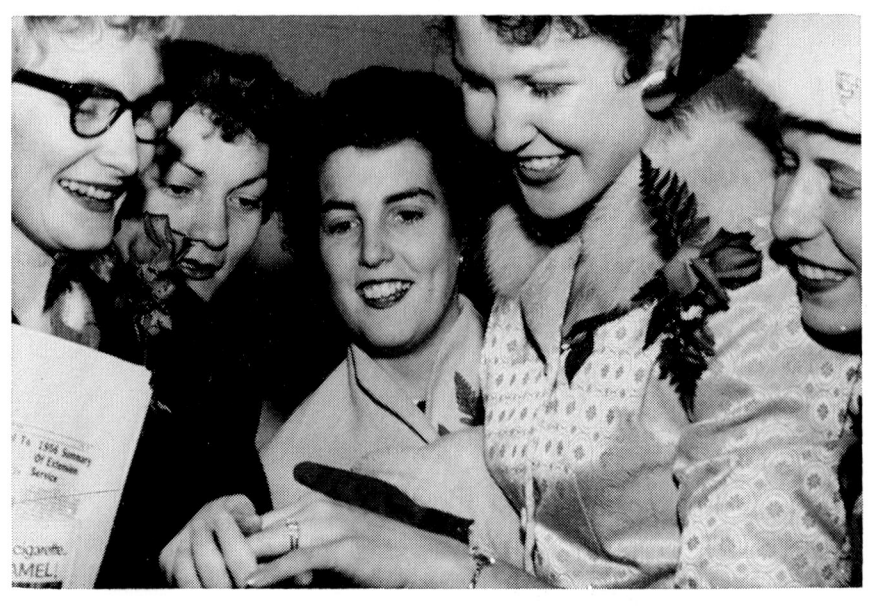

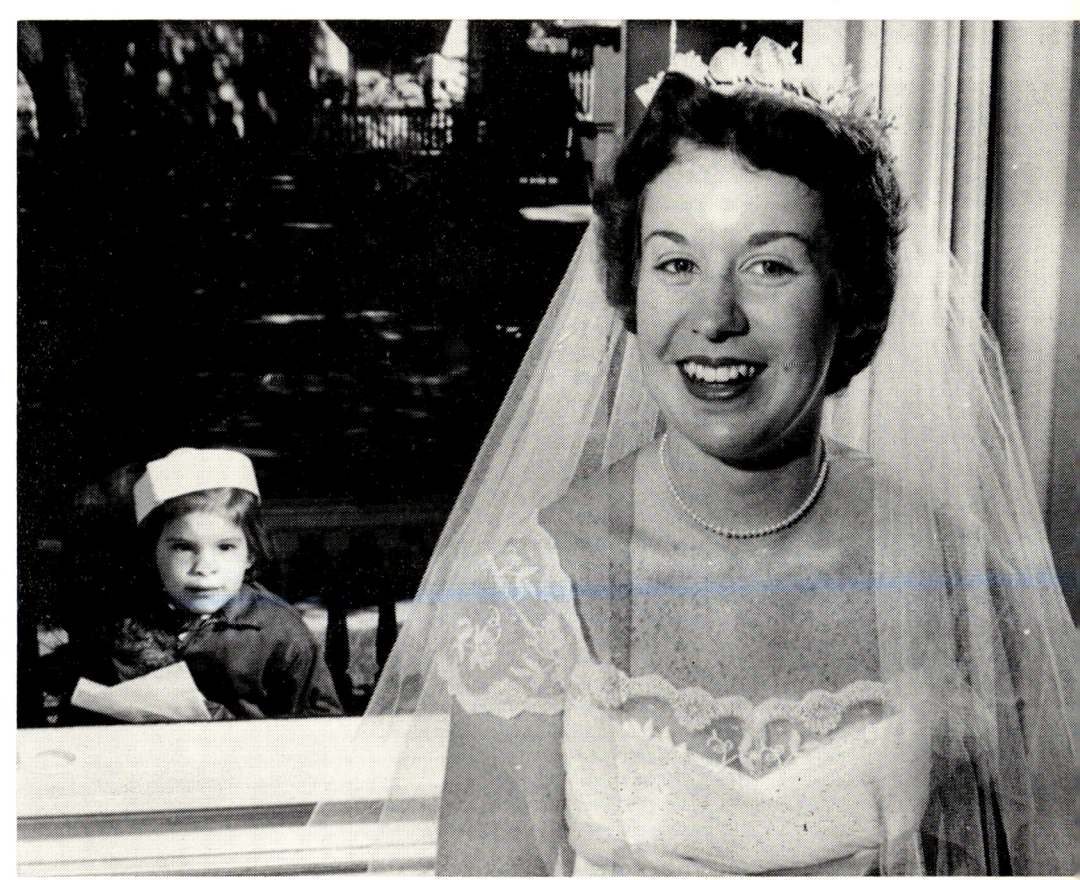

63 A picture of the bride in her beautiful gown can be dignified and still contain the delight of a feature.
*The Milwaukee* Journal

anniversaries, parties and brides-to-be. But all wedding pictures don't need to look as if they came out of an album, portraits can be more than conventional head-and-shoulders shots, people at parties can be organized into interesting groups for pictures.

Many wedding pictures are taken by studios and furnished to newspapers in exchange for a credit line, and studios have determined ideas about how pictures should be taken. And in many communities convention almost decrees that wedding pictures be taken according to time-honored rules. Still — more often can't wedding photographs be informal, news-type pictures, showing the couple leaving the church, or fleeing for their car in a shower of rice, or with the cute little flower girl kissing the groom, or with some such story-telling quality?

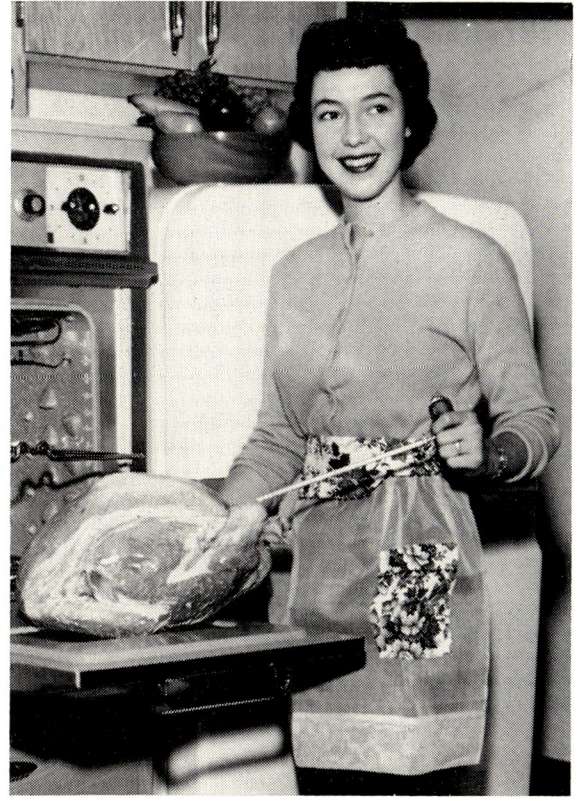

64 This young woman will depend upon the newspaper's foods pages to help her with meal planning throughout her years as a homemaker.

— 49

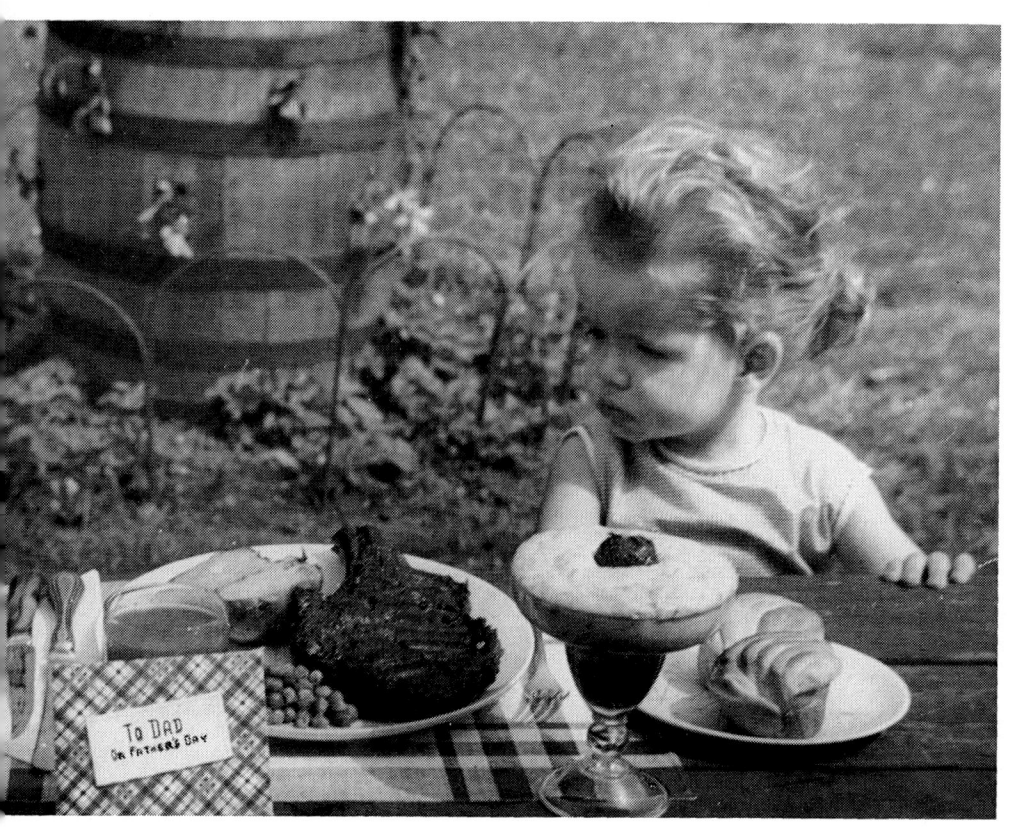

65   Pictures can draw attention to recipes and menus, especially when the photograph contains a human figure like this charming child and a Father's Day dinner that includes a strawberry-barrel dessert. Out-of-focus background emphasizes the subject matter.
*John W. Dougherty for Thomas J. Lipton, Inc.*

Why must golden wedding anniversary pictures so frequently be formal and stuffy? Why not have the couple at ease in their home, or working together in their garden, or petting their dog, or looking lovingly at some of the treasures they have collected in 50 years of living happily together.

Pictures taken at parties can show action, fun, a story-telling situation, an interesting grouping of figures.

Good portraits tell stories in terms of personality, indicate action by means of expression.

**Food Pictures Offer Opportunities**

Because women face a tough problem in planning, buying supplies for, and preparing three attractive and well-balanced meals a day, they have an understandable interest in recipes, stories and pictures about proper diet requirements, attractive table settings and about economical and seasonable purchases of food. In their preparation of meals they find an opportunity to express their love for their families, and they are understandably eager.

For the non-metropolitan paper, food pictures in black and white are difficult to take satisfactorily, and anyway they lack warmth. But every town has many women who are superior cooks, or who have some interesting specialty they make to perfection, or who become locally famed because they successfully take charge of big church or lodge dinners. These women can be pictured in their kitchens in story situation pictures in connection with recipes, bits of advice and cookery lore. Successful hostesses can be pictured planning table decorations and settings. Some wives originated in foreign countries or have lived abroad and can be pictured making exciting foreign foods, especially at Christmas or other holiday seasons.

66   Speaking of recipes, this little girl looks up one for candy. . . .

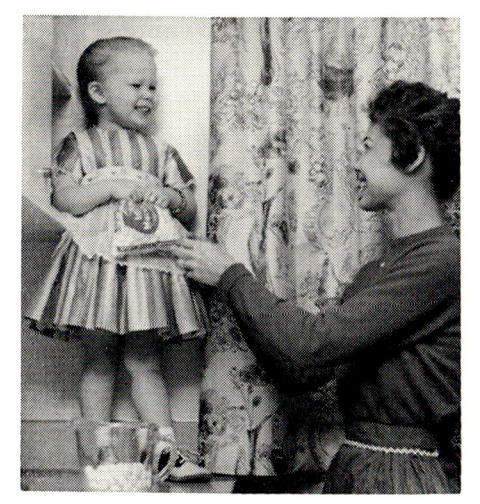

67   Gathers her ingredients. . . .

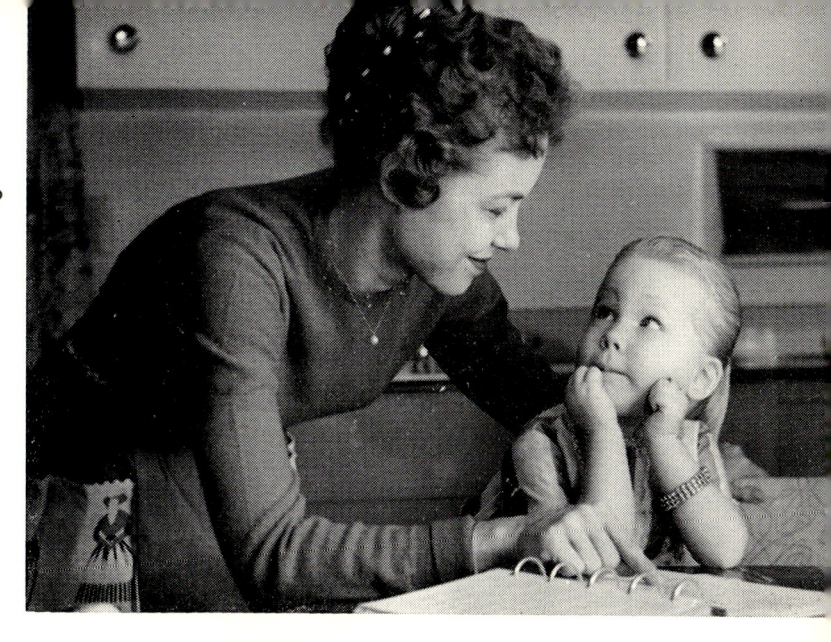

68   Adds a little — quite a little — sugar. . . .

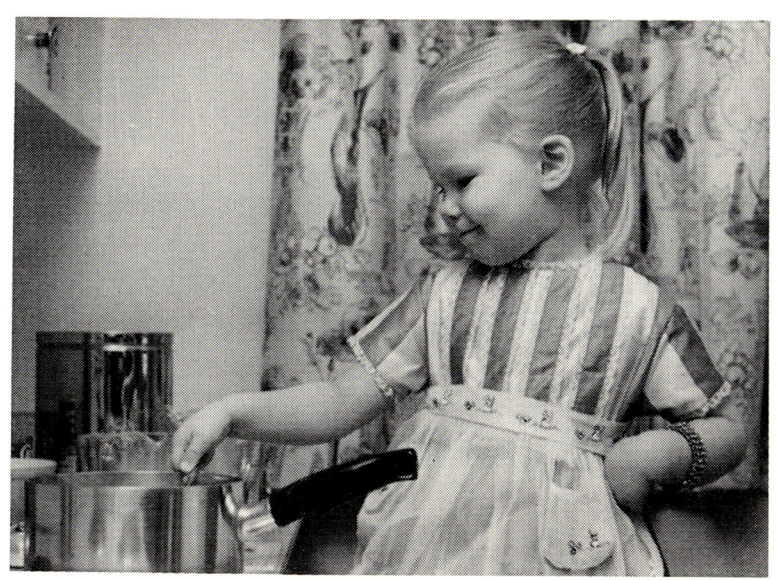

69   Stirs the mixture vigorously. . . .

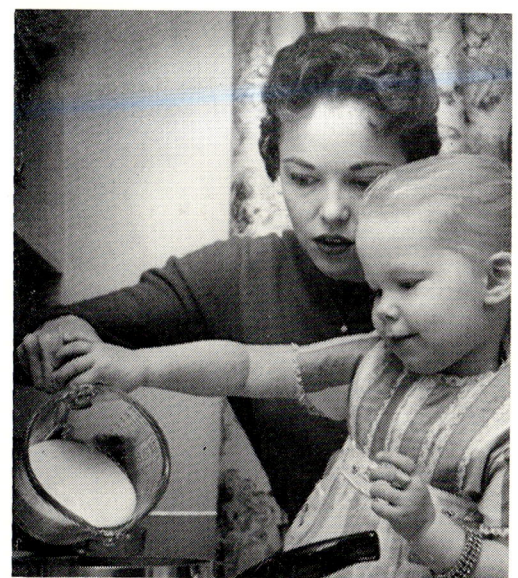

70   And yummy, what a treat!

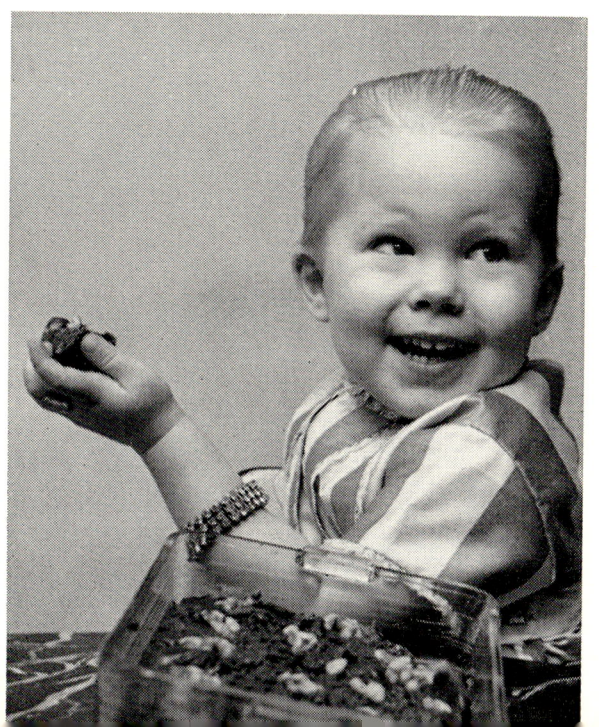

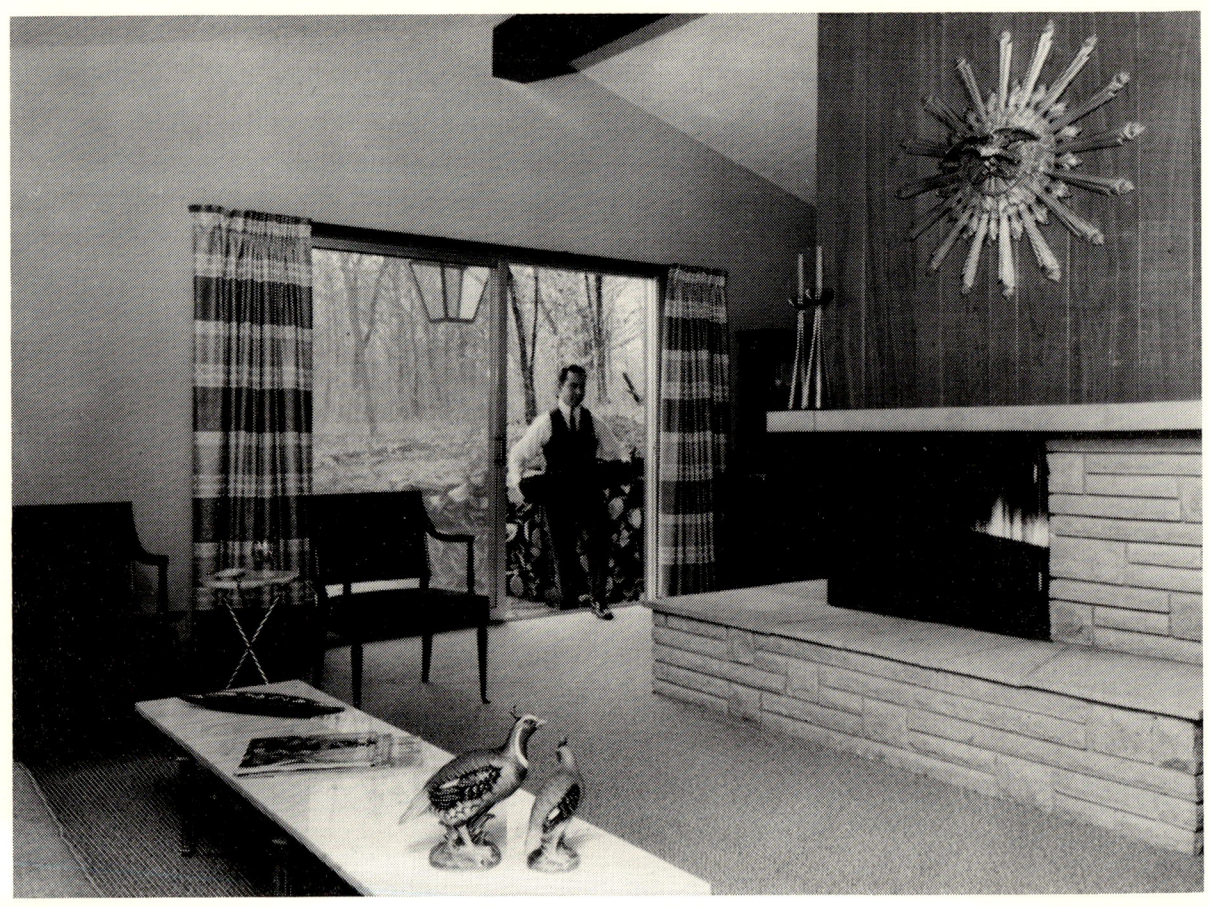

71  The photographer helps readers satisfy their natural curiosity as they enter the homes of others through pictures.
*John McIvor, Cedar Rapids (Iowa)* Gazette

### Room Interiors Reveal Personalities

Almost everybody likes to see the interior of somebody else's home. Perhaps part of this fascination stems from the fact that the arrangement of furniture, the selection of pictures and books, the way a room interior is planned reveal penetratingly the personality of the woman who decorated it. Perhaps the key to success in photographing a home interior lies largely in selecting those aspects of a room which most revealingly depict the personality of its hostess. Intelligently planned pictures of interiors usually include human figures and make warm, exciting news pictures for women's pages.[1]

Some people argue that certain pictures of interiors intended to show decorations or some specific aspect of furnishing are better

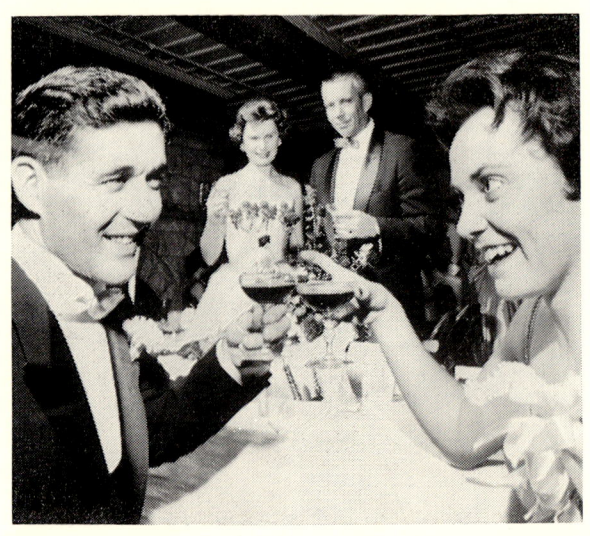

72  Pictures of social affairs can be as gay as the events they depict.
*Photo by Clifford R. Yeich, courtesy of the Reading (Pa.)* Times

---
[1] For an expansion of the idea that rooms and their decorations reveal personality, see *Nonverbal Communication* by Jurgen Ruesch and Weldon Kees, University of California Press, Berkeley, 1956.

without human figures. If the draperies are the reason for taking a picture, they argue, don't include a human figure because it will steal too much attention away from the draperies.

**Fashions Fascinate Women**

Fashions fascinate most women. It's true they can turn to magazines and other media to get their news about fashions. But the local press has the advantage over magazines in the fashion field in that it can picture local fashions photographed on local women and children. In thousands of cities and towns too small to be concerned about professional models, it usually is easy to find personable women of prestige to pose for style pictures in clothing available from local stores. The stores usually are more than happy to cooperate. This can especially well be done in connection with spring or autumn style shows or openings and similar events.

**Advertisers Are Pleased**

But, you may think, it is far too expensive in terms of time, space and effort to take quantities of food, fashion and interior decoration pictures. But look! Your paper makes its living selling advertising. Most important advertising, probably, is of foods, clothing and home furnishings. Your advertisers will be delighted if you do a good job on women's and society pages with attention-exciting pictures in those three areas. After all, women do most of the buying of such commodities. Chances are your pictures will stimulate advertising at the same time they provide good will, greater readership and increased interest in the women's pages on the part of your readers. Your pictures may even help increase circulation.

Some women's pages have successfully included stories about matters of social significance, such as marriage versus career, debates about the desirability of early marriage, problems of older people, plans having to do with the prevention of juvenile delinquency.

Others seem to have made appealing copy from pictures and stories about glamorous and prominent women who range from queens, presidents' wives and moving picture stars to locally outstanding and successful hostesses. Perhaps thousands of women find in such pictures vicarious pleasure and dream fulfillment. Subject matter of this sort opens the way for many excellent story-telling pictures.[2]

---

[2] Six major appeals, the first three suitable for use on women's and society pages, were shown to account for nearly all measured variation in interest in most pictures used in a study, "Women's Interest in Pictures: The Badger Village Study," reported in the Spring, 1953, *Journalism Quarterly*, by Malcolm S. MacLean, Jr., and William R. Hazard.

The appeals were: Idolatry, social problems, picturesqueness, war, blood and violence and spectator sports.

73  Fashion pictures are important on women's pages.
*Bob Weir, Alpha Delta Sigma, Malden (Mass.) Press*

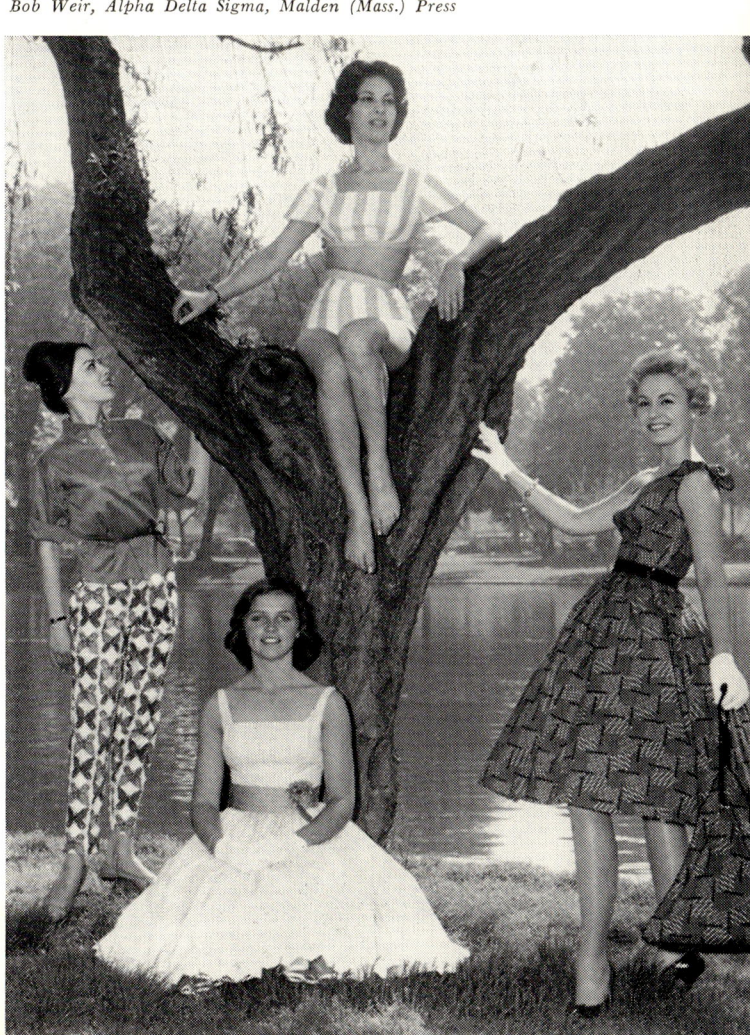

## Chance for Building Good Will

Many clubs, church groups, lodges are grateful for space for their organizations on the society pages. They are especially happy when a picture is used. Space for this sort of thing is limited. But here is a chance to build much good will for your paper.

Use of many pictures of clubs and other groups can help papers in smaller communities achieve their objective of publishing the picture of everybody in town at least once a year. Properly planned group pictures can be interesting.

## How About a Contest?

News photography contests conventionally include categories for general news, feature and sports pictures. Why don't they more often add a section for pictures of special interest to women? Pictures in this realm can be warm, newsworthy, exciting, socially significant and wonderfully important in the building of good will toward a publication both among readers and advertisers.

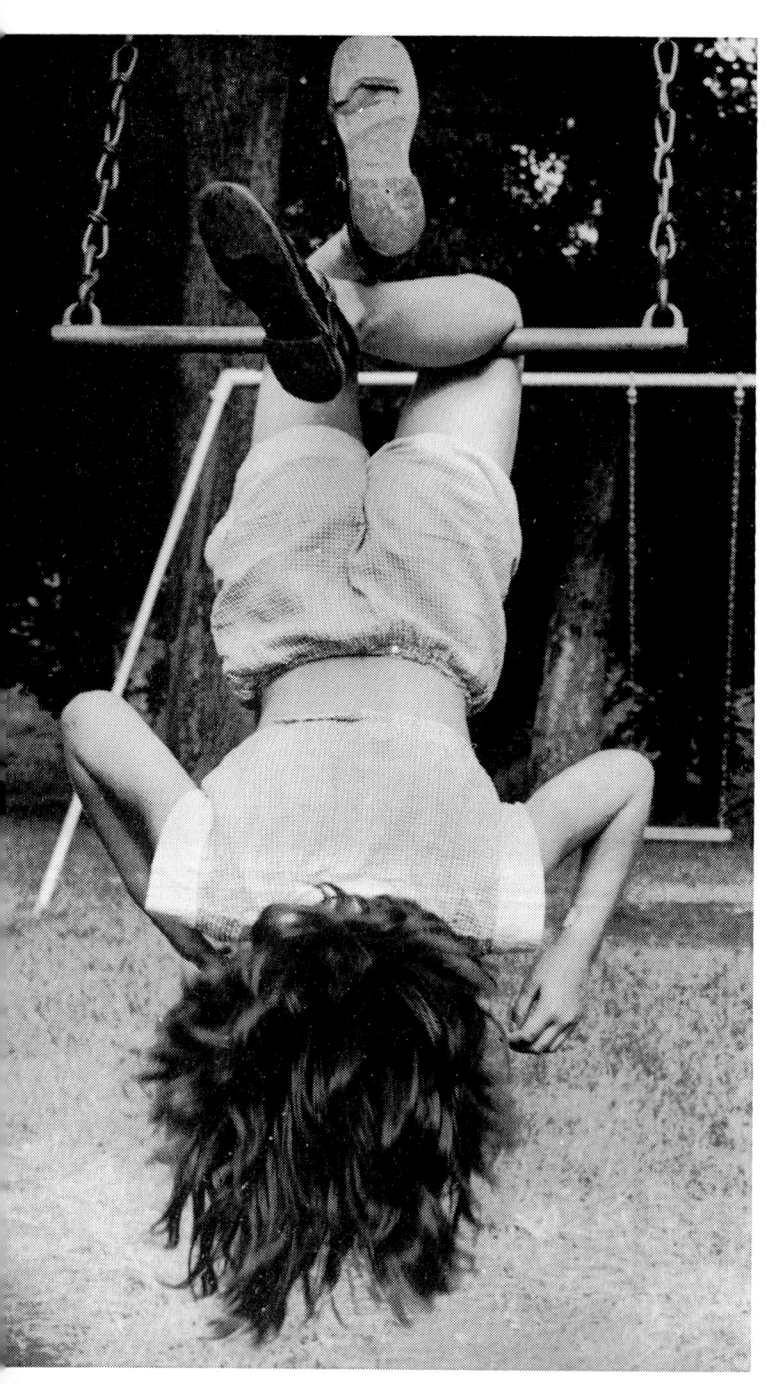

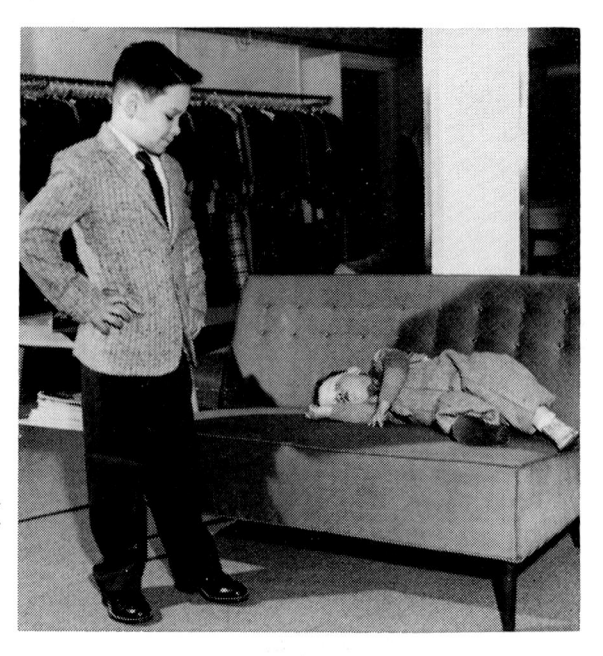

74    Shoes — or the need of them — can be the feature of pictures published by women's pages in support of charities, such as camps for underprivileged children.

75    But for some people, shoes — even big brother's shiny new ones — arouse little interest.
*Davenport (Iowa) Morning Democrat*

CHAPTER 7

# Win Readers With Pictures of Leisure-Time Fun

WHY CAN'T THE UNDOUBTED SUCCESS of sports coverage in attracting readership of probably three-fourths of the men and quite a few of the women be extended to reach a high percentage of those who don't now read sports?

Can't the interests of many of those thousands who don't follow the sports pages be reached by a more active coverage of the hundreds of leisure-time activities now so avidly pursued by vast numbers of Americans? And might not many of the present sports page readers follow this news about recreation other than sports? After all, these leisure-time activities are "sports" in the eyes of those who pursue them.

The wholesome, happy utilization of leisure time has become a major sociological problem in America as working hours are steadily reduced, as the number of still energetic but retired persons is increased, as young people are forced to wait longer to

76 Springtime brings out birdwatchers to see the great migrations. *Iowa Conservation Commission Photo*

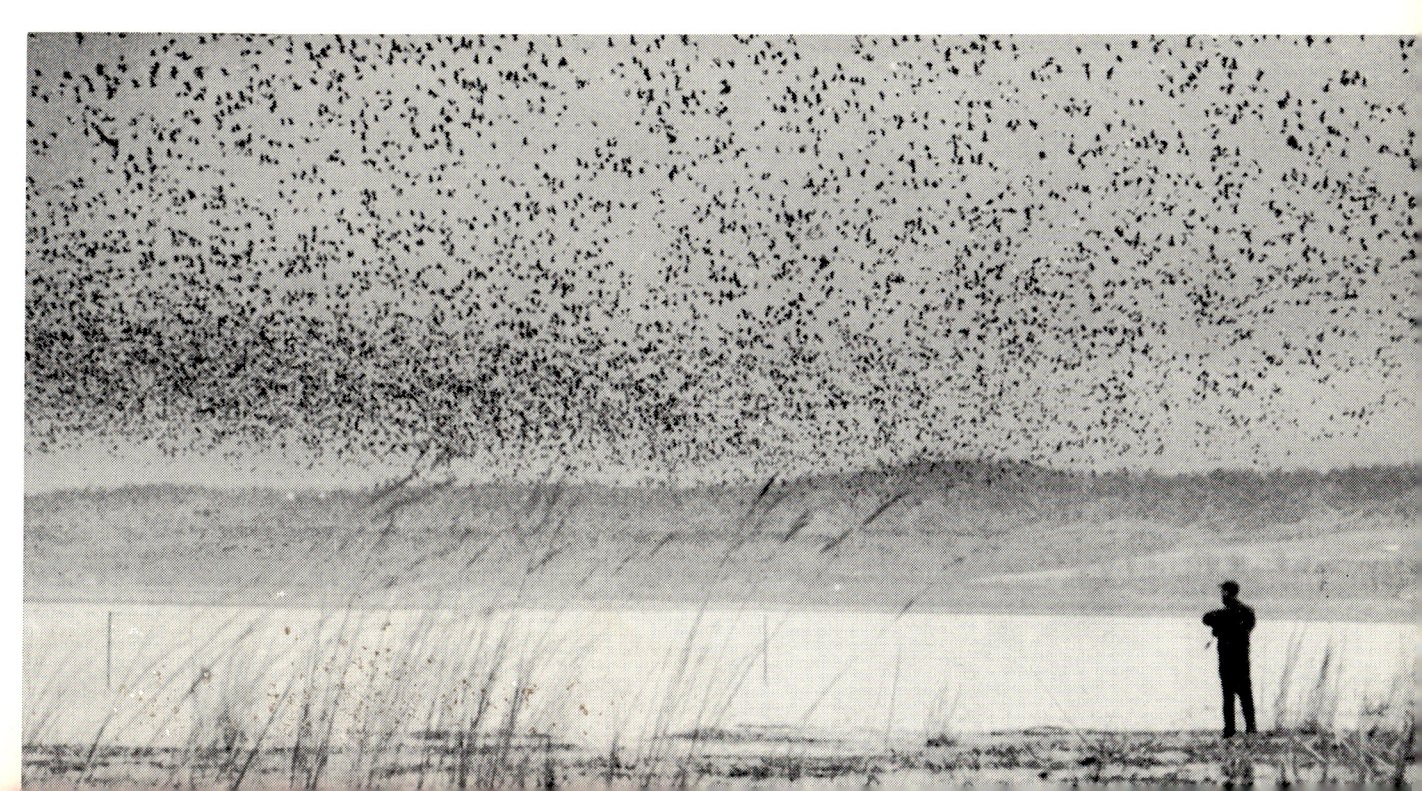

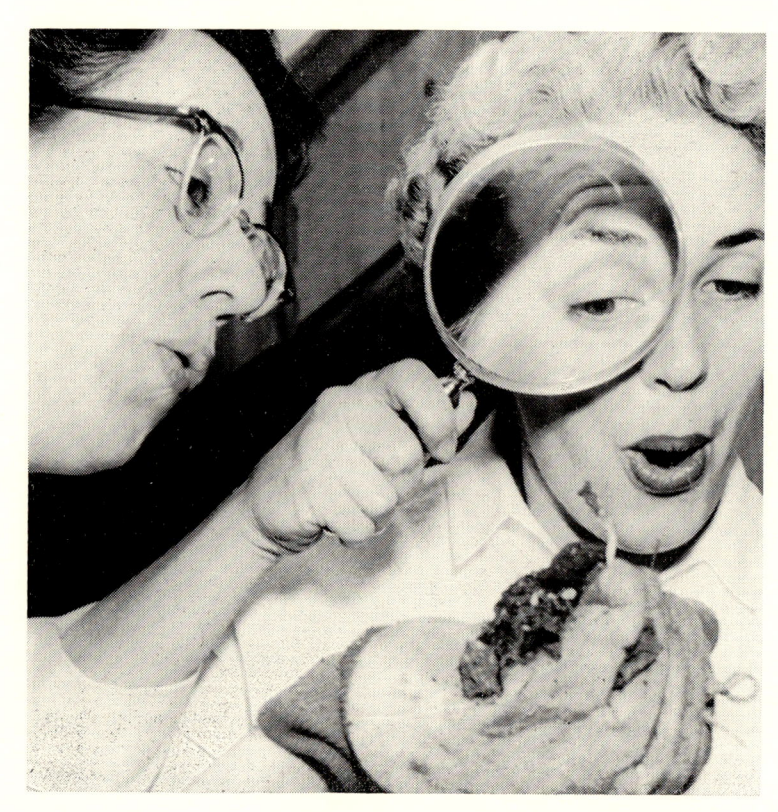

**77** Suburbanites react with wonder to the first garden sprout. . . .
*Davenport (Iowa)* Morning Democrat

start gainful employment and as housework becomes easier and leaves women with more spare time. The amount of leisure time available for Americans probably will continue to increase rapidly with more automation, increased population of working age, greater efficiencies of production and distribution.

**Two Groups Need Leisure-Time News**

Americans with leisure time to spend — and there are millions of them — can be divided into two groups: those who are shopping for activities that might interest them and those who are deeply immersed in hobbies and pursuits already. Both groups might be expected to be interested in news of leisure-time activities. Both groups have considerable money to spend on the cameras, boats, binoculars, paints, tools, books, records, arrows, albums, seeds and other supplies that the leisure-time users want and buy. Sale of such supplies must total a big sum in any sizable town, which suggests that the advertising department has an interest in this kind of coverage. It should increase advertising sales.

Americans today are spending increased amounts of time and money on bird watching, rock hunting, stamp collecting, amateur photography, painting, collecting everything from seashells to salt shakers and antiques, raising pets and hundreds of other diversions.

Thousands have moved to suburbs and have found new joys in gardening, lawns and shrubs. Well-equipped workshops exist in thousands of homes.

Many persons have acquired interests in the fine arts. Art centers have sprung up

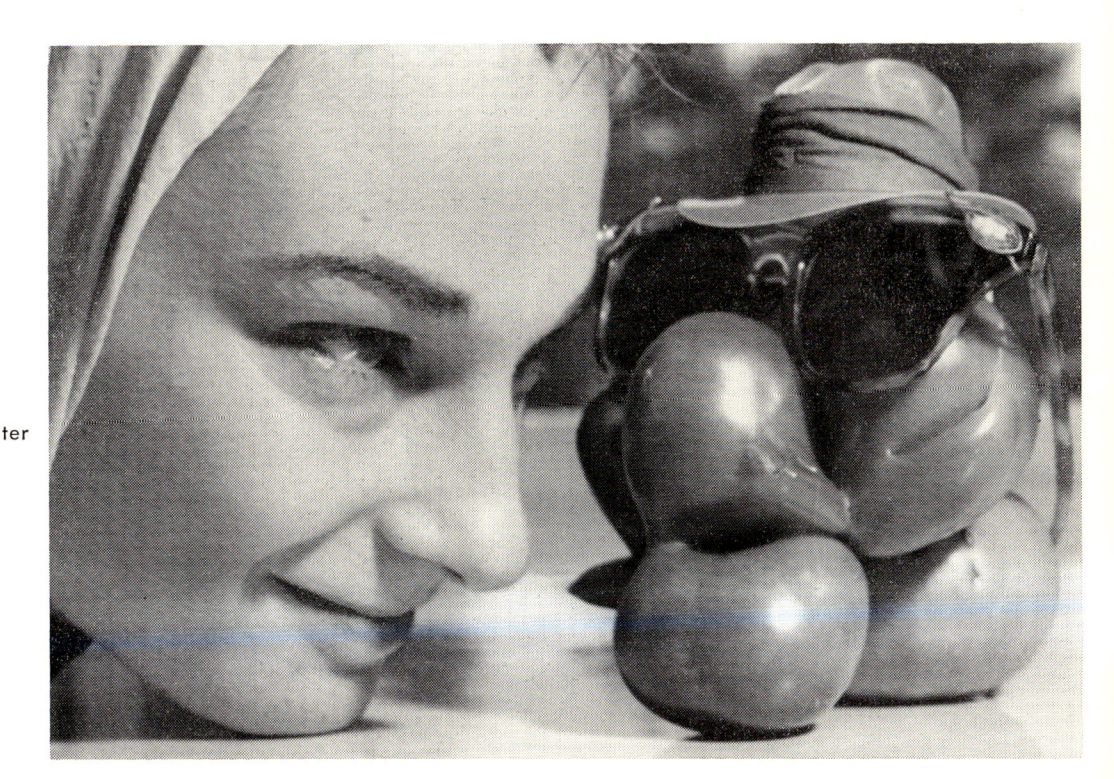

78   And dream of later triumphs with tomatoes.

*Richard Kraus,*
Newsday, *Long Island, New York*

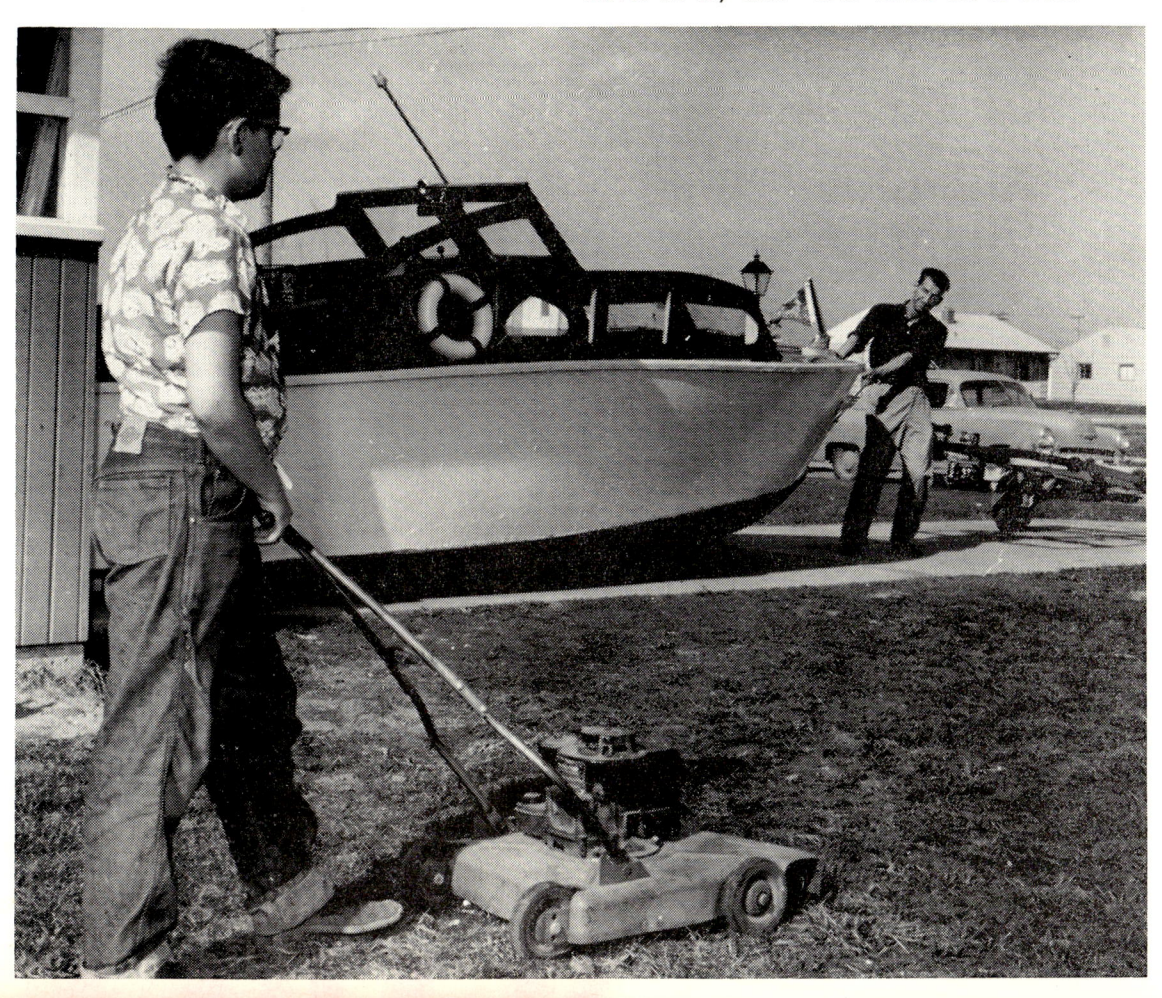

79   As summer comes, the great inland fleet moves on dry land — after lawns are in order.

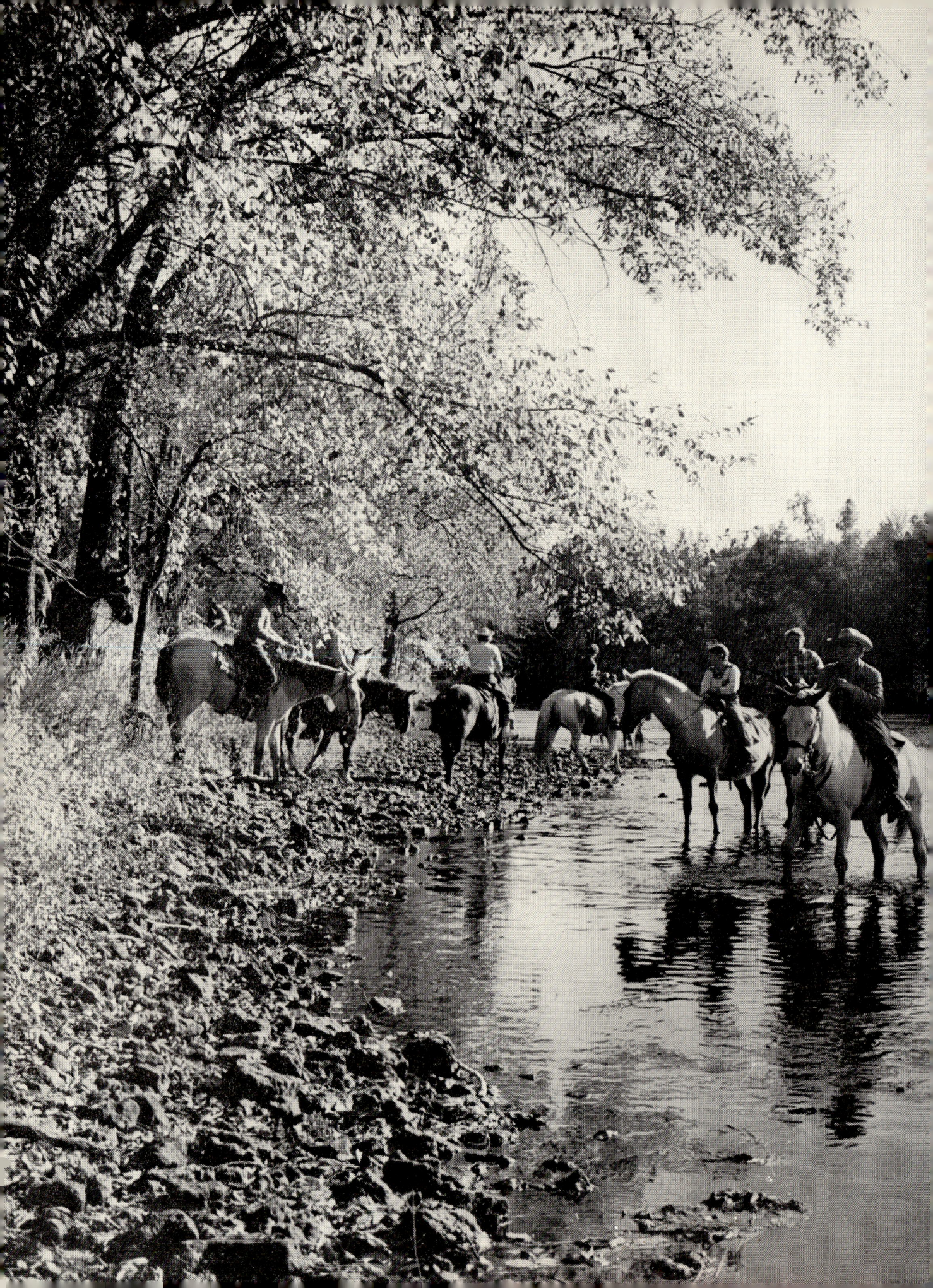

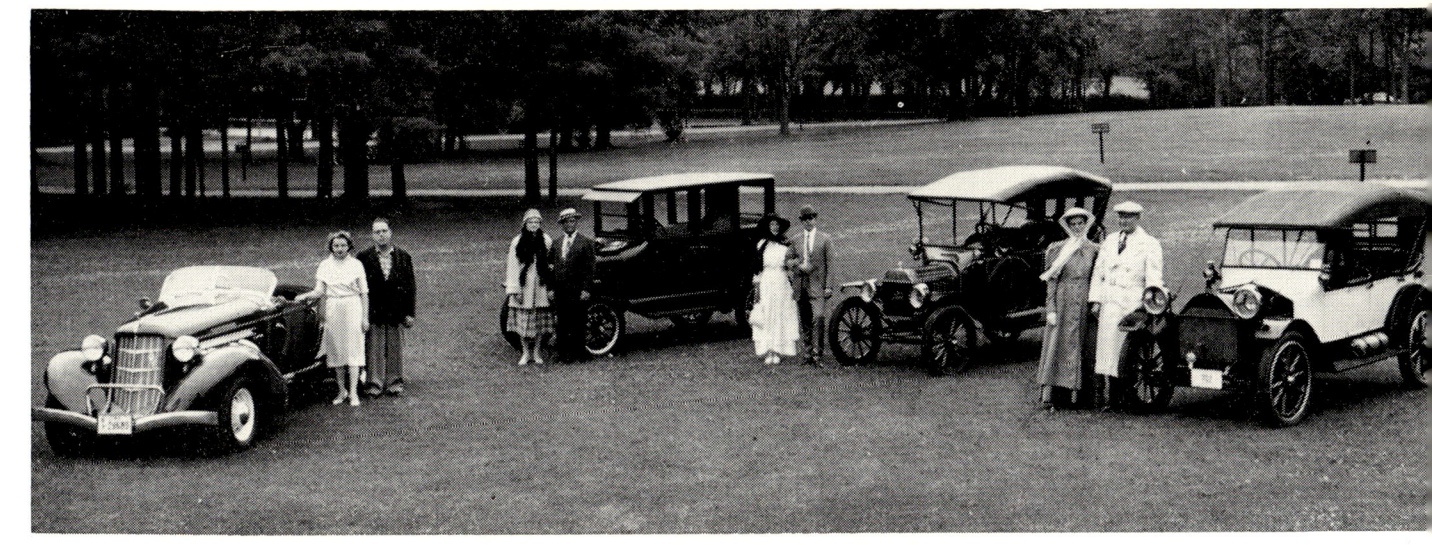

81 Old car enthusiasts stay away from the open roads.

even in comparatively small cities, and many persons attend classes in painting, sculpture and crafts. There is a huge sale of phonograph records. The sale of quality paperback books has zoomed. Amateur drama groups are happily active in hundreds of towns. Camera clubs flourish.

The intensive coverage of major sports certainly pays off for daily newspapers. Coverage of the minor sports is generally well done and pays high returns, unquestionably. But the coverage of professional and regular school and college sports makes possible the use of names and pictures of a limited number of persons only, mostly men and boys. Interest in stories and pictures about these sports is enormous, but they aren't followed by everyone by any means.

**More Names and Pictures Needed**

The number of persons who can be written about and pictured on sports pages is greatly increased when peripheral sports such as archery, horseshoe pitching, checkers and chess, skin diving and fishing are well covered. More and different people take part in such sports. Some of them appeal to people in older age groups more than do football and basketball. In smaller cities and towns where newspapers with somewhat lim-

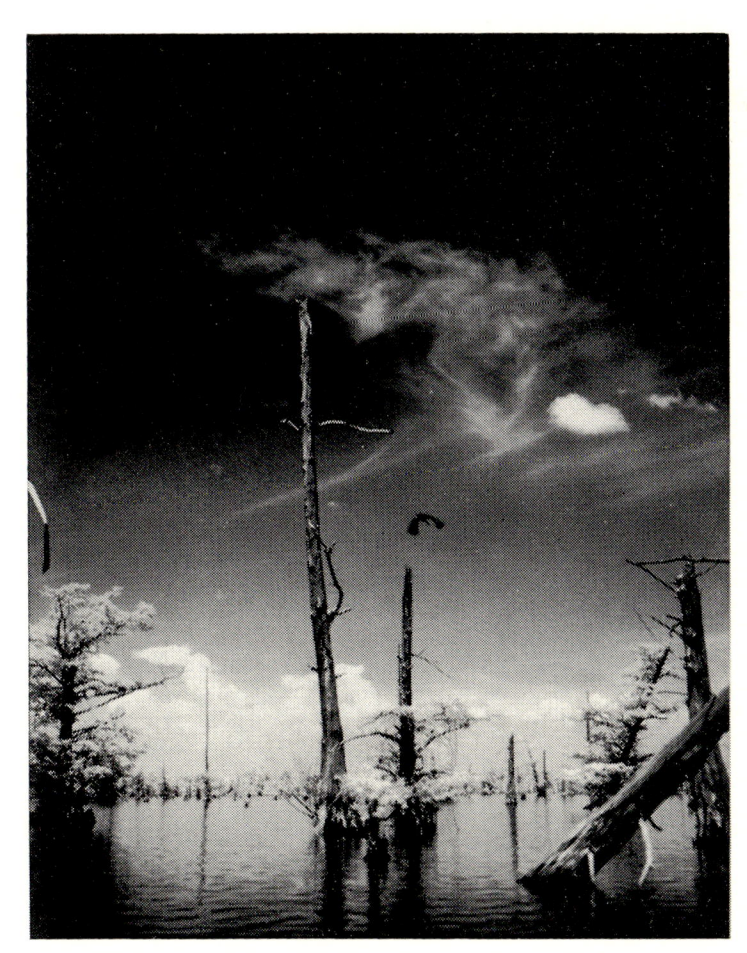

82  Vacationists take to the highways to photograph the trees and landscapes. . . .
*The* Courier-Journal *(Louisville), Thomas V. Miller, Jr*

80   Trail riders may follow the waterways.

ited facilities must compete in big-time sports coverage with radio and TV and nearby metropolitan newspapers, it might seem that intensive coverage of these little sports might yield greater good will and readership than would a too great coverage of big-time sports that can be better handled by competing media. In smaller cities, names still make news, and pictures with names are far better than names alone.

But wouldn't it pay to extend the enthusiasm with which sports are now covered to include many of the things people do in their leisure time for escape from boredom and for the joy and delight they find in such activities? To do so would be to appeal to the interests of a high percentage of the thousands of women not interested in routine sports, to the interest of many older men who have lost interest in sports, and to the interest of some other men who don't follow sports pages. And many who now avidly read sports pages might be interested in these other leisure-time activities too.

Some metropolitan papers have added excellent leisure-time sections to Sunday editions. Many large papers give considerable space to such things as stamp collecting, amateur photography, to reviews of recitals, concerts, art exhibits, lectures, motion pictures, radio and television. Many smaller papers are doing an excellent job in covering the very minor sports, activities and hobbies.

**Greater Coverage Should Pay**

But from looking over large numbers of newspapers, the impression can be gained

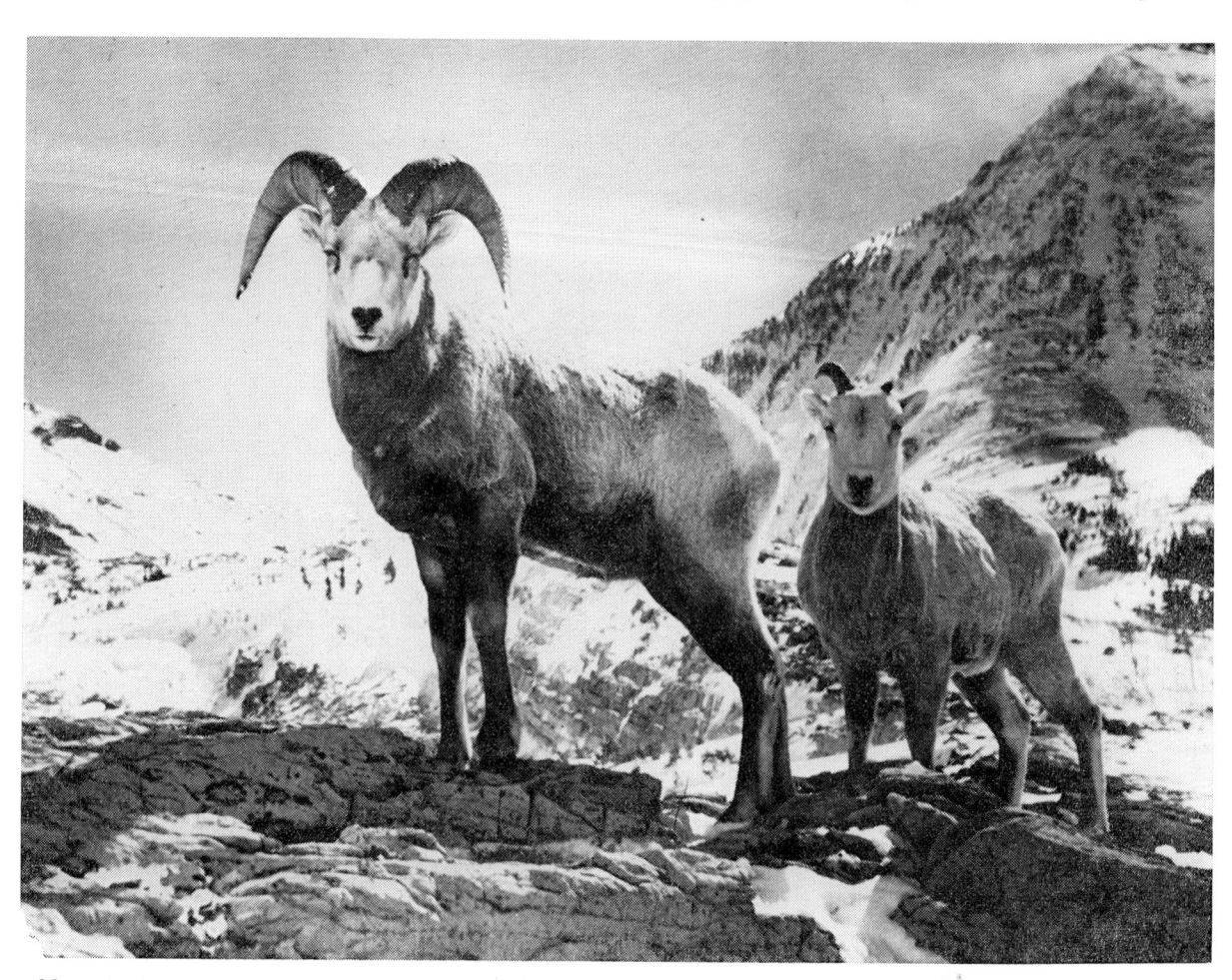

Some drive to national parks to watch the wild animals .... *Mel Ruder for the* Hungry Horse News

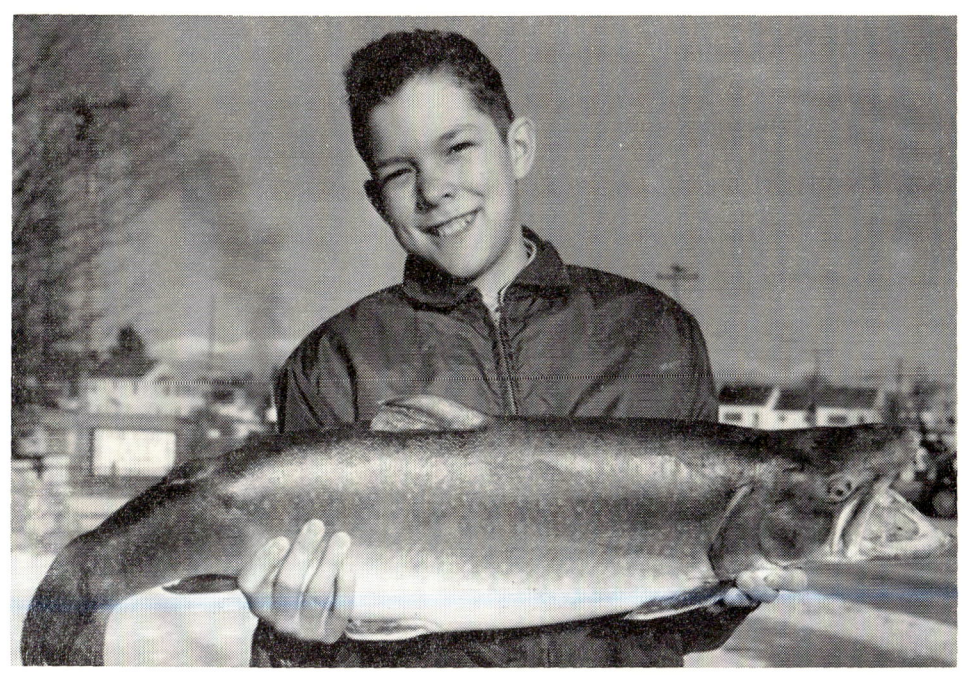

84   Or go fishing in high altitude lakes.    *Mel Ruder for the* Hungry Horse News

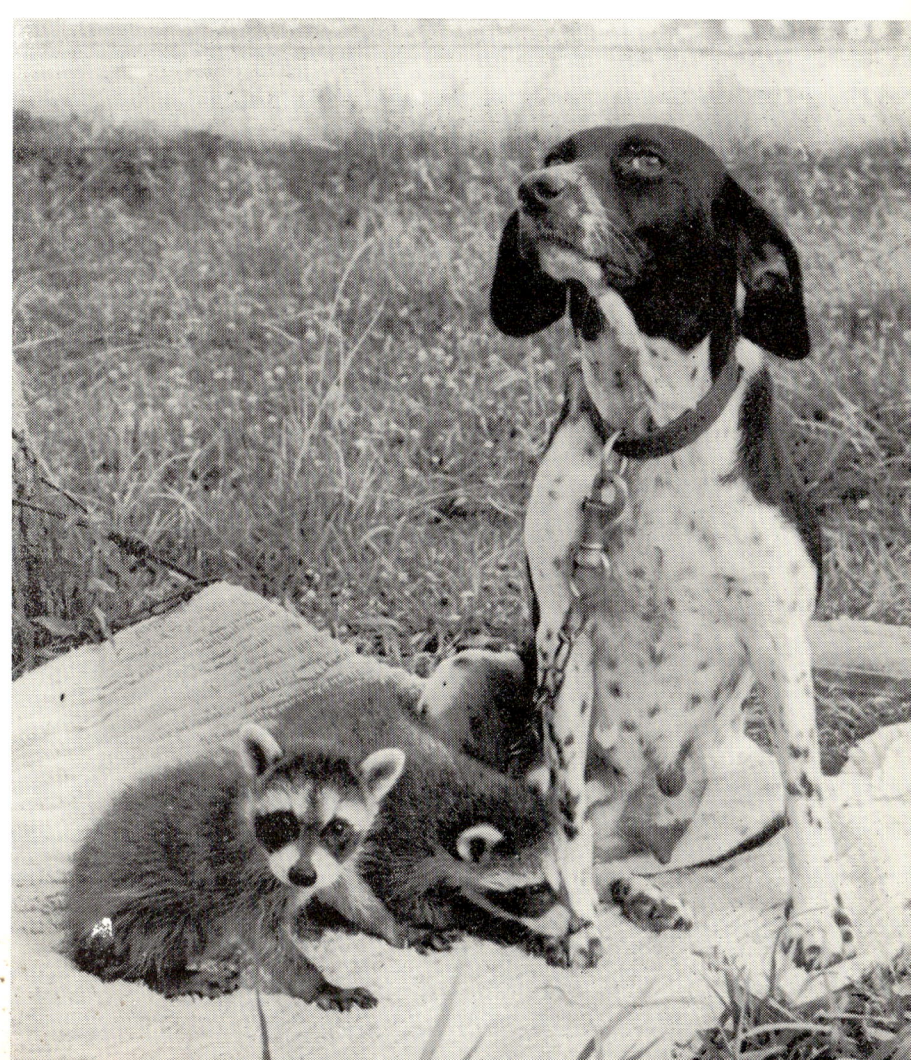

85   Sportsmen marvel at this hound, scourge of all coondom, whose mother instincts got the best of her and made her rear these orphans.
*Johnnie Quinn,*
The Gazette, *Ville Platte, La.*

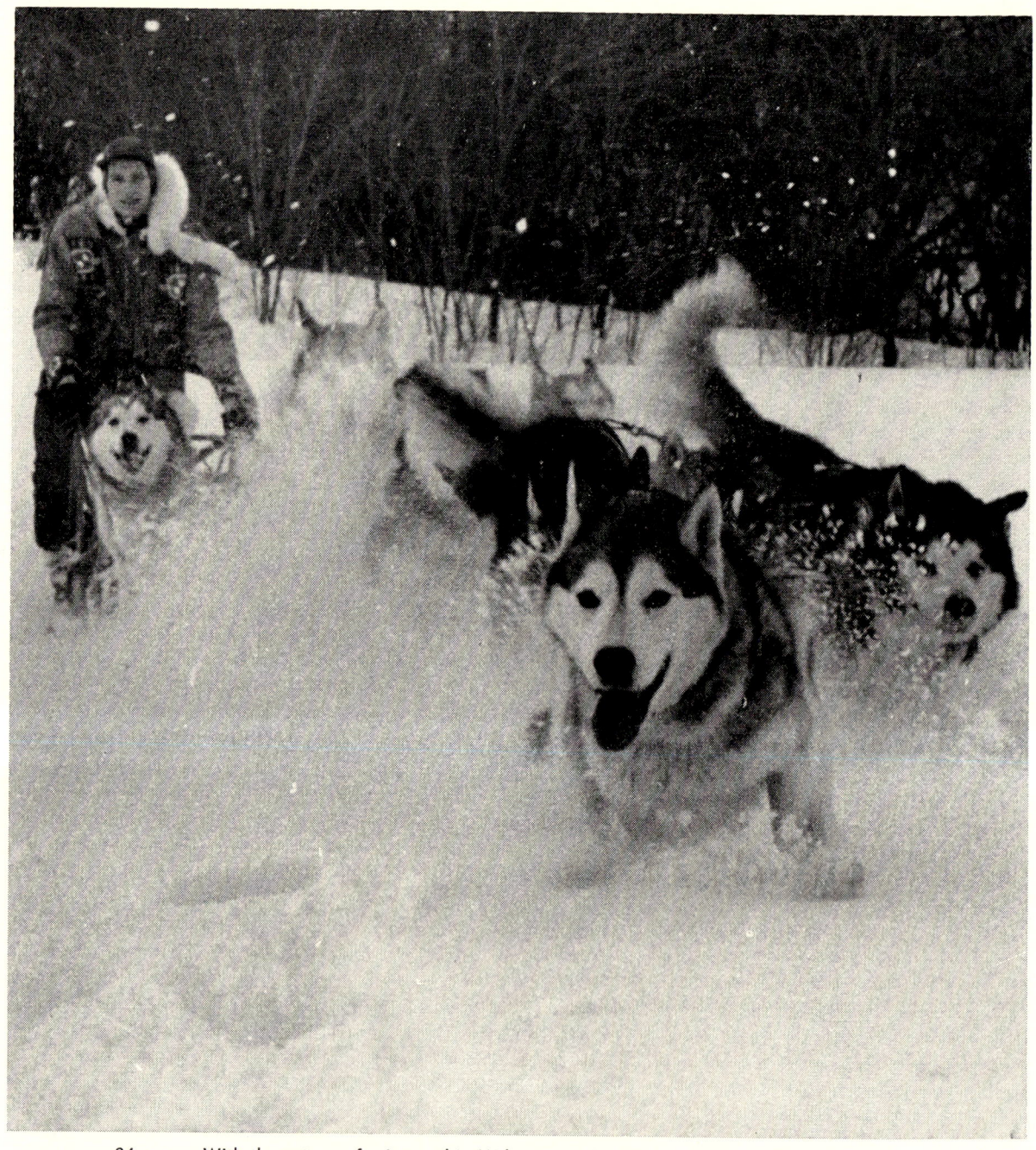

86   With the return of winter, this Midwesterner gets out his trusty dog team. . . .

that many publications slavishly follow old news formulae, valid a few years ago, essentially good today. But these papers might find that the large-scale development of leisure time, its activities and its need for activities, offers opportunities for a kind of coverage that would attract more readers, build greater good will and interest among readers. If this increased readership and good will were attained, it would please all advertisers. Some merchants who supply the needs of leisure-time activities might increase the amount of advertising they buy.

The very nature of many leisure-time activities suggests picture coverage. Bird watchers are as interesting as the creatures they pursue with their glasses. Amateur painters can be photographed with the scene they are producing as background. Archers can be dramatic — are sometimes pretty. Amateur dramatists should certainly look dramatic. All of such activities are full of photo possibilities.

**Why Not Sponsor Photo Contest?**

Why not give the amateur photographers a break by sponsoring a contest for them? Such contests turn up some interesting winning pictures for publication. And if amateur photographs run to children, cats, dogs, flowers and autumn scenes with falling leaves, it could be that such things are what a large number of people really want to see in pictures.

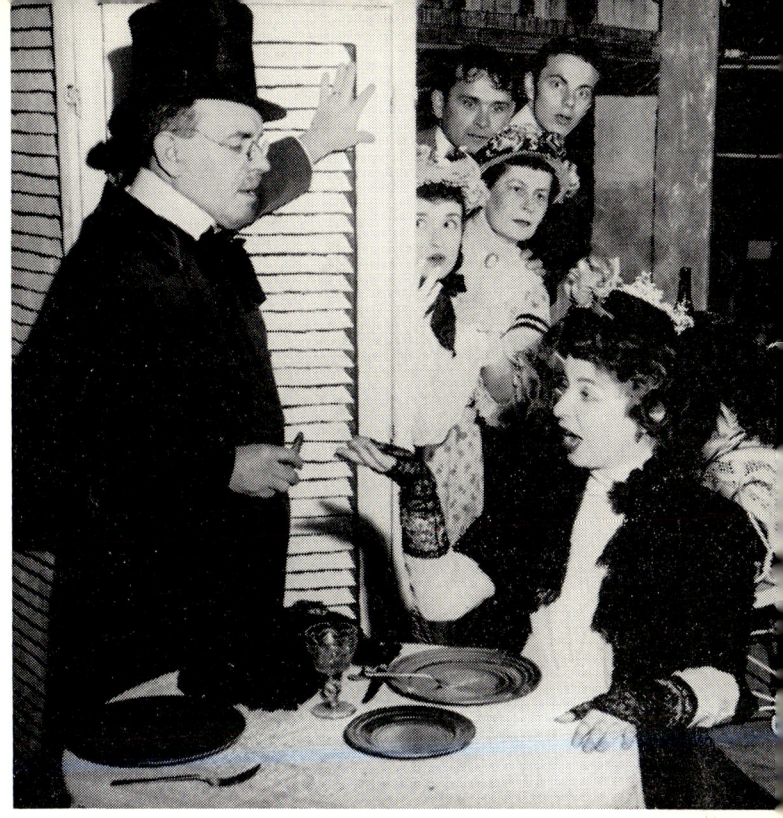

87   While indoors, amateur theatricals get under way again.
*Carl Franks, Cedar Rapids (Iowa)* Gazette

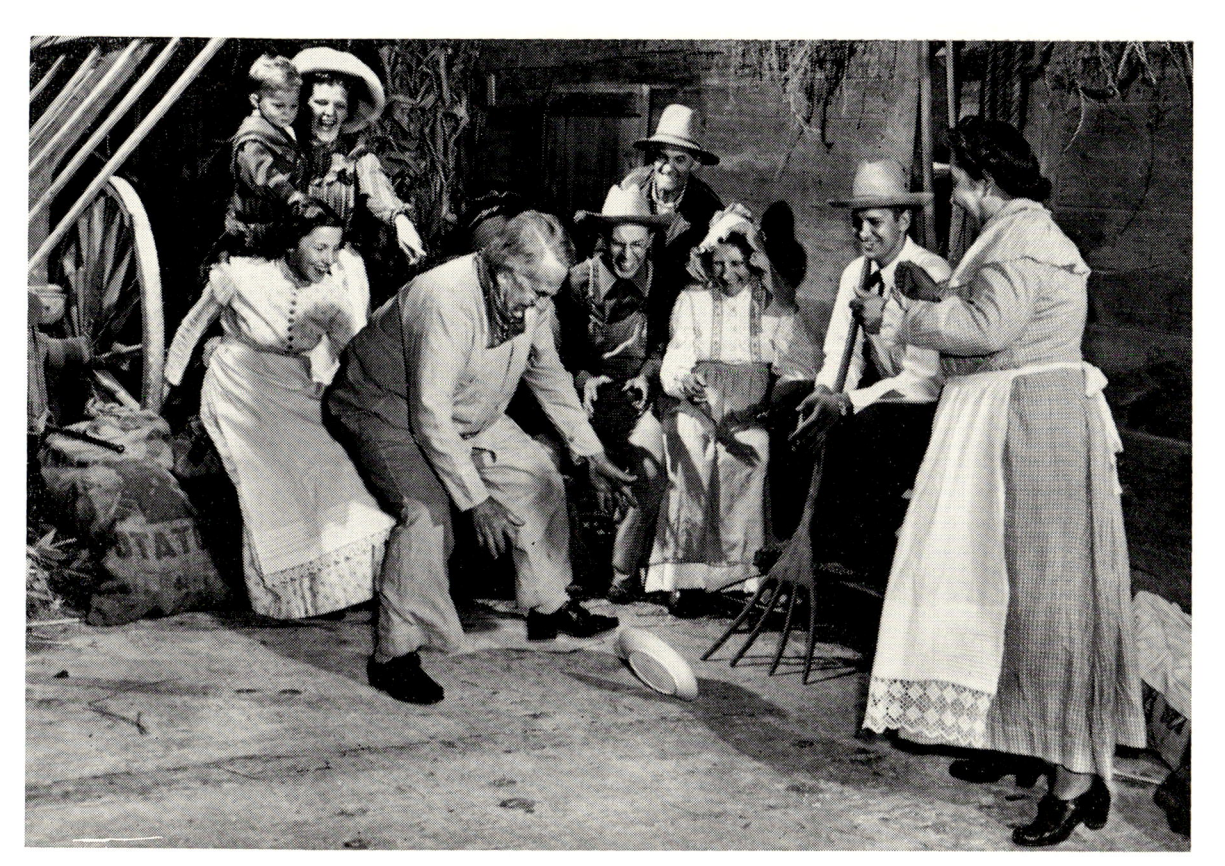

88   Traditional games like this one played by Pennsylvania Dutch folk provide enjoyment for participants — and for those who see such pictures in the papers.
*Photo by Clifford R. Yeich*

— 63

CHAPTER 8

# Pictures to Lure Young Readers

THE FIRST BATCH of Americans reared against a background of television are now in their mid-teens, and it remains to be seen whether members of this group ever will acquire a lasting taste for newspaper reading. Unless they do, newspapers will have lost important ground to electronic communication.[1]

As supplements to their intensive television fare, these young people have turned to radio, comic books and moving pictures rather than to anything that requires the effort of reading. If they've noticed newspapers at all, it's probably because of comics or photographs, or in the case of boys, sports.[2]

That the growth of non-readers of newspapers is especially heavy in the younger age brackets was revealed by a study that noted a general increase of non-readers of newspapers.[3]

Unfortunate as it may be, there seems to be considerable evidence that many schools have not done a good job of teaching reading skills to a large group of students, nor have the schools succeeded in instilling in youngsters a growing interest in public affairs or a deep appreciation of history as background for the developing story of their nation and of the world — interests and appreciations that could result in avid reading of newspapers.

**Must Arouse Interest**

Even if television has not stunted interest in reading, and if the quality of education in grade and high schools is generally higher than some studies indicate, a problem of gaining for newspapers the interest and readership of youths still remains. Children cannot be expected to read newspapers extensively. If they are to acquire this interest as they approach maturity, their attentions must be attracted favorably to newspapers and what they have to offer.

When — and if — newspapers capture this approval of the oncoming generation, the papers not only will assure themselves of

---

[1] That newspapers face a tremendous challenge to supply worthwhile and interesting news to a younger generation is a point of agreement between the authors of this book and an opinion expressed by Norris G. Davis and Sue Watkins in a three-part article, "Teen-Age Newspaper Reading" starting in the July 23, 1960, *Editor and Publisher*. But after years of experience with astonishingly poor answers to current affairs quizzes given college students, the authors of this book question the high teen-age readership figures in the Davis-Watkins study, despite its impressiveness. The study does include much interesting and stimulating material.

[2] A study by Wilbur Schram and David M. White, reported in *Journalism Quarterly*, June of 1949, seemed to indicate that young readers are introduced to newspapers by their pictorial contents. Among readers 10 to 15 years old, comics are most read items in papers followed by news pictures and public affairs cartoons, the study showed. Members of that group read news far less than they did the pictorial features.

[3] The study was made by Dan E. Clark & Associates, Inc., and reported in the July 16, 1960, *Editor and Publisher*.

continued readership but also will introduce to young people a source from which they can gain information they must have to function intelligently as members of an enlightened democratic society. Radio and television, with some magnificent exceptions, are doing only a superficial job in this area yet.

If newspapers can honestly claim high readership by young people, advertising salesmen will not only have better total circulation figures to show advertisers but also will have an impressive argument to present to some advertisers. With their new independence, young people have considerable buying power, and obviously their voices are influential in deciding what brands of products their parents buy. It would seem that verified claims of high interest in newspapers by young people might help sell more advertising, especially in such categories as automobiles, radio and television, clothing and entertainment.

A number of magazines directed toward teenagers already have appeared on newsstands to exploit the circulation and sales potentials of this group. Looked at from the adult viewpoint, some of them seem rather fine, most of them empty and silly, some of them downright obnoxious. But all of them will compete with newspapers, along with radio and television, for the attention of this age group.

89    American youth loves sports and its symbols.

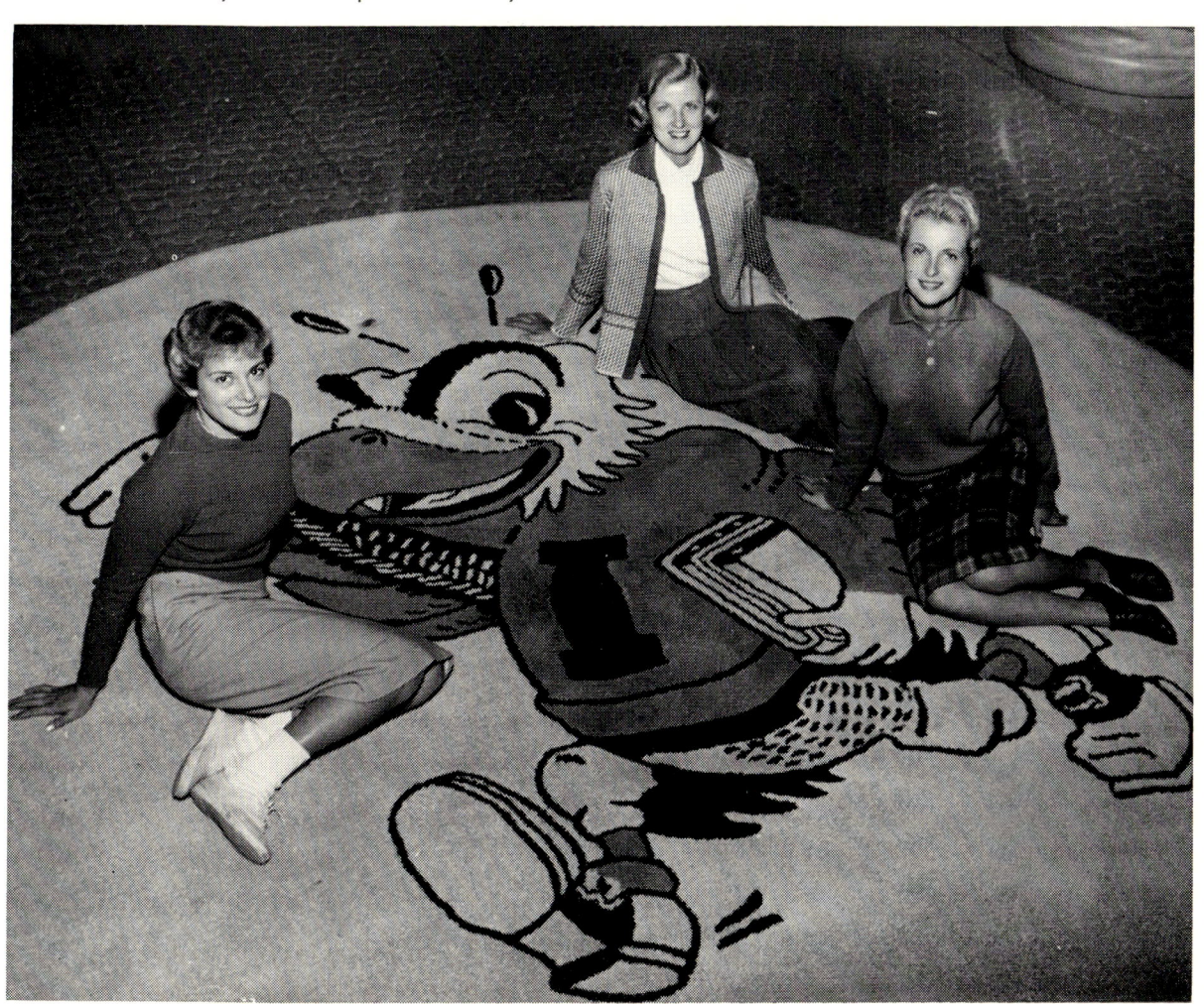

**Two Suggestions Made**

How can newspapers vigorously attempt to capture the readership of this developing group?

Two suggestions might be helpful:

1. Include in newspapers more matter of immediate and vital interest to young people.
2. Make copious use of pictures in the presentation of this material. The television generation hasn't troubled much yet about gaining information by the comparatively difficult method of reading. Why should these people be expected to change their habits all at once?

If material of real interest to them is presented in the form in which they are used to obtaining facts and ideas, they might be expected to start looking at newspapers. Once their interests are aroused, it might be hoped they will start reading the more adult content of newspapers, especially if it, too, is simply and interestingly written and well illustrated.

What is the material that might be expected to appeal to this group, in addition to comics, sports and entertainment news now probably somewhat read by them?

Automobiles are so deeply entwined in the emotional lives of the young that they deserve special treatment from the viewpoint of youths. To them, cars are objects of affection and seem to symbolize freedom and maturity and escape.

Because cars seem so essential, they become for young people a major problem. To buy and maintain an automobile deeply

90     A parade is fun for everyone, from any angle.

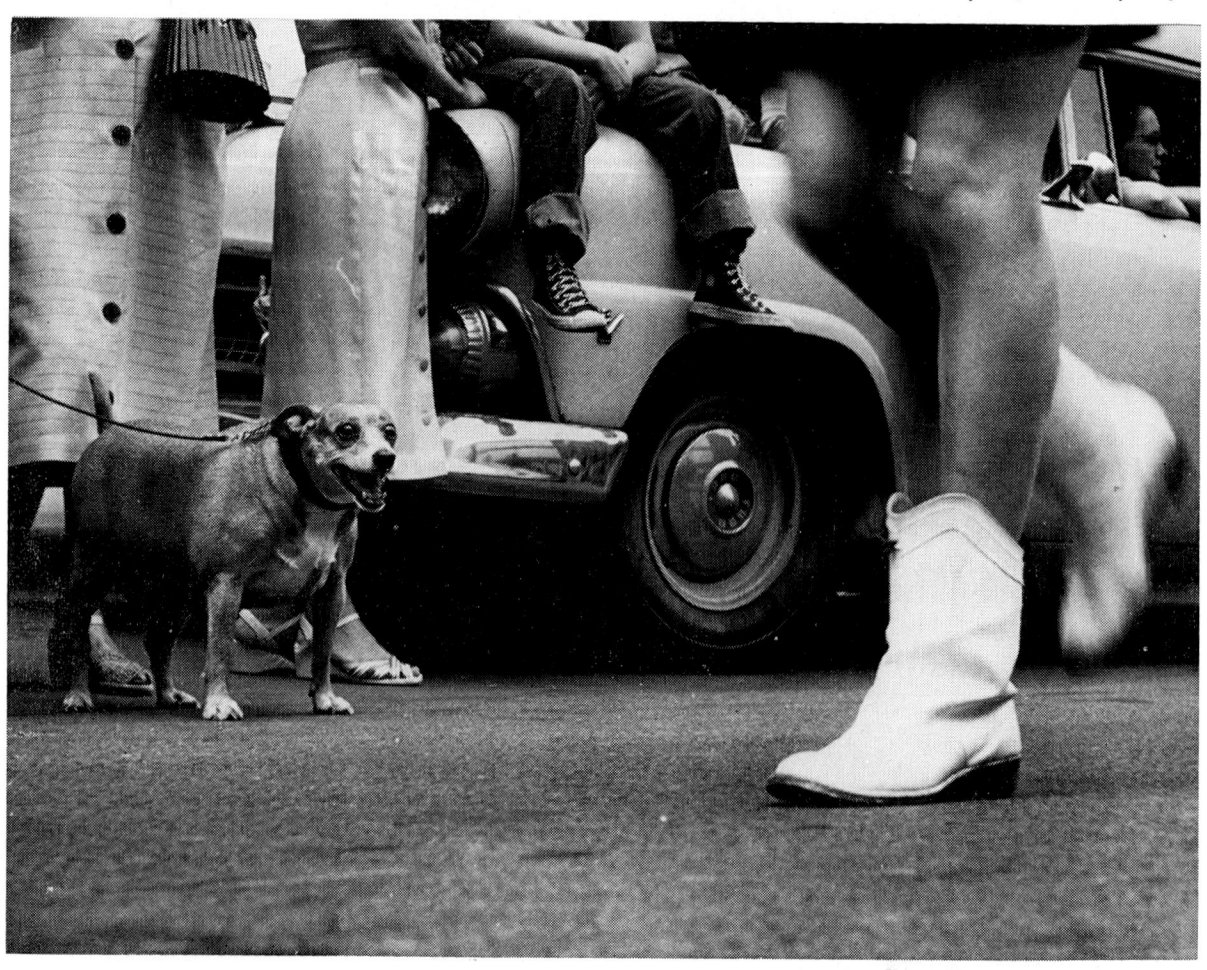

66 —

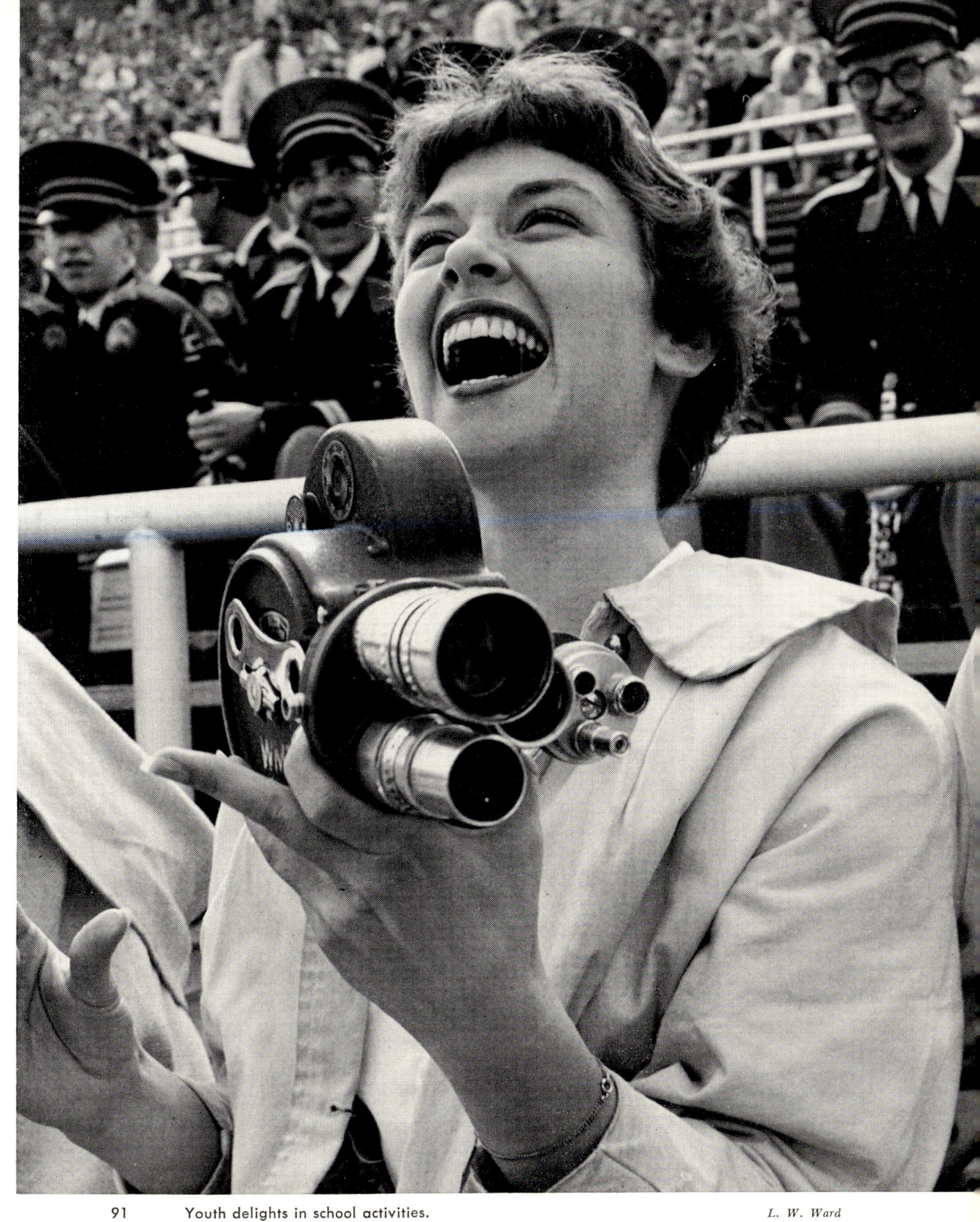

91    Youth delights in school activities.                                L. W. Ward

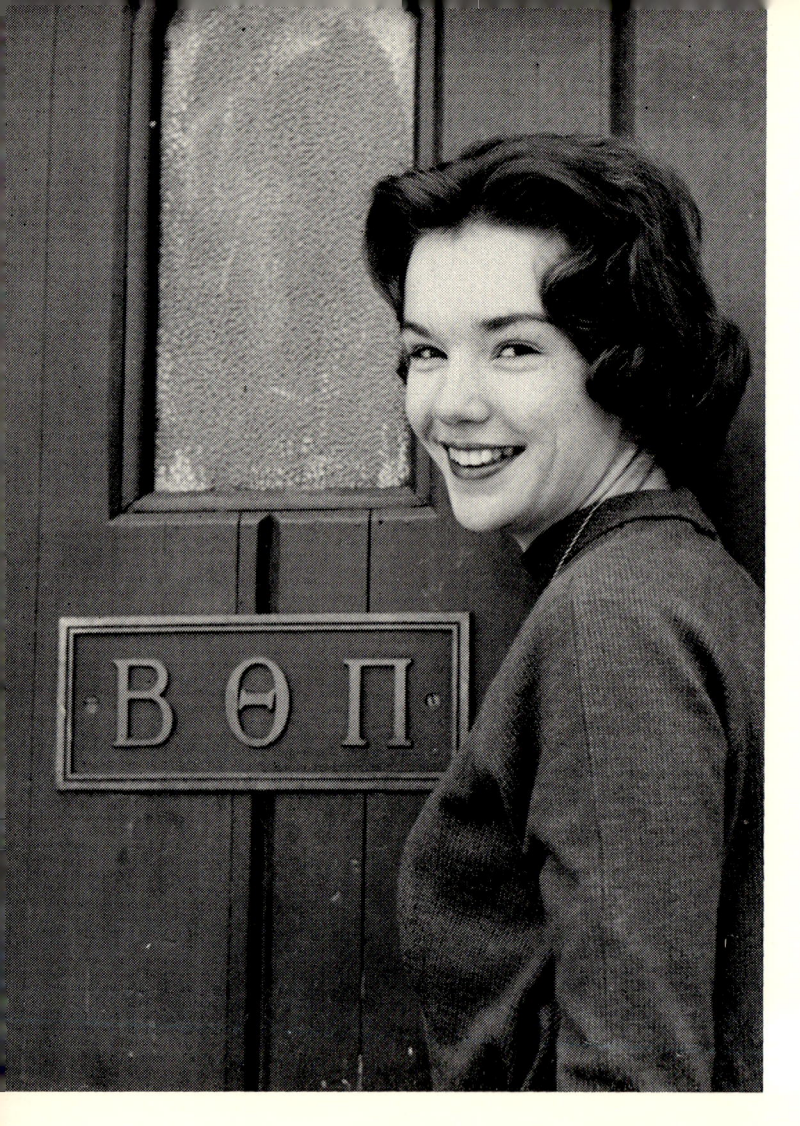

92    Folks at home appreciate pictures of their young collegians.
*L. W. Ward*

taxes the resources of most young people and often their parents. Many are willing to sacrifice school and college for the sake of an automobile. In addition, the impetuousness of youth in driving often involves young people with police; studies indicate that ownership of a car often cuts down grades; much pressure is brought on young people on grounds of their "moral" behavior in and around automobiles.

When young people are so preoccupied with automobiles, and to some extent motorcycles, scooters and motor boats, pictures and stories about motors quickly suggest themselves. Conditions of the secondhand market, how to make repairs and remodel, ideas for trips, traffic regulations, sponsored drag strips, driver training, discussion of problems related to cars — things of that sort should have appeal. They can be expected to read the stories about automobiles prepared for adults, too, but they could be especially appealed to by material written for their age group.

**Vital Information Wanted**

To seek youth readership by means of lurid appeals to sex involves grave moral problems. But because young people start to date and marry young today, they have a legitimate interest in discussions of early marriage and sociological and moral problems concerning courtship and marriage. While material of this sort must be handled with great care because of intensity of feeling and strongly conflicting viewpoints about it, with restraint and good taste it can be used. Interviews with officials, clergymen, psychologists, sociologists, social workers and others can yield stories that not only have high readership appeal but that contribute needed information to young people. With taste and restraint such stories can be illustrated.

Youths face demanding vocational problems. Each one has to decide whether he

93   High school girls enjoy sports participation — well, most of the time.
*George Brownlee, Kingfisher (Okla.) Times and Free Press*

should finish high school, go on to college. If he doesn't go to college, what kind of work should he seek and what jobs will be more rewarding in terms of money and satisfaction? If he goes to college, which one should he select, what should he take, what kind of career aim toward after graduation? Because of today's early marriages, these vocational problems are especially urgent. They suggest possibilities for many stories. With pictures, they can be interesting — both to young people and their parents.

Might greater pictorial coverage of high schools and colleges pay off in terms of greater readership by young people? School activities, in addition to sports which usually are well covered, are endless, vigorous and vitally interesting to students. They abound with picture possibilities. And the beauty about pictures of young people and their activities is that with their action and their attractiveness they appeal to the general readers as well as to students and their parents.

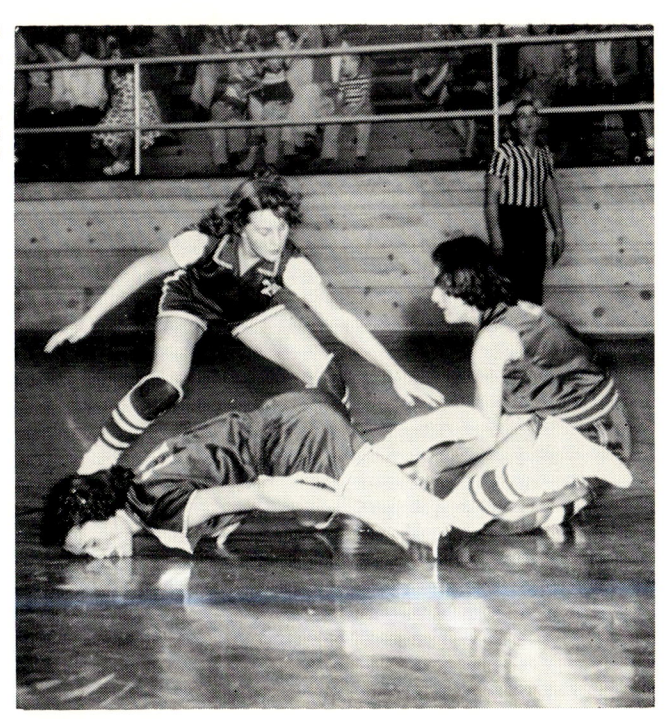

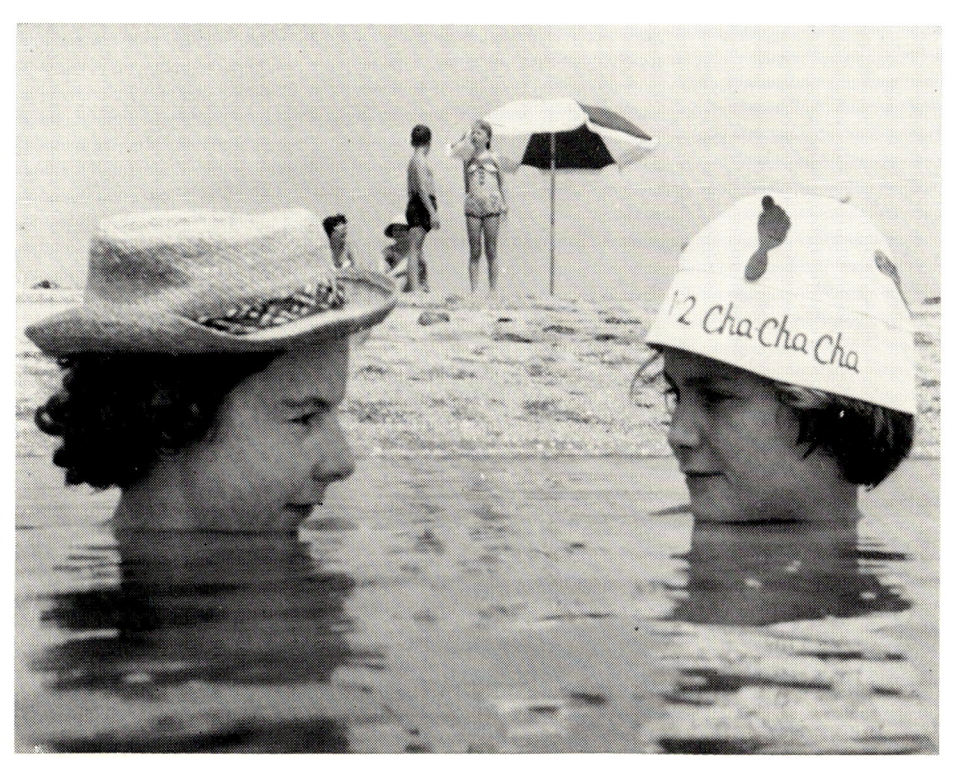

94   The beach offers chances for good pictures of young people — including some gag shots.
*Harvey Weber, Newsday, Long Island*

— 69

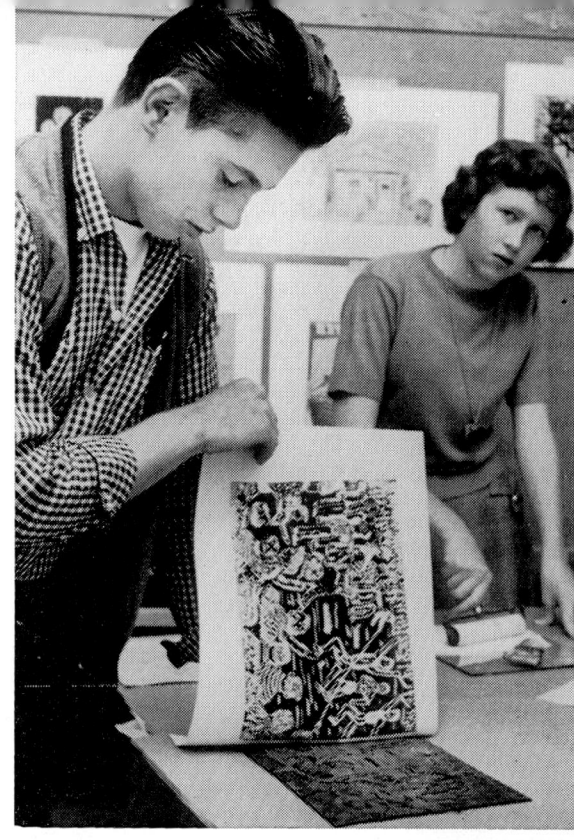

95   Some young people are engrossed in art activities.

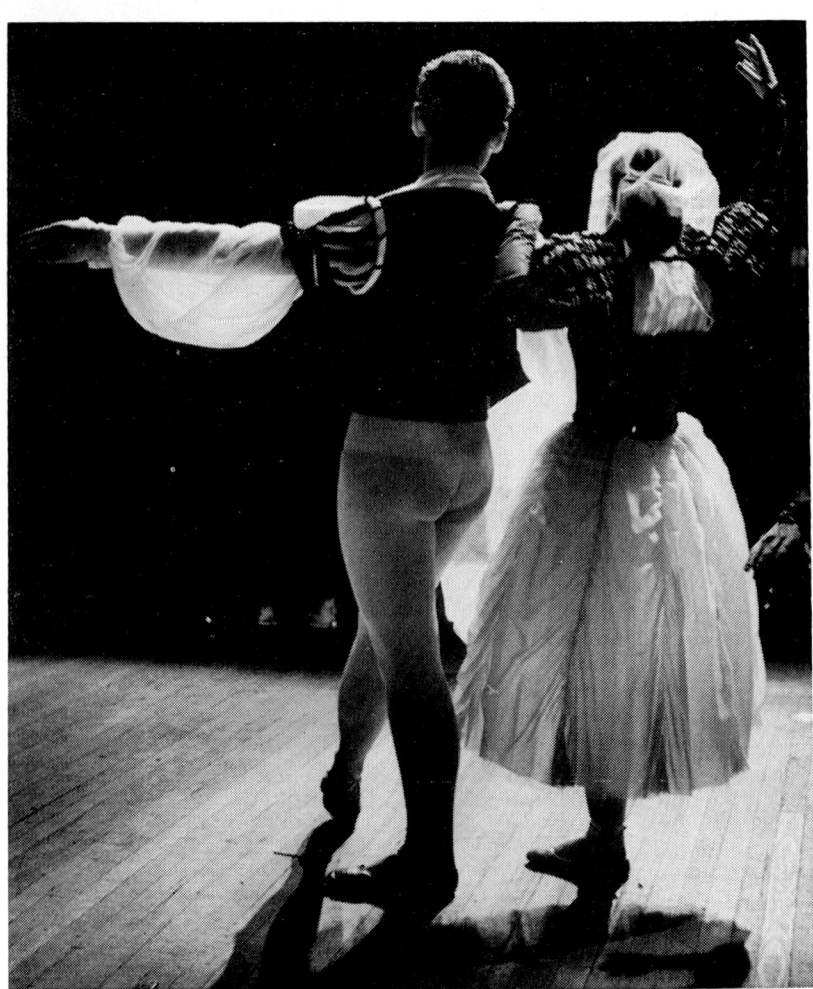

96   Amateur stage productions provide good picture opportunities. Only the stage lights were used in taking this back-lighted picture.

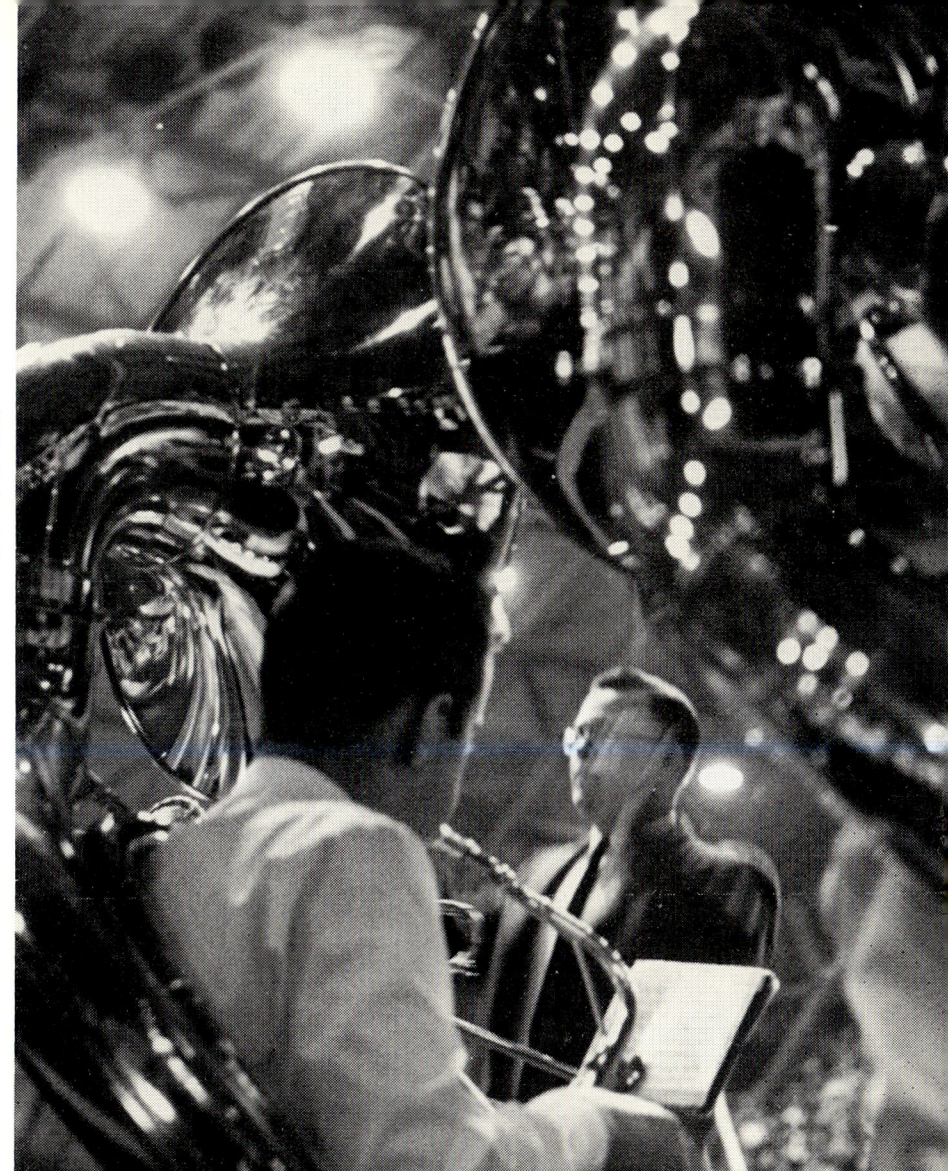

97  Music can be a wholesome outlet for youthful exuberance. Normal light creates an effect that would have been lost had a flash been used.
*Cliff Ganschow*

**Many Organizations To Cover**

In addition to school affairs, there are many youth organizations such as those sponsored by churches, lodges and including 4-H clubs, YMCA's and similar groups. Their activities provide many picture ideas.

Obviously, too, there is the whole world of swimming, golf, tennis, horseback riding and sports that may be touched on sports pages but are participated in by many whose achievements don't usually result in stories on sports pages. Some of this activity is school associated, some is separate from schools. All of it offers good picture ideas.

Teenage styles in clothing may seem casual and peculiar to adults, but they are important to youths — and are often picturesque. Fashion pictures at a rather informal level, including some passing fads, should make good pictures when displayed on local boys and girls. Such pictures should please some advertisers too.

Certain popular arts are of great interest to this group. Popular music, dancing, radio-TV could be better covered from the youth viewpoint perhaps. In cities with art centers and some serious music, more young people might be lured into reading about them and into a real interest in them if they more frequently were covered in simple words and in good pictures instead of, as sometimes

98   Dancing is an art, too.

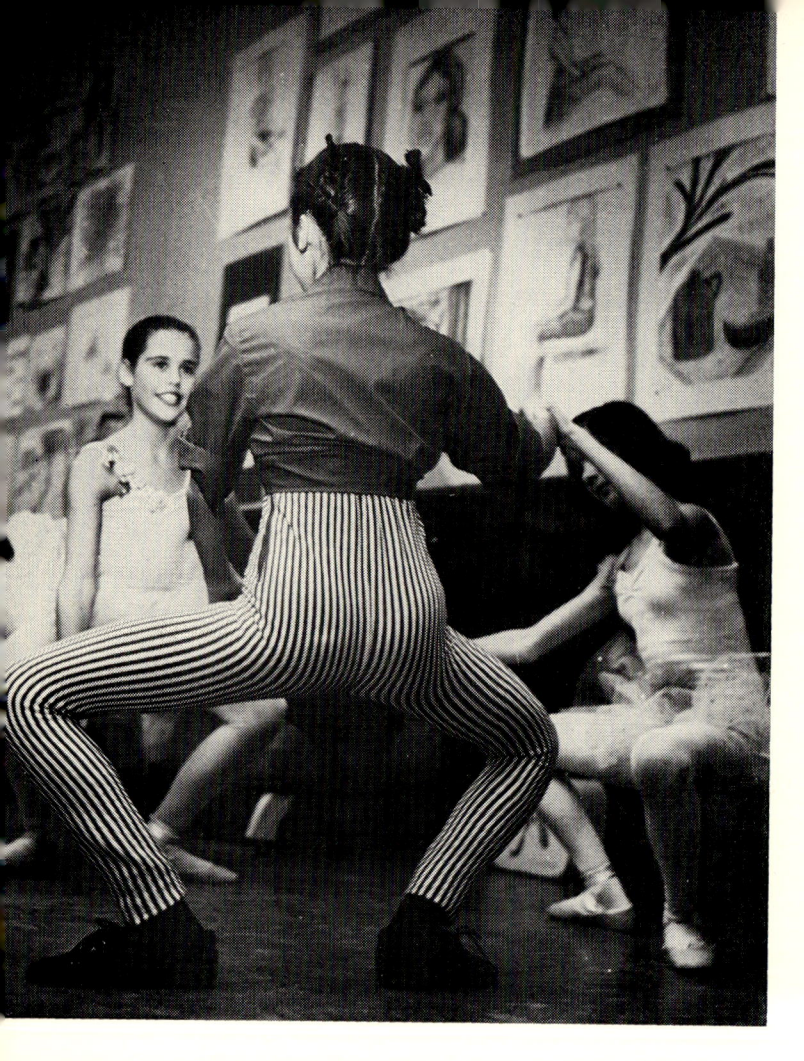

happens, in verbose criticisms written by somebody with a pompous ambition to display his special learning. A really modern library with music rooms, art exhibits, and a clever selection and display of good books can yield pictures and stories of interest to some young people.

**Resent Delinquency News**

Teenagers, even the overwhelming majority of well-behaved ones, seem to resent the amount of coverage given to juvenile delinquency. But that is one of the things in newspapers they seem to read. Problems involved in reporting such material, loaded as it is with moral and ethical considerations, must be solved in terms other than the desire to please any special group.

If material planned to attract readership of youth is to succeed, it must avoid a tone of condescension that sometimes mars efforts to do that sort of thing. Nobody, especially a young person just beginning to feel his oats, wants to be patted on the head and told to listen while Daddy, who knows everything, explains just how things are today.

Above all, pictures should play an essential part in attracting members of the television generation.

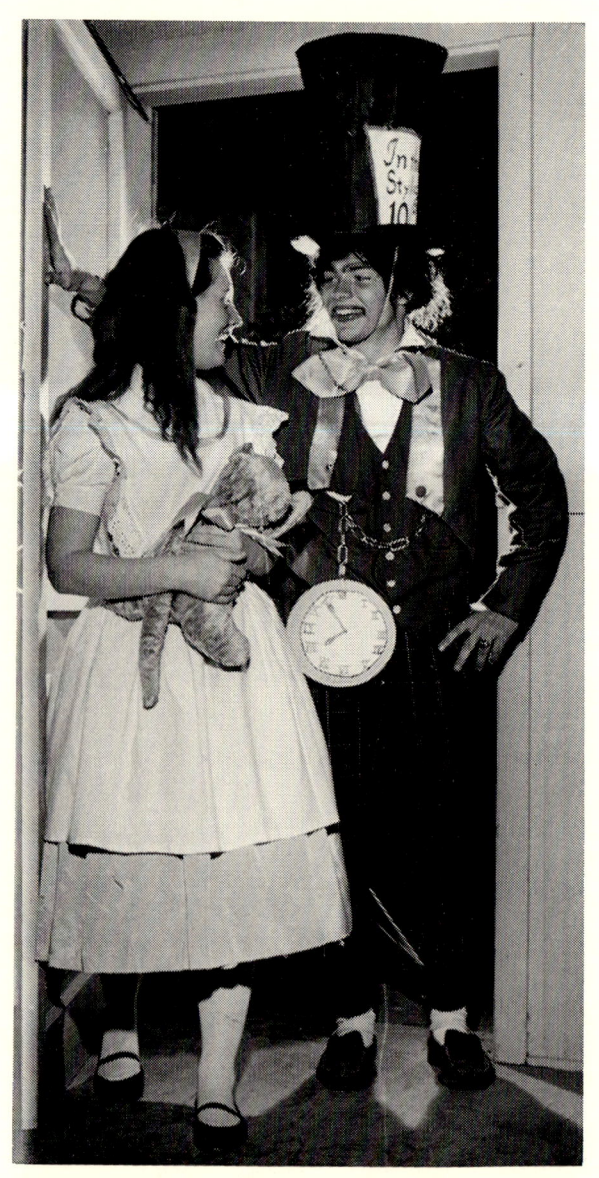

99   Costume parties provide fun for the photographer as well as the guests.

— 72 —

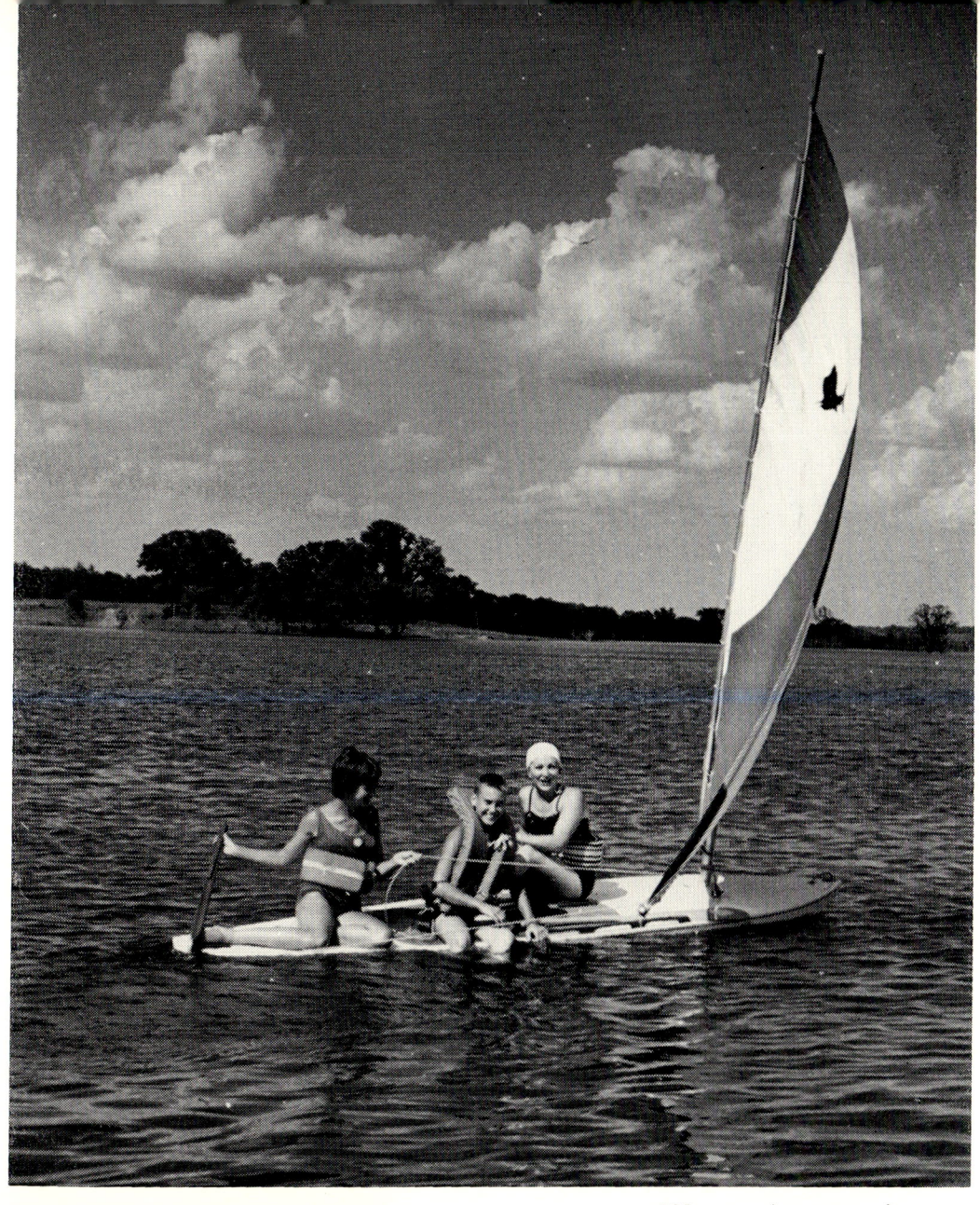

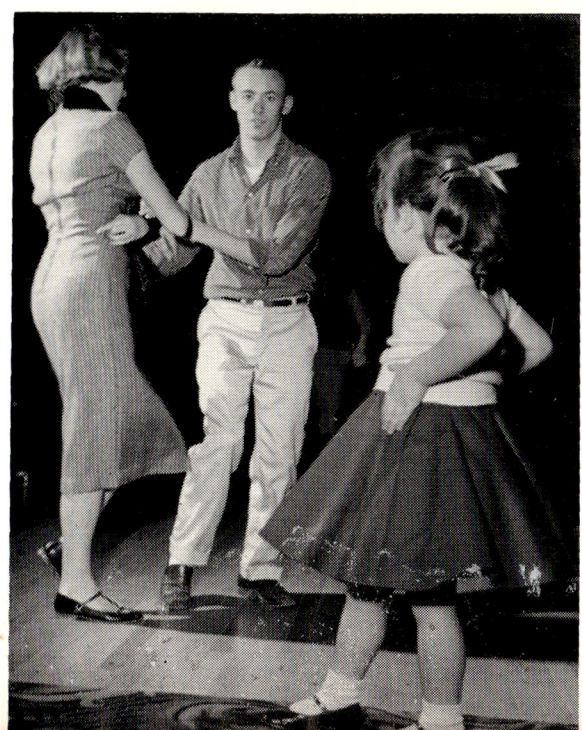

101   A summer sky, a sparkling lake, and a sailboat manned by a happy crew provide good summer subject matter for the photographer.

L. W. Ward,
*Cedar Rapids (Iowa)* Gazette

100   Dancing, ballroom style attracts the young — and the very young.

— 73

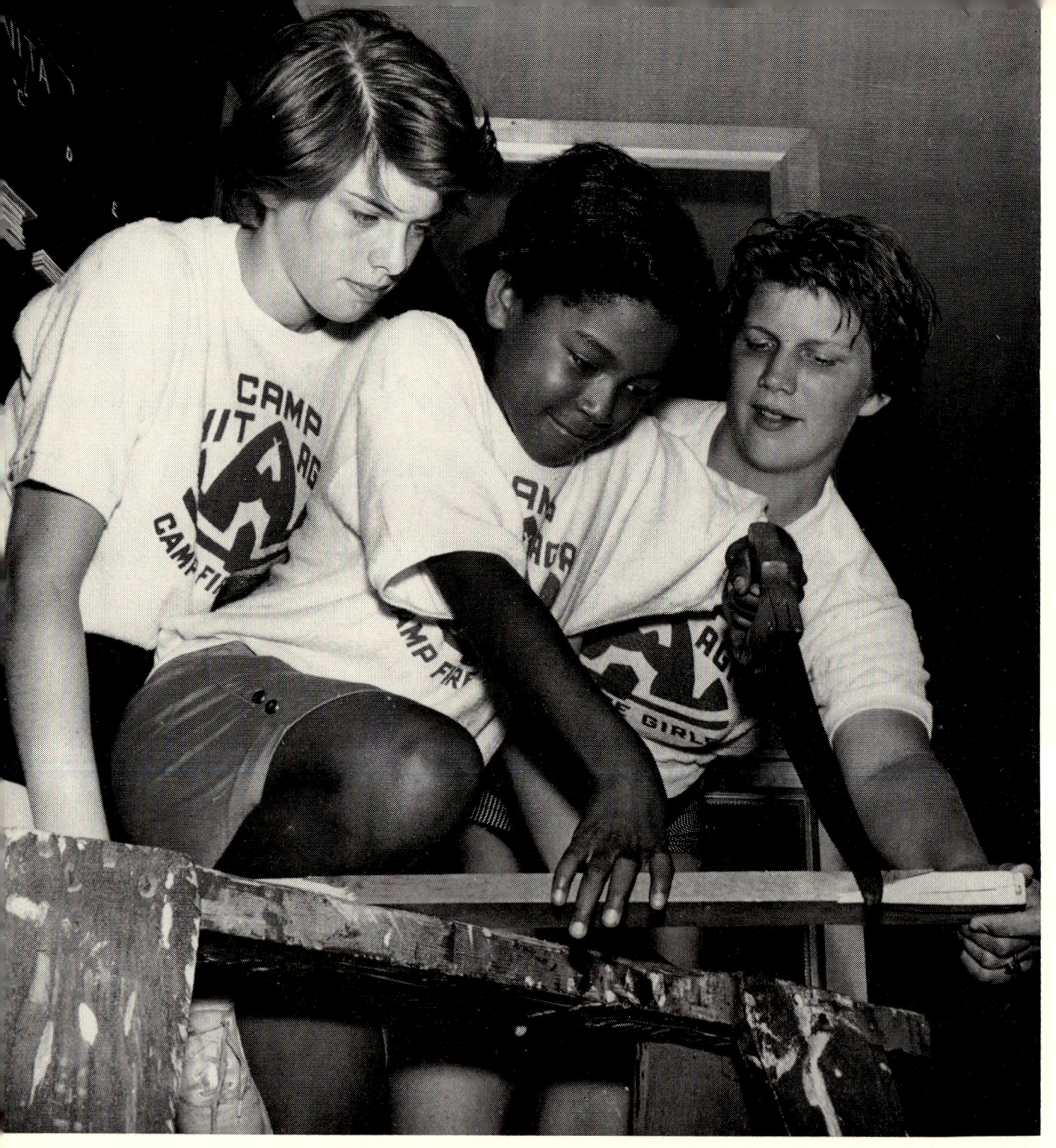

102    Even very young teenagers start developing a favorable attitude toward the paper that publishes pictures of their activities.

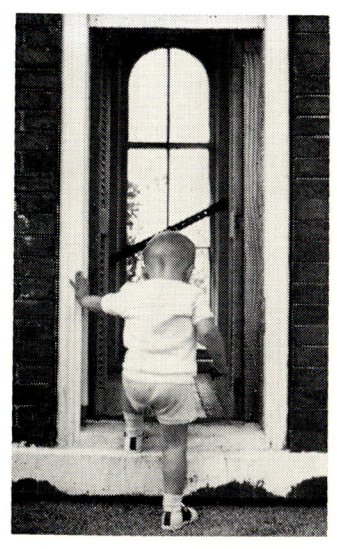

*Charles H. Cox*

PART 2

# How Pictorial Organization Increases Appeal

CHAPTER 9

# The "Organized" Picture—Does It Really Pay?

Just as a news reporter must organize the facts he gathers into a neat, orderly and effective word story, so should a news photographer order the elements in his pictures in the most effective way possible.

A well-planned, organized picture is easier and more pleasant to look at than is a disorganized one.

It's easier to grasp the meaning or understand the story a picture is intended to convey if the photograph is simple and is orderly.

The way the elements in a picture are put together is called composition. It can create an emotional reaction on the part of most viewers in addition to that evoked by the subject matter shown, or can enhance or detract from the impact of the reaction.

The purpose of good composition is to make pictures have the greatest possible impact, make them do their jobs in the most effective way. Beauty isn't the basic purpose of composition, although good composition is essential in creating a picture that generally would be considered to have beauty, whatever that abstract quality may be.

**Does Good Composition Pay?**

Are people in general really sensitive to good composition and do they react favorably to it? Or is the public reaction to a news photograph based almost entirely on its subject matter and perhaps on photographic quality?

Because no definitive answer to such questions exists, these arguments may be stimulating:

1. Subject matter is by far the most important factor in a news photograph. It only stands to reason that good technical qualities in a photograph and its reproduction are important.

2. Without question, some people enjoy and respond to good composition in pictures a great deal more than to casual or disorganized ones. Because art is widely taught in schools, is a source of interest and enjoyment to thousands, is practiced on an amateur basis by many Sunday painters and photographers, this group is much larger than many news photographers and editors might realize.

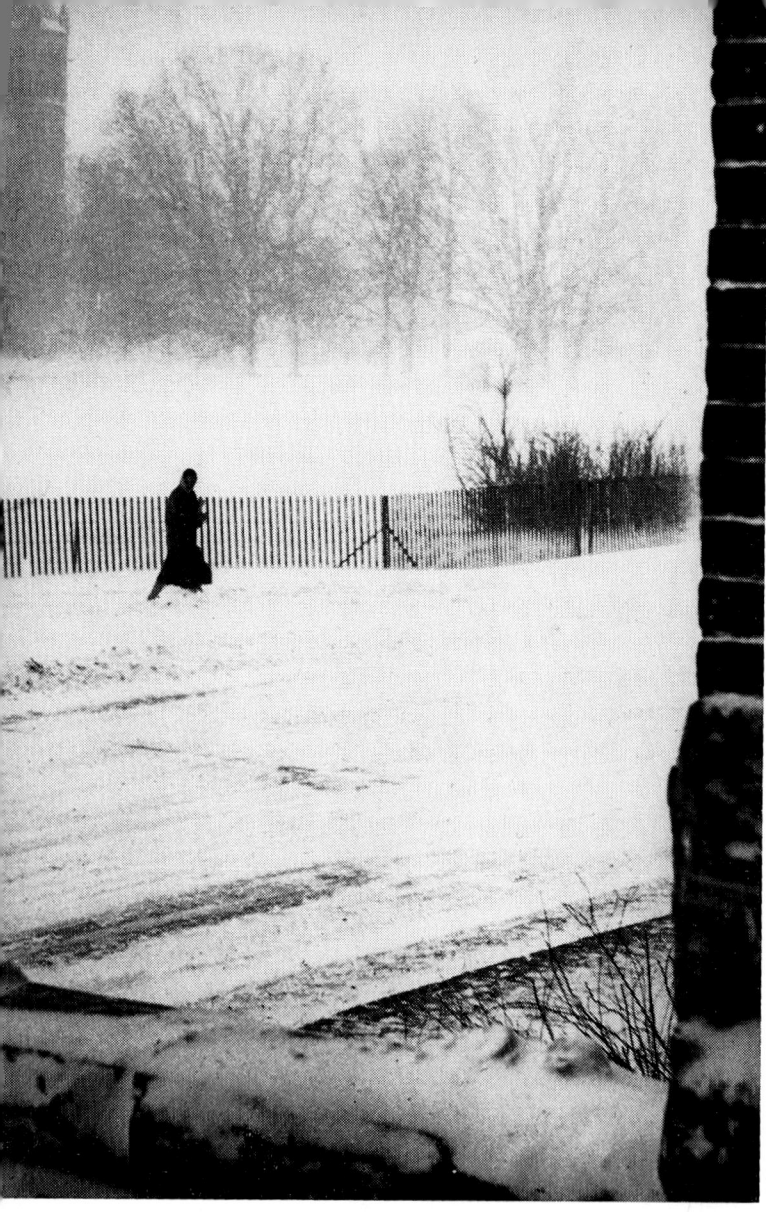

**103** This picture framed by brick and wall was more popular than . . .

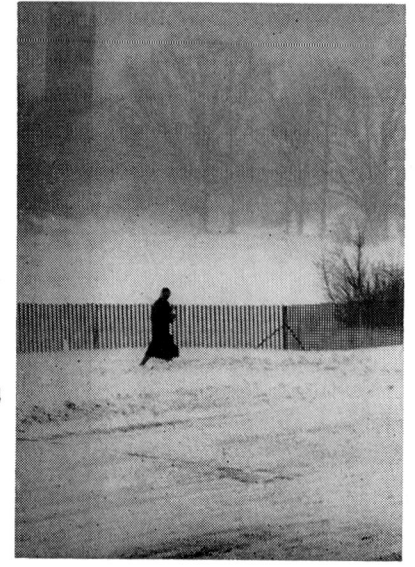

The same picture without frame.

**104**

3. A probably much larger group of persons without any training or experience in art react sensitively and favorably toward pictures that are neatly and cleverly organized. This is possible because good composition basically is not a set of rules devised by artists for the private use and pleasure of artists. Rather, good composition is the intelligent application of a knowledge of how most people react to the way the elements of a picture are put together. Much of the knowledge was found by trial and error and by intuition by artists through the centuries, but much of it has been and is being verified by scientific research.

### Science Probes for Answers

Some aspects of good composition contribute significantly to the general appeal and meaning of photographs. This is indicated by a study revealing that framing makes pictures more dynamic and third dimensional.[1]

In this study, 5 mature persons with some art training, 17 students with some training in art, and 18 students without any training in art viewed this pair of pictures, one framed (Photo 103) and the other with the frame eliminated (Photo 104).

> 5 out of 5 experts preferred the picture showing brick and stone frame. (Photo 103.)
>
> 28 out of 35 students preferred the framed picture. (Photo 103).
>
> 15 out of 17 students with some art training preferred the framed picture. (Photo 103).
>
> 13 out of 18 students without art training pre-preferred the framed picture. (Photo 103).

The same group viewed a second pair of pictures (Photos 105, 106) with different croppings.

> 5 of 5 experts preferred the closely cropped picture. (Photo 105.)

---

[1] Ganschow, Clifford, "A Study of the Contribution of Certain Compositional Factors to Photographs' Effectiveness." Unpublished report in journalism, Iowa State University, 1960.

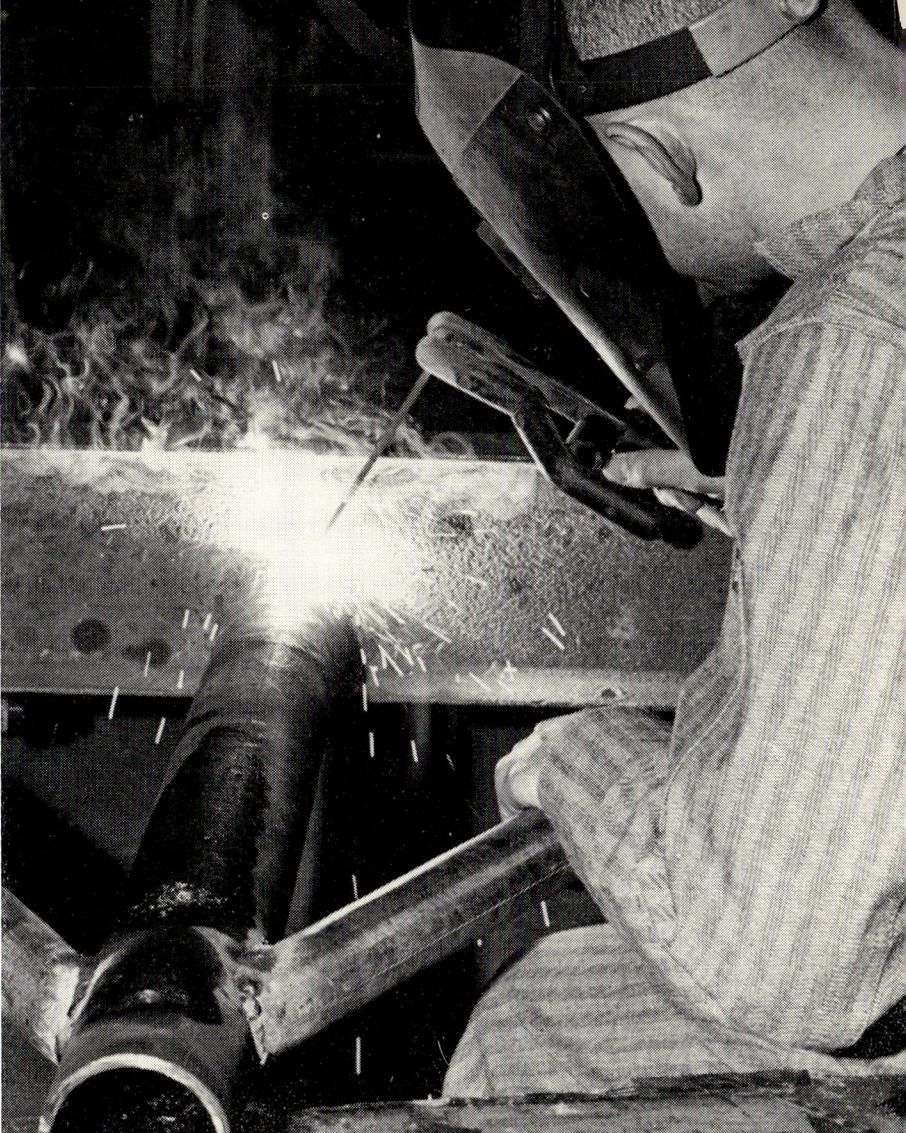

105   The closely cropped picture at right, centering on action, was approved by more viewers than was the full shot (below) showing far more area.

106

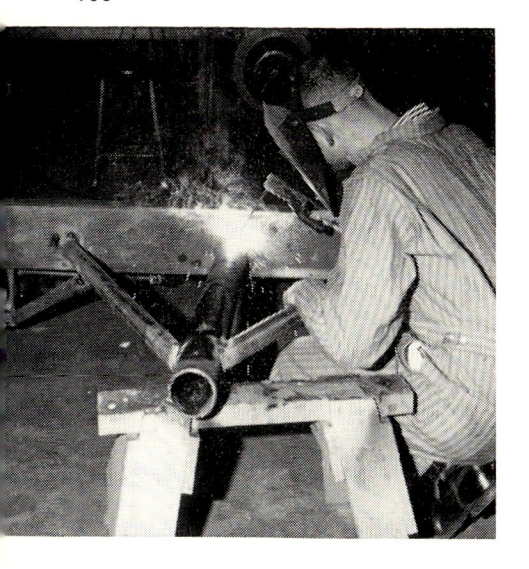

30 of 35 students preferred the picture closely cropped. (Photo 105.)

15 of 17 students with some art training preferred the closely cropped picture. (Photo 105.)

15 of 18 students without art training chose the closely cropped picture. (Photo 105.)

Limited as is this study, it does indicate that the question of whether good composition is of value in pictures for newspapers and other general circulation publications can be answered by research.[2]

[2] Another study of interest is that made by Kaz Oshiki, *Effects of Smiles, Subject Arrangement and Lighting on Reader Satisfaction From Pictures of Groups of People.* Unpublished Master of Science thesis in journalism, University of Wisconsin, 1956.

A good working assumption, based on experience and tentative results of research, is that good organization of a news picture considerably enhances its effectiveness. For the magazine or publication with a circulation largely among persons with at least some little contact with art, there seems little question but that good composition can be a very great factor in improving the effectiveness of pictures.

The next few chapters are devoted to some simple and basic suggestions about how to create well-organized pictures. The bibliography suggests references that provide more detailed and profound ideas about pictorial composition.

CHAPTER 10

# Balance Makes Pictures Look Comfortable

BALANCE IS JUST A MATTER of making pictures look comfortable. Nobody likes to look for long at an object that seems about to fall. There is something discomforting about an object that looks unstable. Unless a picture is to give something of the feeling one suffers when he looks at a dish of gravy tottering on the edge of a table above a beautiful

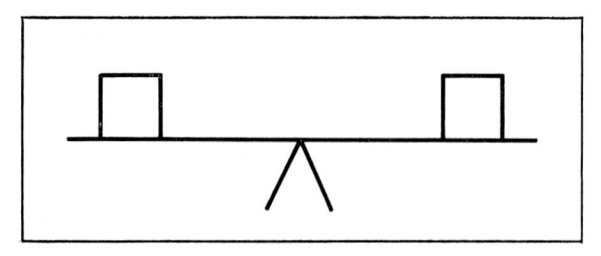

Figure 1

rug, the elements of that picture must be so distributed that it looks stable and at ease.

A photographer can achieve balance in his picture by a skillful management of several factors. Different kinds of balance are possible.

**Formal Balance**

Formal balance in a picture is achieved when elements on both sides of the picture are of equal weight. The idea can be diagramed as in Figure 1 by showing equal weights on both sides of a centrally placed fulcrum. Formally balanced pictures look somewhat static and unexciting, but have dignity. Photo 107 is an example.

Formal balance, of course, does not demand that a picture be symmetrical. Symmetrical pictures, in which both sides are exactly alike, are seldom used. Some painters, when they have sought great dignity, have used symmetrical balance for crucifixion scenes or for pictures of gods or great heroes. A photographer, in order to obtain a special effect, might want to take a symmetrical or essentially symmetrical picture, but almost never. Usually, such pictures seem too formal and static. Photo 107 is nearly symmetrical.

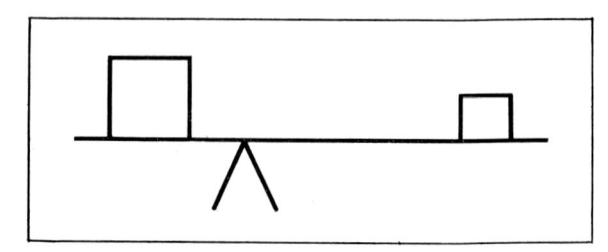

Figure 2

**Asymmetrical Balance**

Asymmetrical balance seems more interesting than does symmetrical balance, usu-

107  Nearly symmetrical pictures are seldom used, but they can achieve great dignity.

ally, and is vastly more often used. Figure 2 illustrates asymmetrical balance as does Photo 109. The fulcrum in Figure 2 is not at the center of the board, but the resulting imbalance is compensated for by unequal weights on the board. The total effect is of balance.

**More Complex Aspects of Balance**

But many factors enter into making a picture balanced. An object far from the center of a picture has more weight than one near the center, as is demonstrated in Figure 2 and Photo 111. An object in the

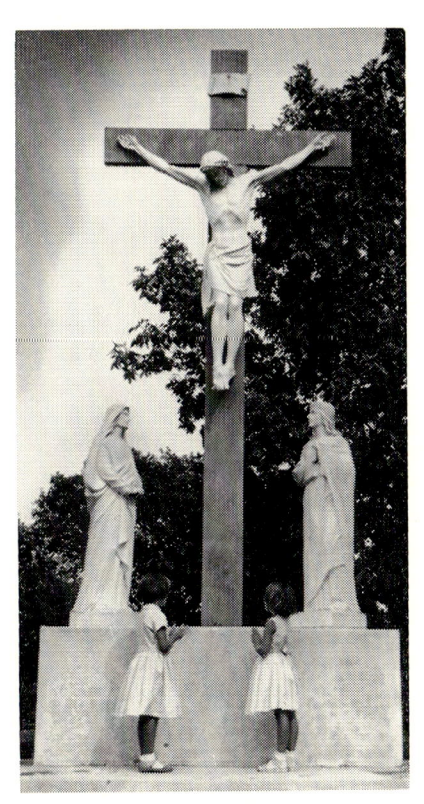

108  This picture is formally balanced, creating a scene in keeping with the attitude of prayer.

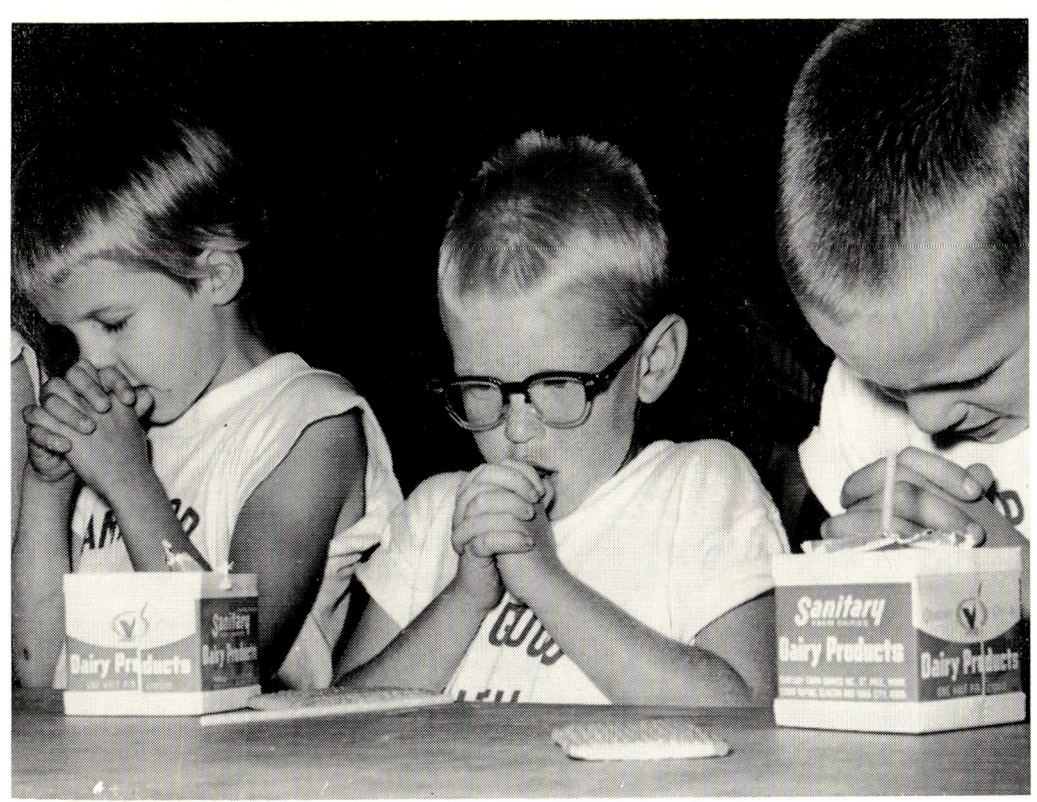

— 81

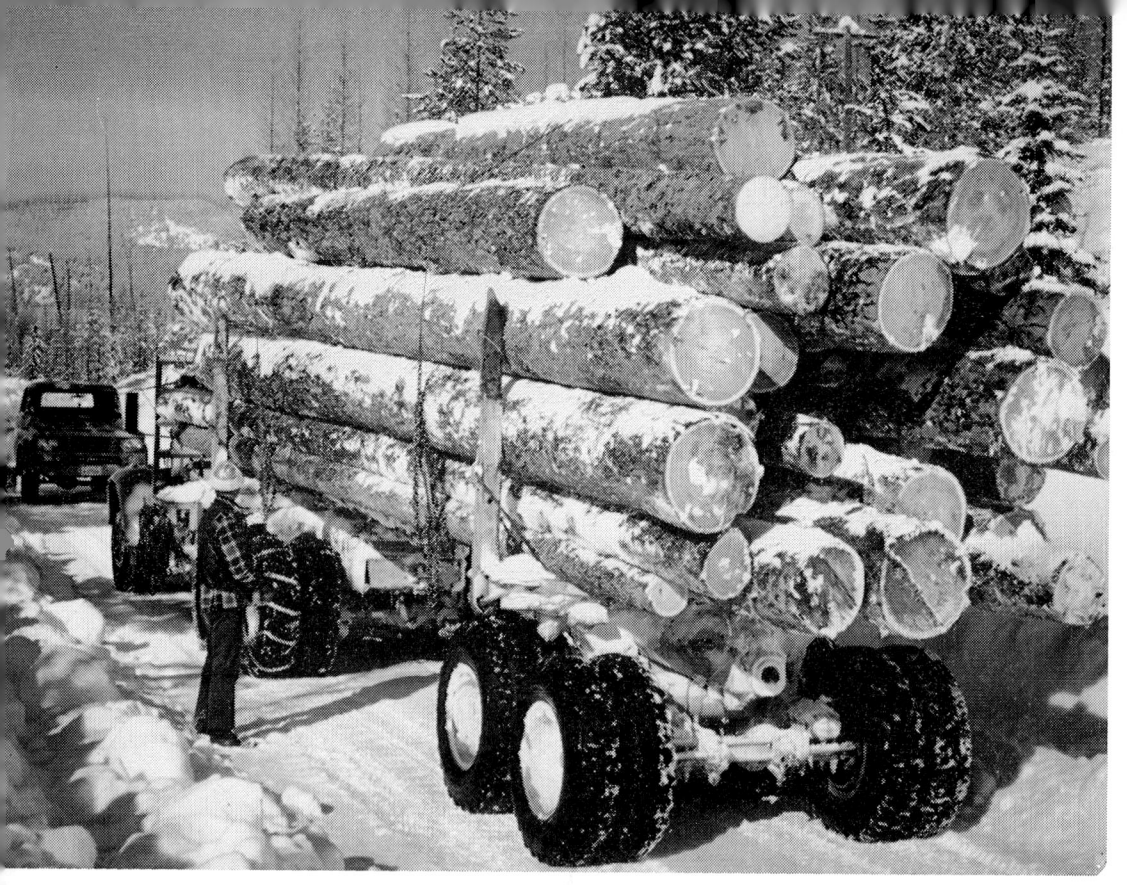

109    The looming rear of this load with its round log ends and round rear wheels (repetition with variation of circles) creates great weight slightly to the right of center. This weight is nicely balanced by the horizon and sky in the upper left and by the second truck and front end of the log truck.

*Mel Ruder Photo for* Hungry Horse News

110    The impressive bulk of the cat is balanced by the rat, his whiteness and intent expression, the light spot on the table top, and by the fact that the left canister looks considerably larger than the partly hidden one on the right.

*Bruce Roberts, staff photographer,*
*Charlotte* Observer

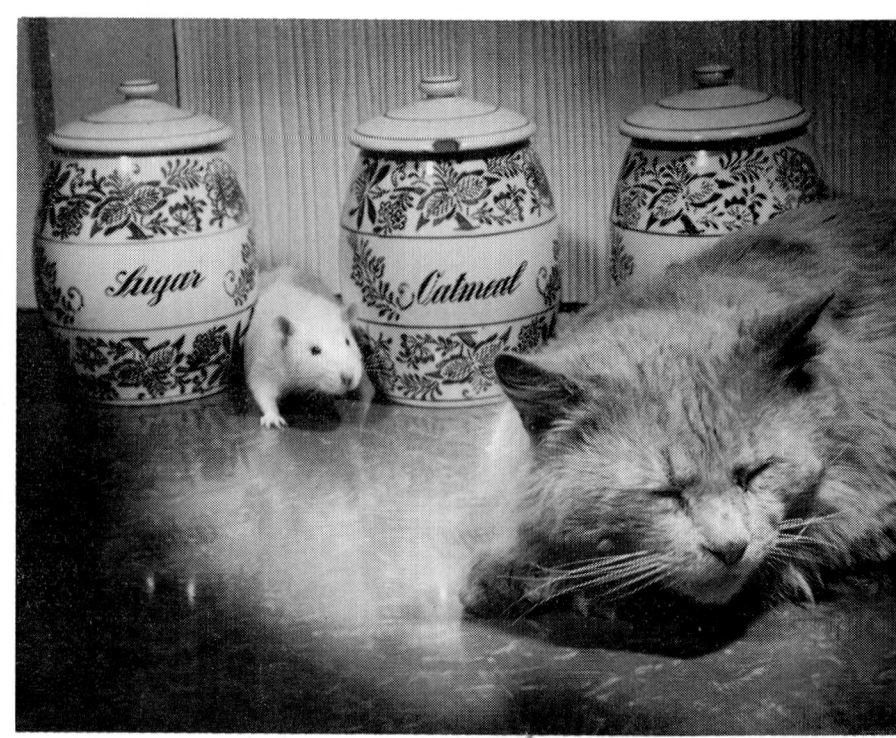

82 —

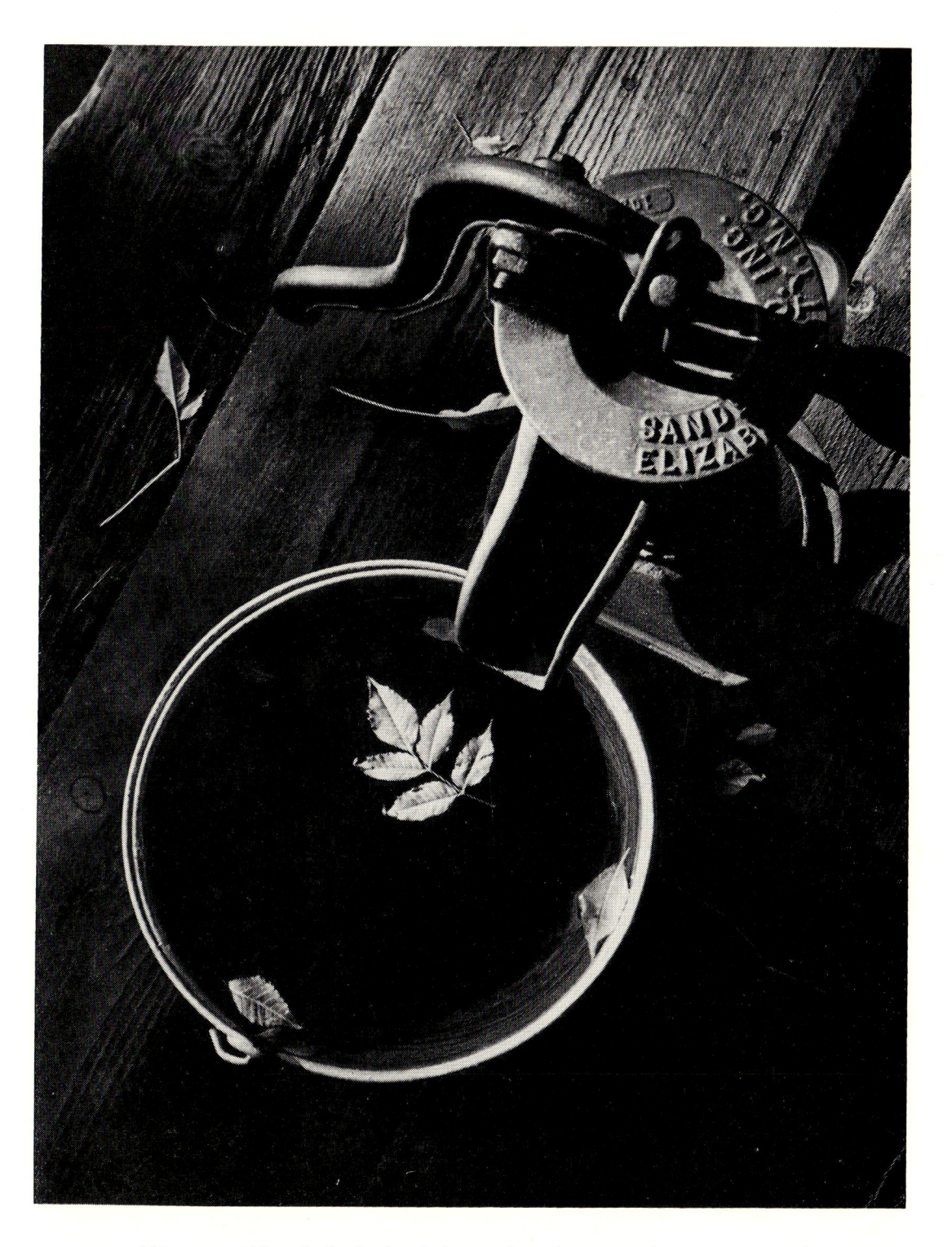

111    Although the bucket is larger than the pump, this picture is nicely balanced. This is true largely because while most of the bulk of the bucket is left of center, part of it is right of center to be added to the weight of the pump. The leaves, masses of light and dark, further act to achieve balance. Notice the textured areas, the interesting repetition of circles and of leaf forms.             *Bruce Roberts, staff photographer, Charlotte* Observer

— 83

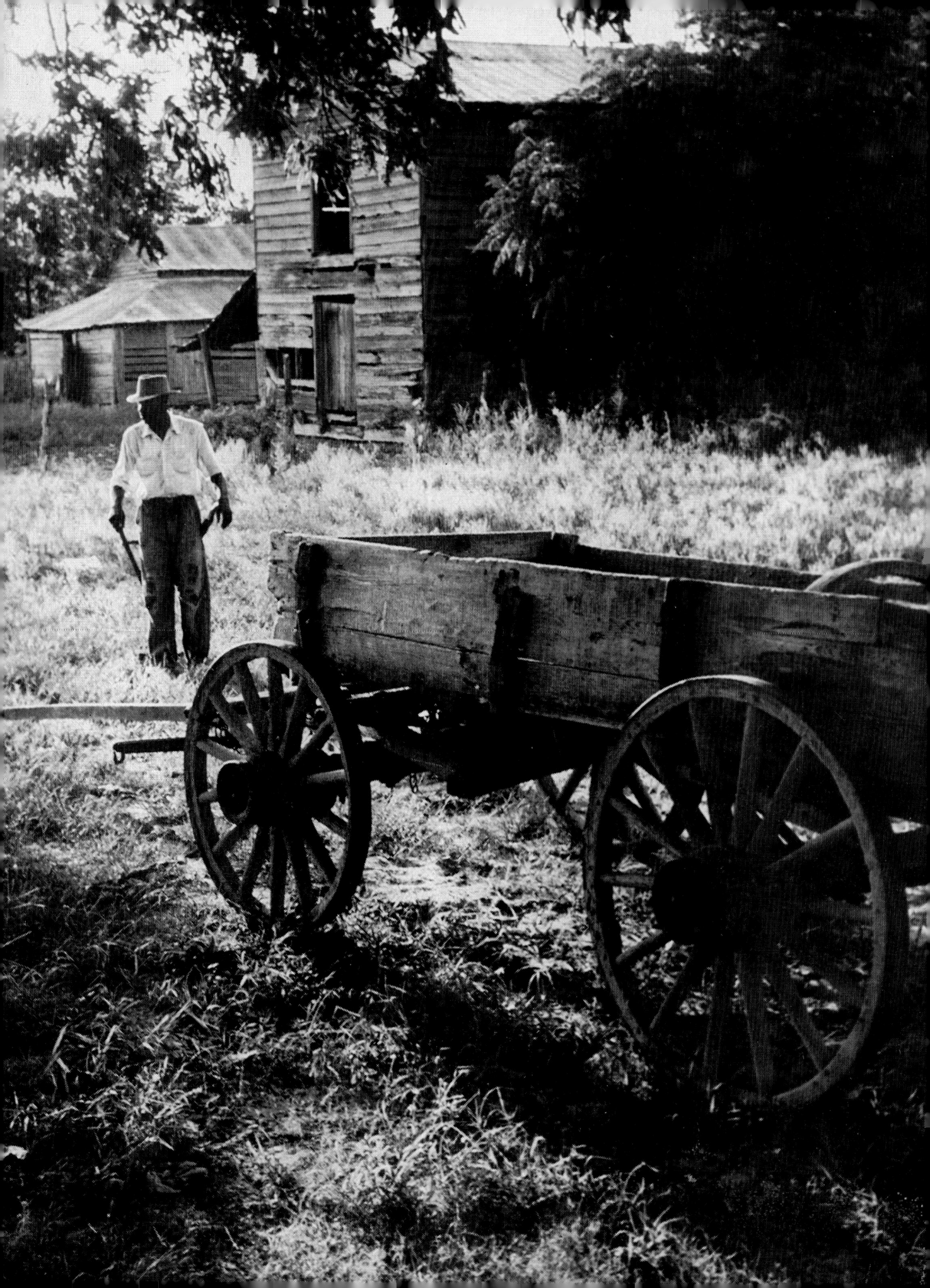

112    In spite of the great weight of the wagon in the lower right, the picture on the facing page is well balanced, both horizontally and vertically. Balance factors include the interest of the human figure and the lightness of the area around him, greater seeming weight of objects in the upper part of the picture, and the fact that part of the wagon's bulk is left of center.
*Bruce Roberts, staff photographer,* Charlotte Observer

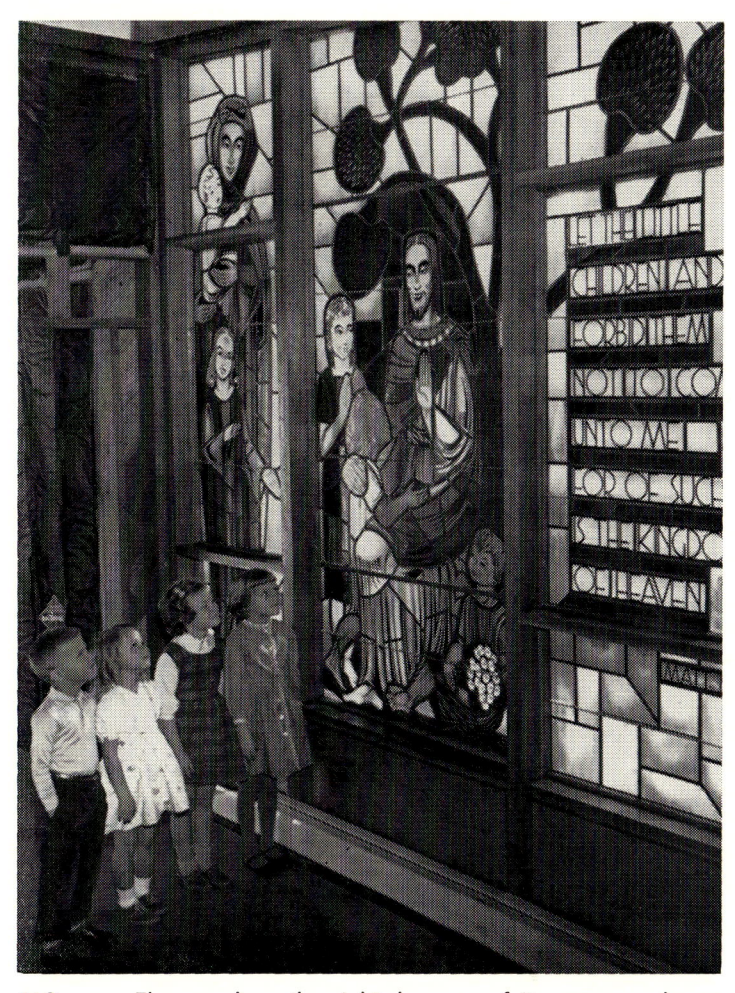

113    The panel on the right, because of its nearness, looms much larger than the one on the left, but the difference is compensated for by the weight of the living children plus the unfinished work behind them.    *Mel Ruder Photos for* Hungry Horse News

upper part of a picture seems heavier than one of the same size in the lower part of a picture, as shown in Photo 112.

Isolation seems to increase weight of an object. In a picture showing a man sitting alone among a great stretch of empty seats in a theater, the man seems to carry more weight than his size or the distance from the center of the picture seem to indicate. Photo 114 demonstrated this point.

The intensely interesting quality of an object may give it extra compositional weight. For instance, in the photograph of a helicopter lowering a rescue rope to a man stranded on a rock offshore from a great cliff, the interest in the human being and his fate seems greatly to increase the compositional weight of the comparatively small aircraft and figure in relation to the vast bulk of the towering cliff. Both the human figure in Photo 112 and the children in Photo 113 illustrate this point.

Regular shapes seem to have more weight than do irregular ones. Objects on the right-hand side of a picture seem to have a little more weight than do objects of the same

— 85

size on the left-hand side of a picture, perhaps because people in western cultures read from left to right.

Within a picture, the direction that certain figures, shapes and lines seem to be moving become important to balance. For instance, the image of a person may be walking in a direction, or eyes may be staring in a direction. The shape of some objects creates feelings of movement. When such directed forces exist within a picture, they upset balance if considered on the basis of size alone.[1]

**Problems of Balance Made Simple**

The big thing for a news photographer to remember is that to give a feeling of "rightness" and comfort to a viewer, a picture should be balanced.

---
[1] A simple but helpful discussion of balance is contained in *Image Arrangement* by Louise Haz, the Haz Book Co., Pittsburgh, 1956. A much more complex but a rewarding discussion of balance is presented in *Art and Visual Perception* by Rudolf Arnheim, University of California Press, Berkeley, 1957. Some ideas for this chapter have been drawn from these books.

An understanding of the factors that are essential to the achievement of pictorial balance will be helpful in turning out compositionally good pictures. But a photographer can move toward the production of better-balanced pictures without stopping to make a complete analysis of each photograph he produces.

If he will keep testing his own feelings for balance as he looks at the ground glass of his camera, or at the easel as he prints, or at the prints as he considers final cropping, he probably will start improving his pictures.

Some day you may, for a special effect, want to produce a picture that deliberately is off-balance. But almost always your pictures will be greatly more pleasing to most people if you are successful in achieving a feeling of balance in them. Certain pictures, such as landscapes, architectural photographs and many others, usually will fail to achieve fully their desired results unless they are successfully balanced.

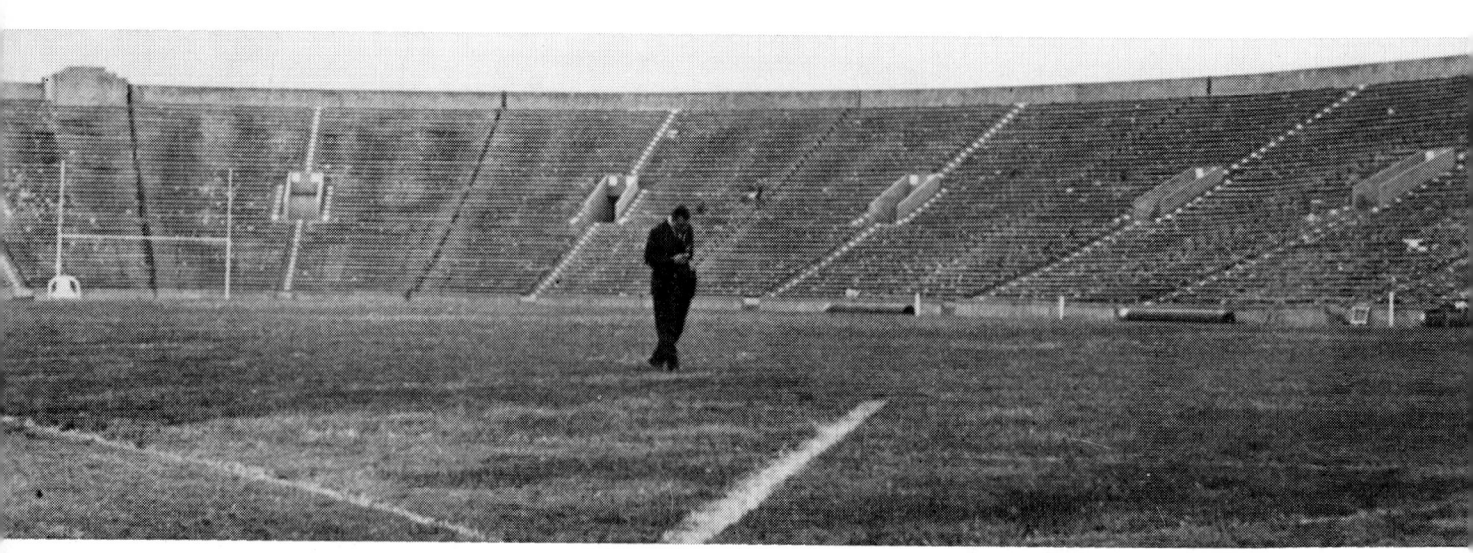

114   Isolation seems to increase the apparent weight of an object. Notice how relatively large the man's figure looks here against the vastness of the empty stadium.   *Cliff Ganschow*

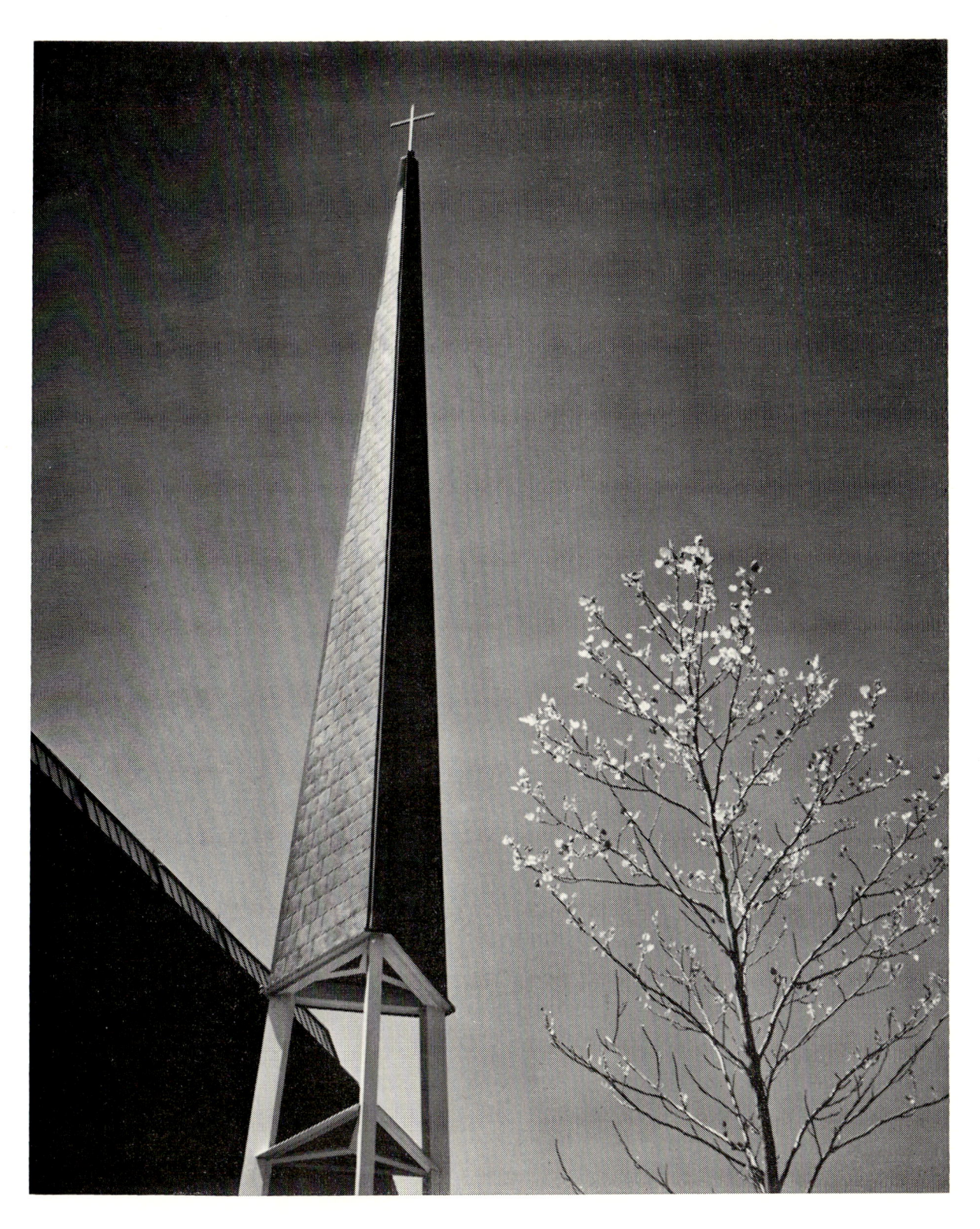

115   In this picture of tree and spire the eye seems forced to move in a triangle to unify the composition. A nice feeling of balance is achieved.
*Fort Wayne* News-Sentinel *Photo by Carl R. Hartup*

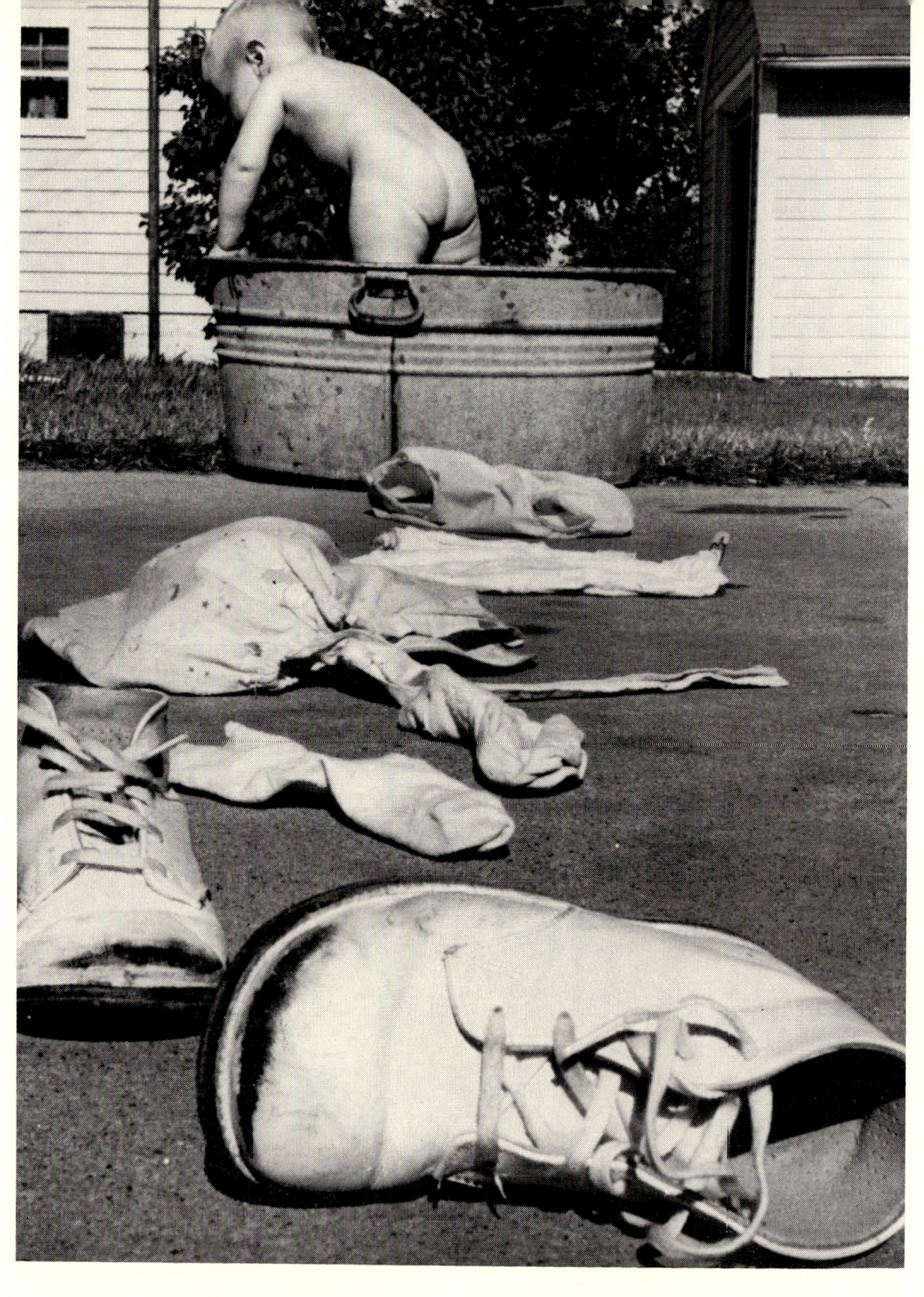

116   The eye works through an orderly picture in a guided way. Here it follows a line of clothing back from the huge, eye-catching shoe in the foreground to the real center of interest in the tub.

*Lowell Georgia, Green Bay (Wis.)* Press-Gazette, *staff photographer*

CHAPTER 11

# Shapes, Lines and Curves As Picture Elements

SHAPES, LINES AND CURVES are important elements basic to planning orderly pictures that create desired effects. A photographer has considerable control over the way these elements behave within the pictures he takes.

Although infinite numbers of kinds of shapes, lines and curves exist, some of the interesting ones that frequently are available in subject matter to be photographed are:

1. Vertical lines that tend to give an impression of dignity when they dominate a picture, as in Photo 117.
2. Horizontal lines which, when dominant in a picture, as in Photo 118, tend to make it serene and quiet.
3. Lines which, because they seem to be falling, suggest instability. They can be used to create a feeling of movement in a picture because they are restless. Photo 119 is an example.
4. Angles that seem to recede from the flat surface of the picture give the impression that the picture has depth, as in Photo 120.
5. A triangle that seems to lie flat on a picture, as does the tent in Photo 121, looks stable.
6. Opposed diagonals seem to produce a feeling of struggle and conflict, as in this picture of a house leaning in one direction, while the trees point the other way, Photo 122. But opposed diagonals can combine to form stable patterns when the opposing lines seem to support each other, as do the ladders in the fire picture, Photo 123.
7. Some curves can create the same feeling of pictorial depth as did the angle in Photo 120. The curving road in Photo 124 creates this feeling of depth.
8. But some curves seem to lie flat on a picture surface. For instance, a curved iron ornament will seem to lie flat against the brick of the fireplace, in the picture of a house taken from directly or nearly directly in front of the structure.

Sometimes two or more adjacent shapes in a picture seem in the eyes of the viewer to merge and form a new shape. This new shape must be considered as a factor in composition. How this happens is demonstrated in Photo 125 and Figures A and B.

Sometimes several shapes within a picture will combine and recombine in several ways, as in Photo 125. If you will learn to see, in the subject matter you are about to photograph, what may emerge as the result of combinations of other shapes, it will help you in planning better pictures.

An ability to see these possible combinations also will help you avoid some of the embarrassments that result from such things as an entire shrub looking like wild hair growing from a woman's head in what was

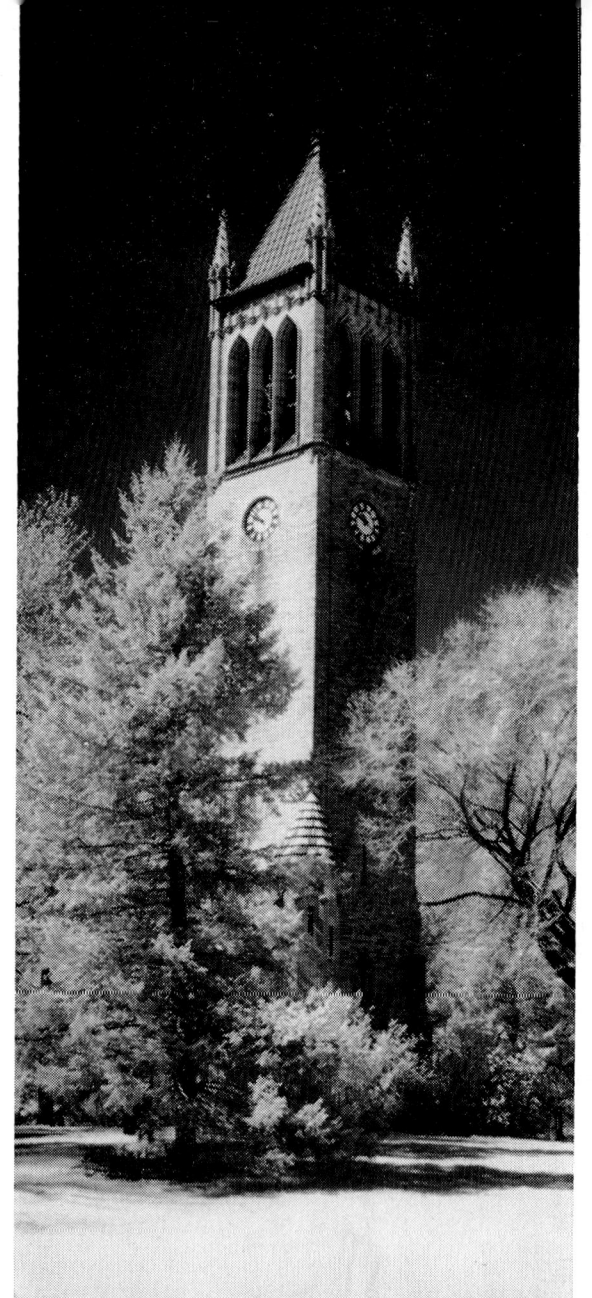

**117** Vertical lines tend to give a picture dignity.
*Iowa State University Photo*

intended to be a dignified portrait. Such unfortunate combinations have ruined many an otherwise good news picture.

The areas between shapes in a picture are shapes, too, and must be so considered in planning a picture. It is often possible to give extra impact to your subject by clever utilization of "blank space."

**Summary About Shapes**

Shapes that enter into careful planning of a picture include those:

1. Of the objects pictured;
2. That develop when two or more objects combine to form new shapes;
3. That are formed by the spaces between other shapes;
4. That are created because an object's image sometimes breaks down into more than one shape, as when a box in a picture may be seen as the whole object or one side may be seen alone as a square or rectangle;
5. That develop by other means such as by areas of texture, areas of light or dark, or are formed by lines, real or subjective, or by other means.[1]

[1] A good treatment of shapes as picture elements is contained in *Photo-Vision* by Ray Bethers, St. Martin's Press, Inc., New York, 1957.

**118** Horizontal lines, when dominant, create an impression of serenity. A yellow filter brings out the billowing clouds. *Rodney Fox in* The Iowan

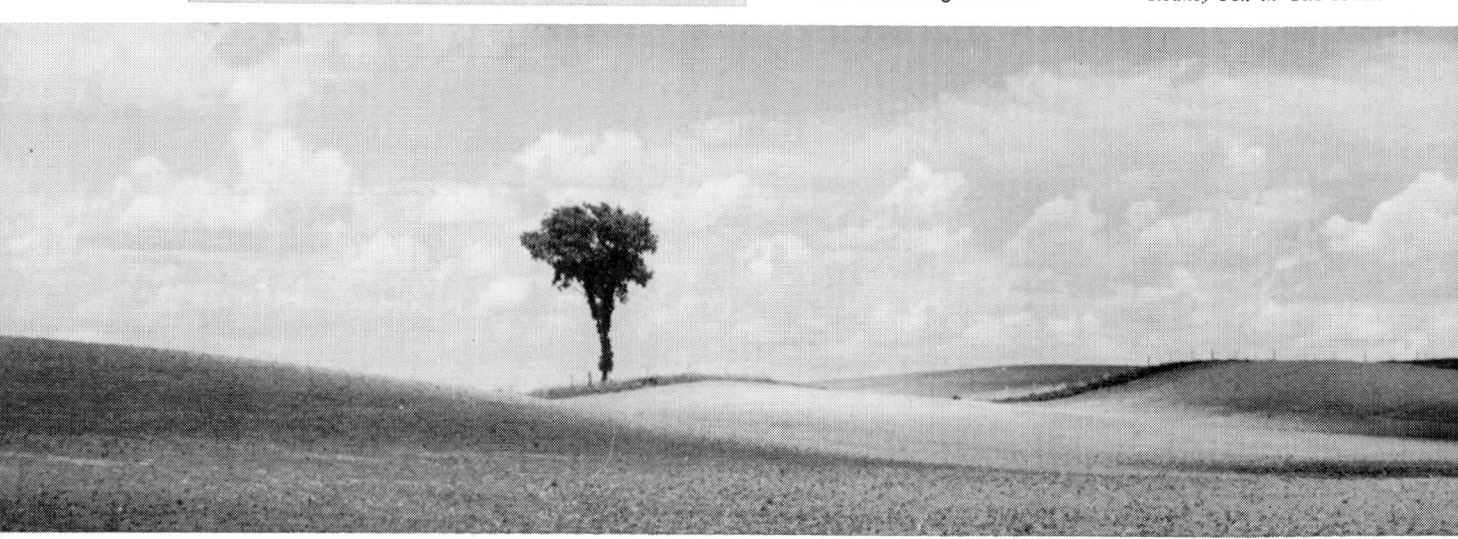

90

119　When a line varies from the perpendicular, as does this vapor trail, it suggests a restlessness and instability.

*Lowell Georgia, Green Bay (Wis.)* Press-Gazette, *staff photographer*

120 Angles that seem to recede from the flat surface of the picture give the impression that the picture has depth.

*Iowa State University Photo*

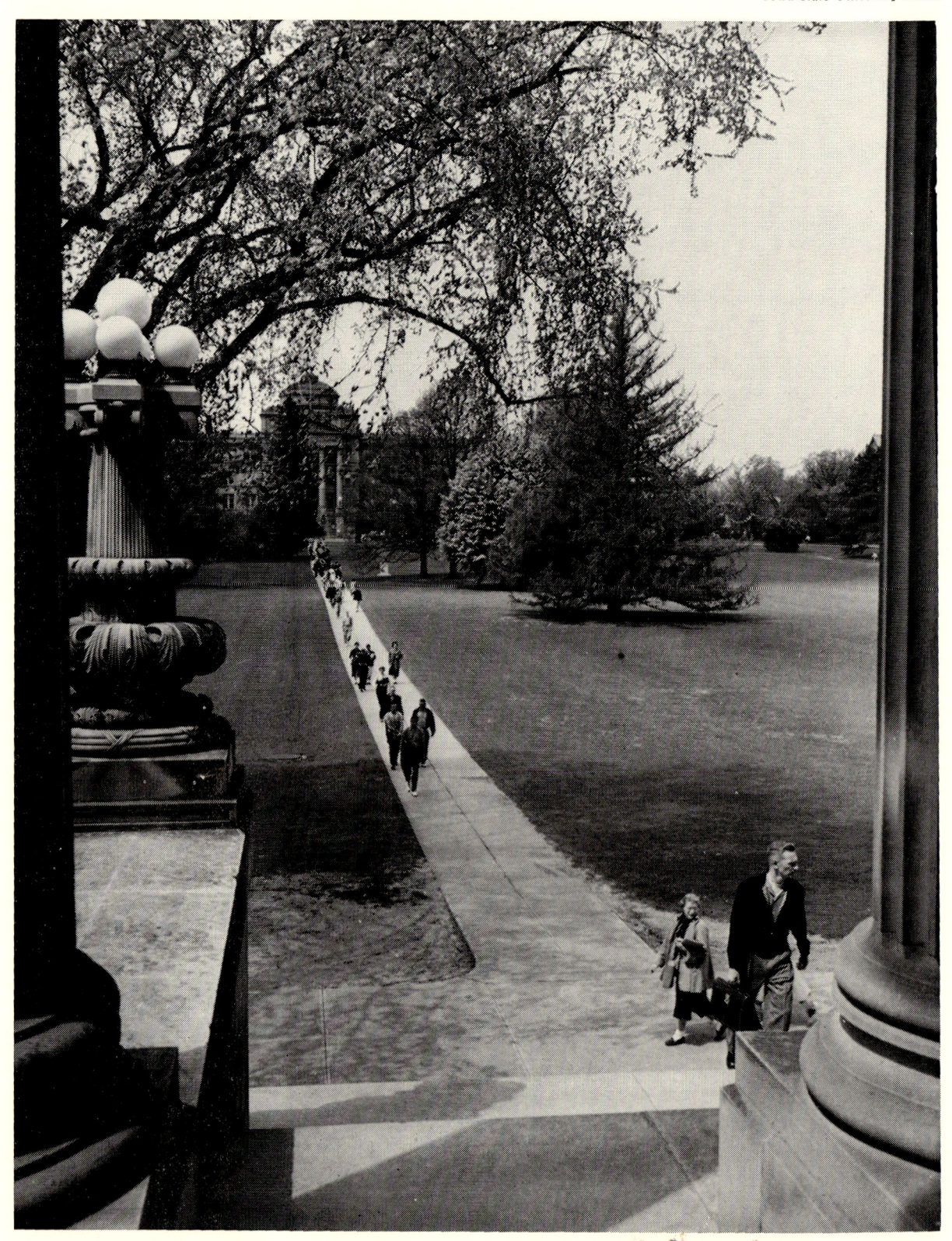

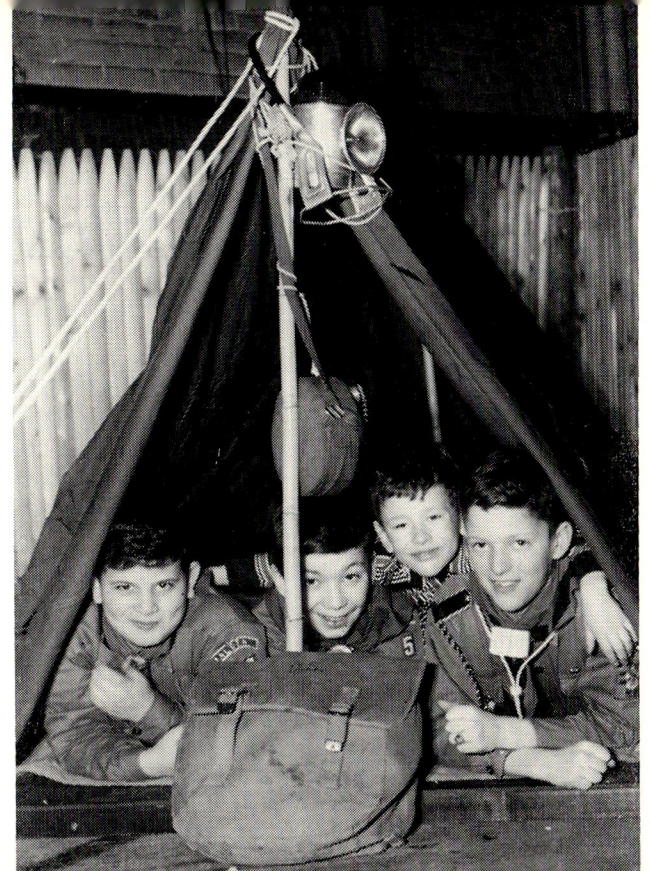

121   But a triangle that seems to lie flat on a picture looks stable.

*Bob Weir, Alpha Delta Sigma, Malden (Mass.)* Press

122   Opposed diagonal lines produce a feeling of struggle and conflict.

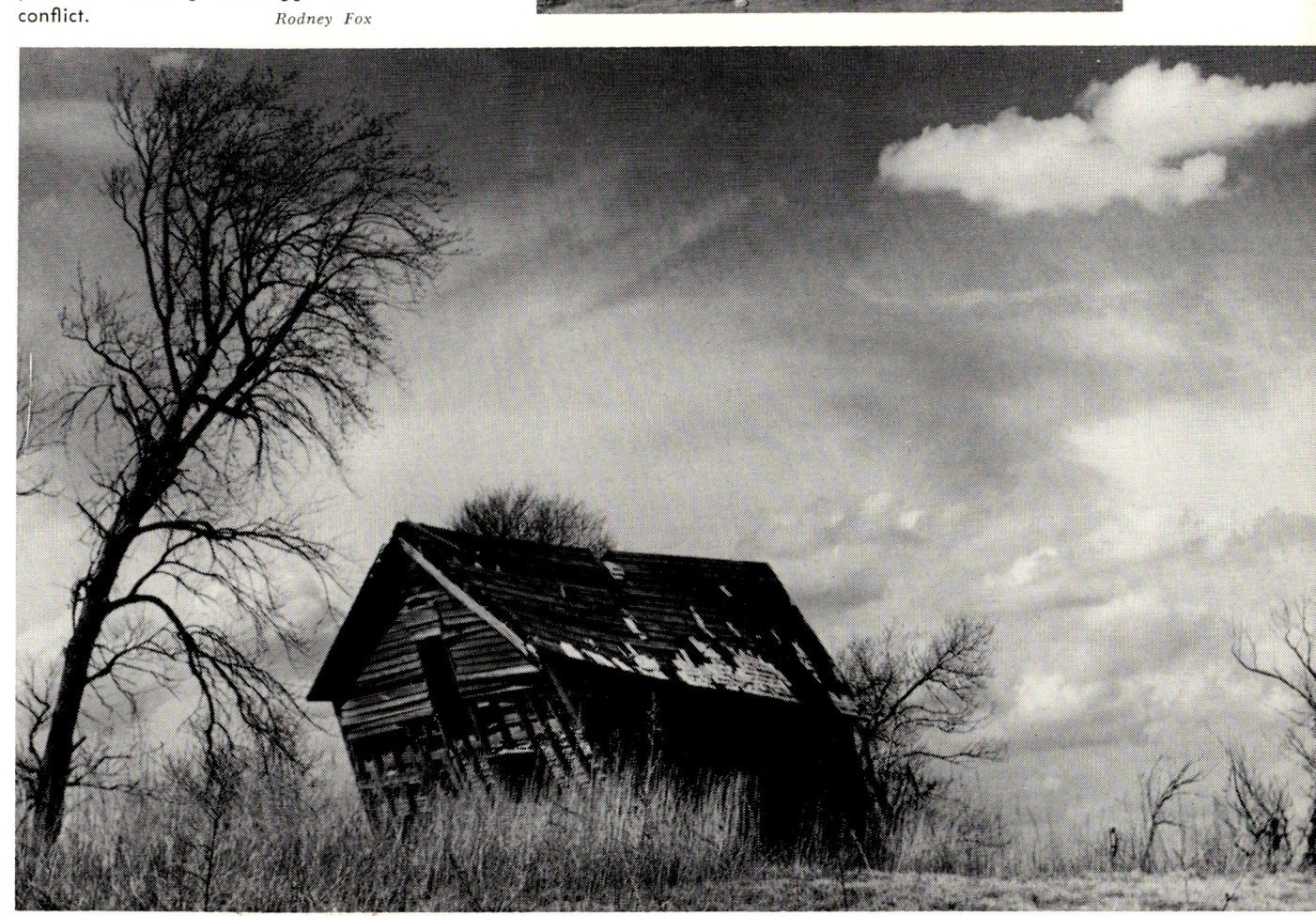

*Rodney Fox*

— 93

**Outside Shape of Picture Called Format**

The outside dimensions of a picture or the exterior shape of a picture is called its format. The contents of a picture should be adapted to its format. A long, horizontal object or line dominating a picture looks better in a long, horizontal format, as in Photo 118.

When a vertical object or other vertical materials dominate a picture, it looks better in a vertical format, as in Photo 117.

**Lines To Guide Eyes Through Picture**

Eyes work through an orderly picture in a guided way, and lines can be used to control and direct eye movement. Points of interest, even the center of interest, can be made more important by the crossing or implied crossing of lines, and the same method can be used to decrease the importance of centers of interest. A fine example of guided eye movement through a picture is provided by Photo 116.

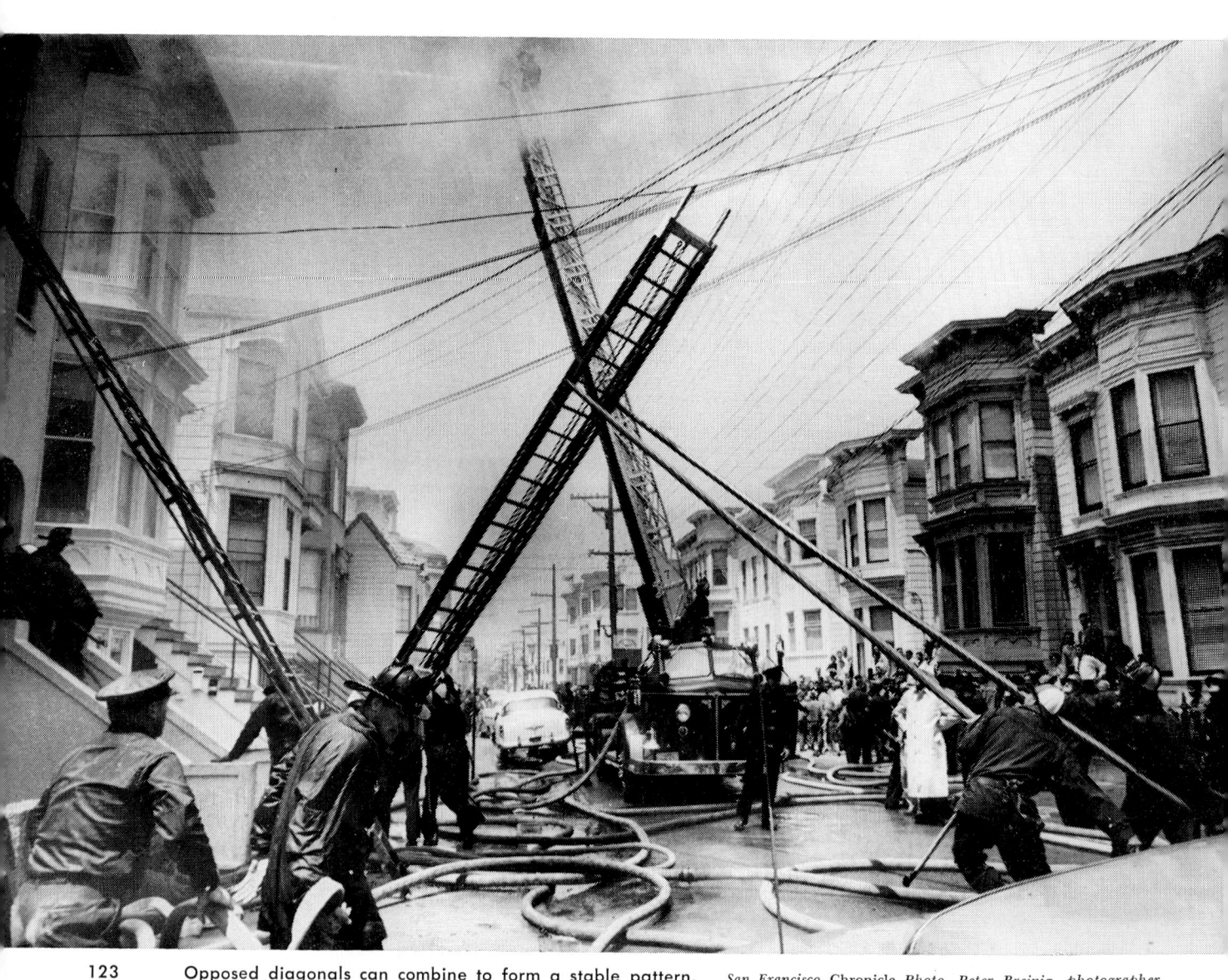

123  Opposed diagonals can combine to form a stable pattern.  *San Francisco* Chronicle *Photo, Peter Breinig, photographer*

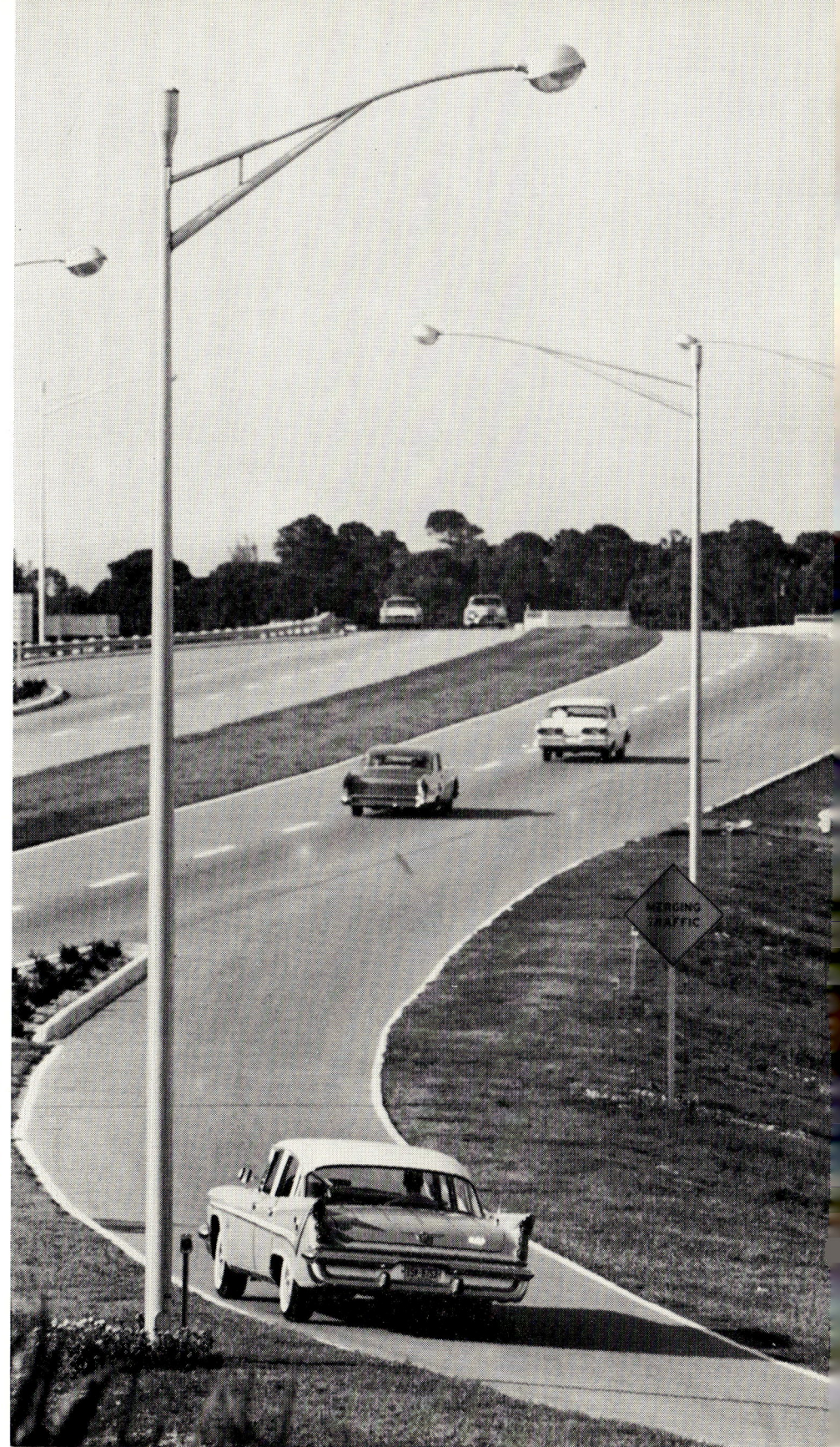

124  Some curves can create the same feeling of pictorial depth as did the angle formed by the sidewalk in Photo 120.

Home and Highway *Magazine, published by Allstate Insurance Companies*

125 All four major shapes in this picture, the three persons and the big teeth, at second glance seem to merge into a new shape, nearly triangular free form. How they do this is illustrated in Figures A and B. Recognition of these abstract shapes by combination of other shapes helps photographers plan their pictures.

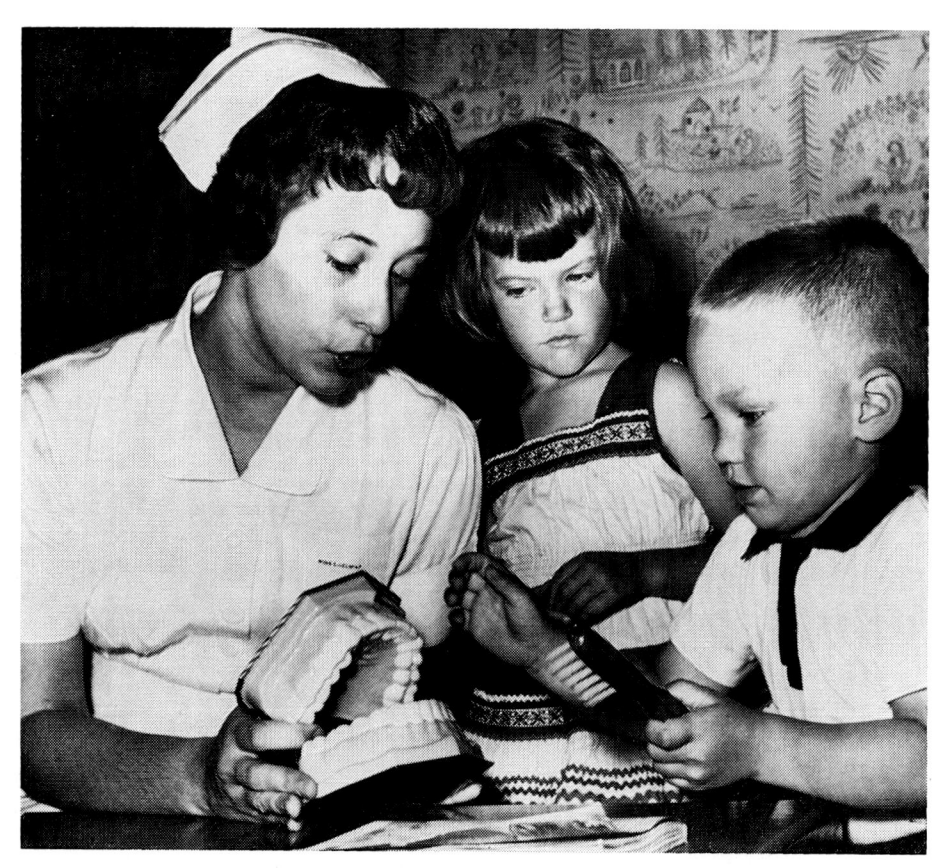

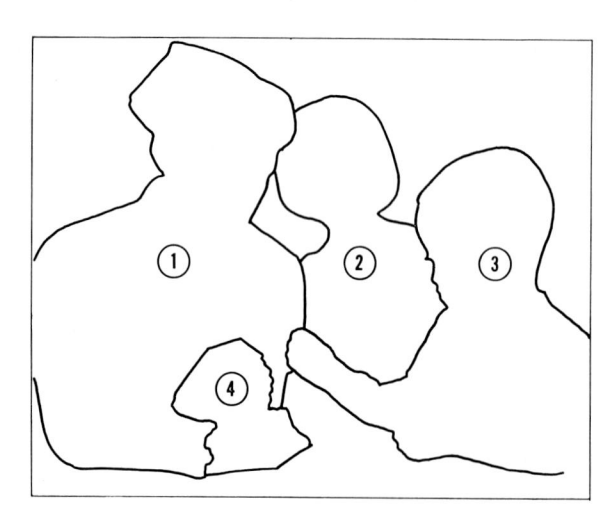

FIGURE A

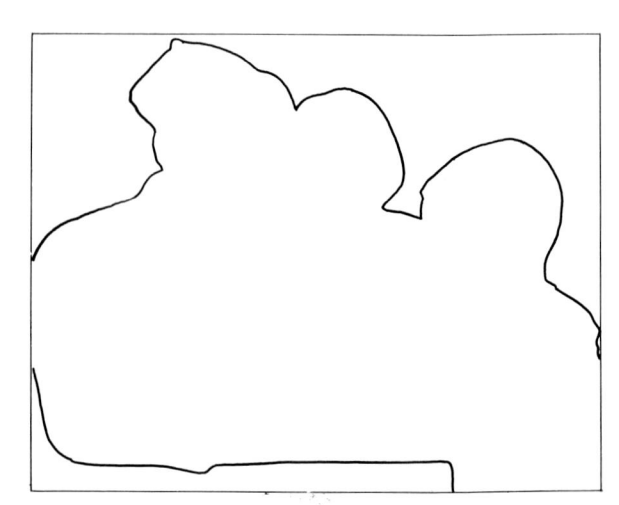

FIGURE B

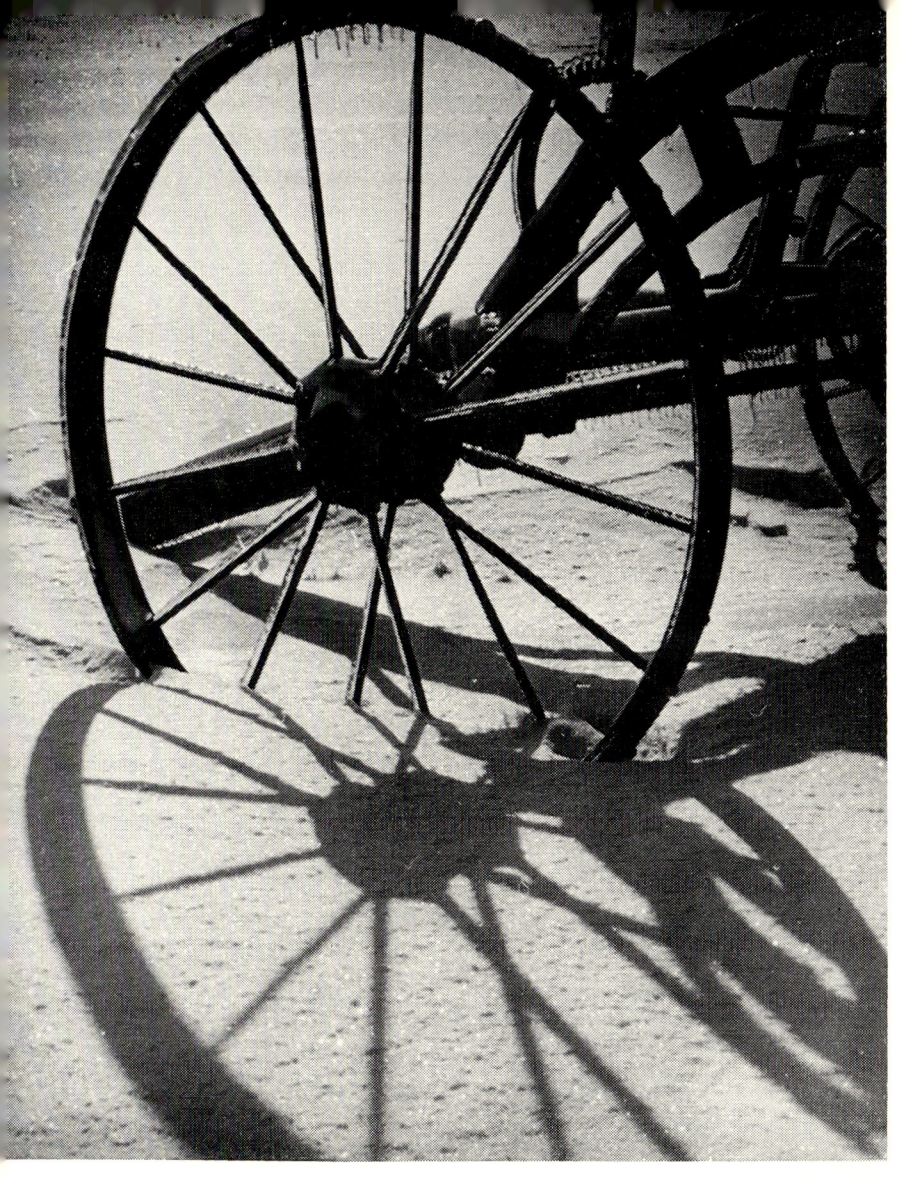

*How lines and shapes can be used to create exciting pictures is demonstrated in these photographs of wires, wheel, and weeds. Backlighting was used in all the shots.*

126  The wheel shape is repeated in variation by its shadow, and the two combine to form a new shape. The shadowy corners—produced in the darkroom—help balance the picture.

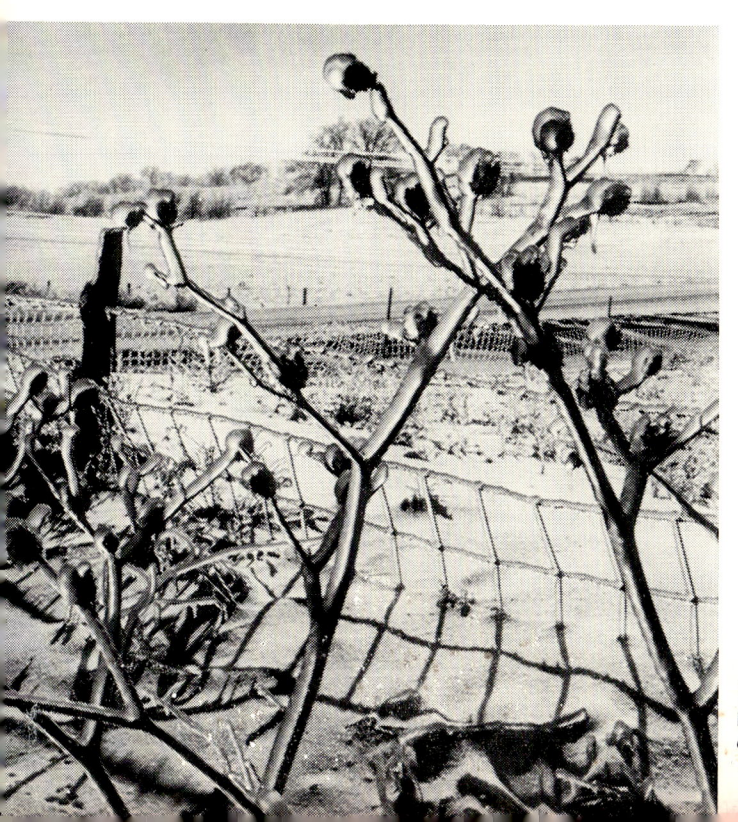

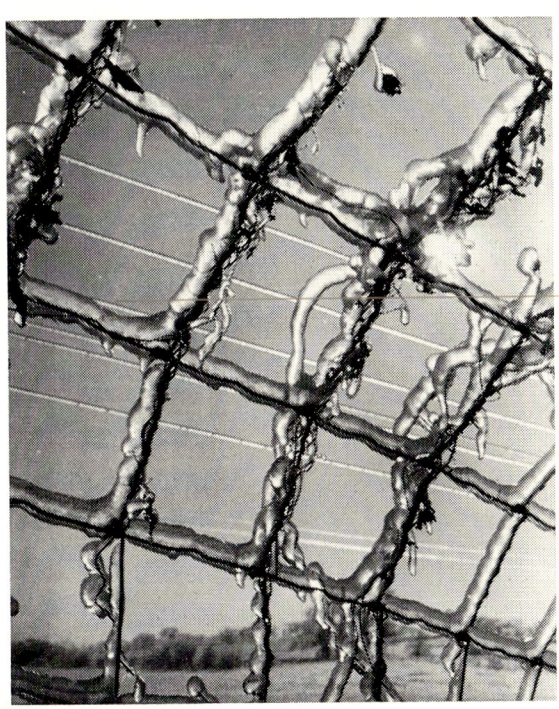

127–128  The eye can see the woven wire as a pattern, it can look at individual rectangles, or it can combine the rectangles in a great many ways.

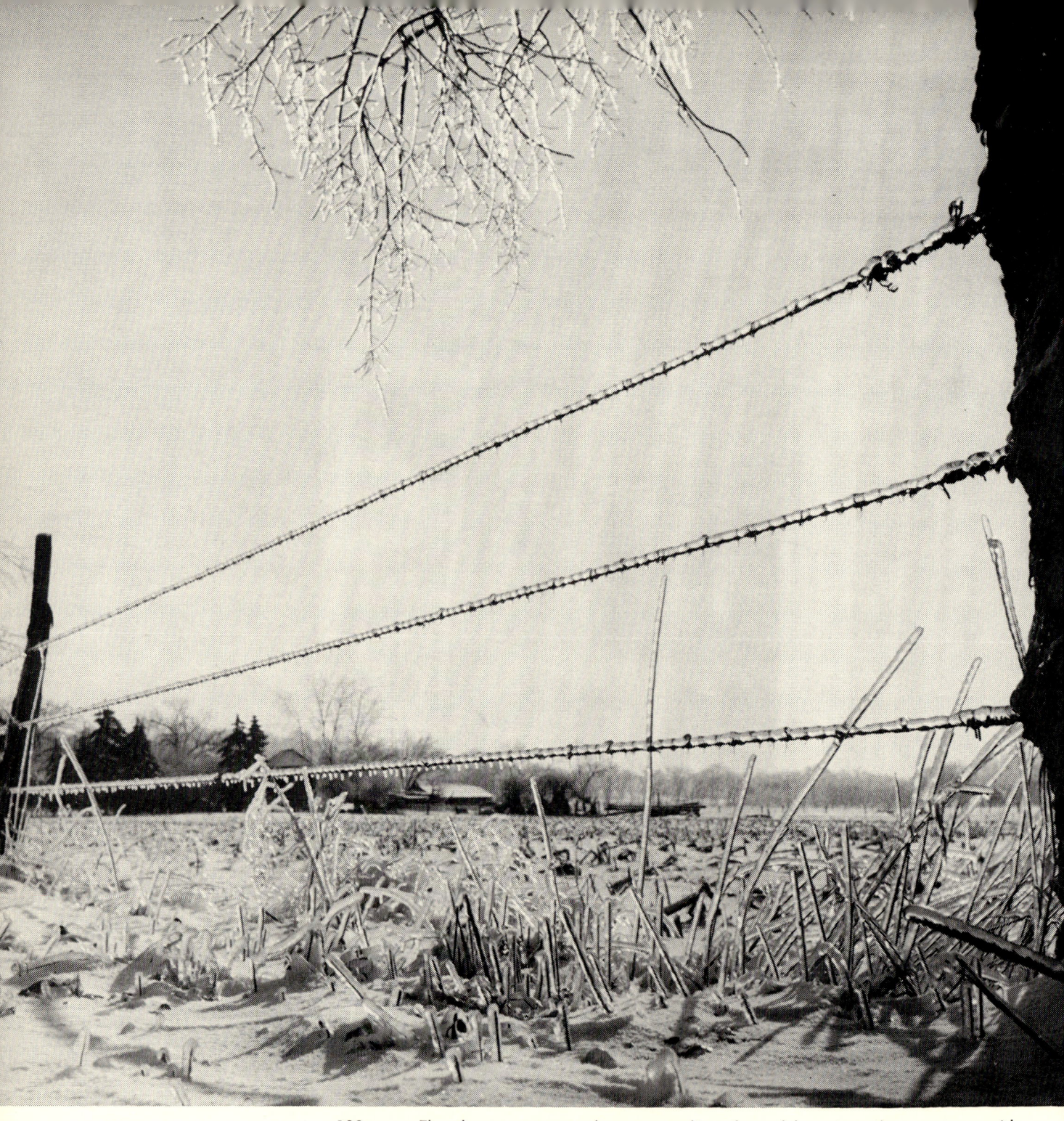

129   The observer can see three strong lines formed by wires; the two trapezoids they form; the repeated post forms; almost identical shapes in the sky and in the foreground, but varied by different textures.

CHAPTER **12**

# Repetition, Rhythm and Pattern Give Pleasure

DISCOVERING SOMETHING FAMILIAR can be delightful. When you're lost and trying to find your way, a familiar landmark gives you pleasure; when you are shopping in a store among a bewildering array of products, you grab for one marked with a familiar brand; when you see a familiar face among a crowd of strangers, you feel excitement, joy if it is the face of a friend.

You can give the viewer of your pictures the delight in finding the familiar by repeating certain elements in your photograph. If

130 Reflections provide obvious repetition with some variation. *Lowell Georgia, Green Bay (Wis.)* Press-Gazette, *staff photographer*

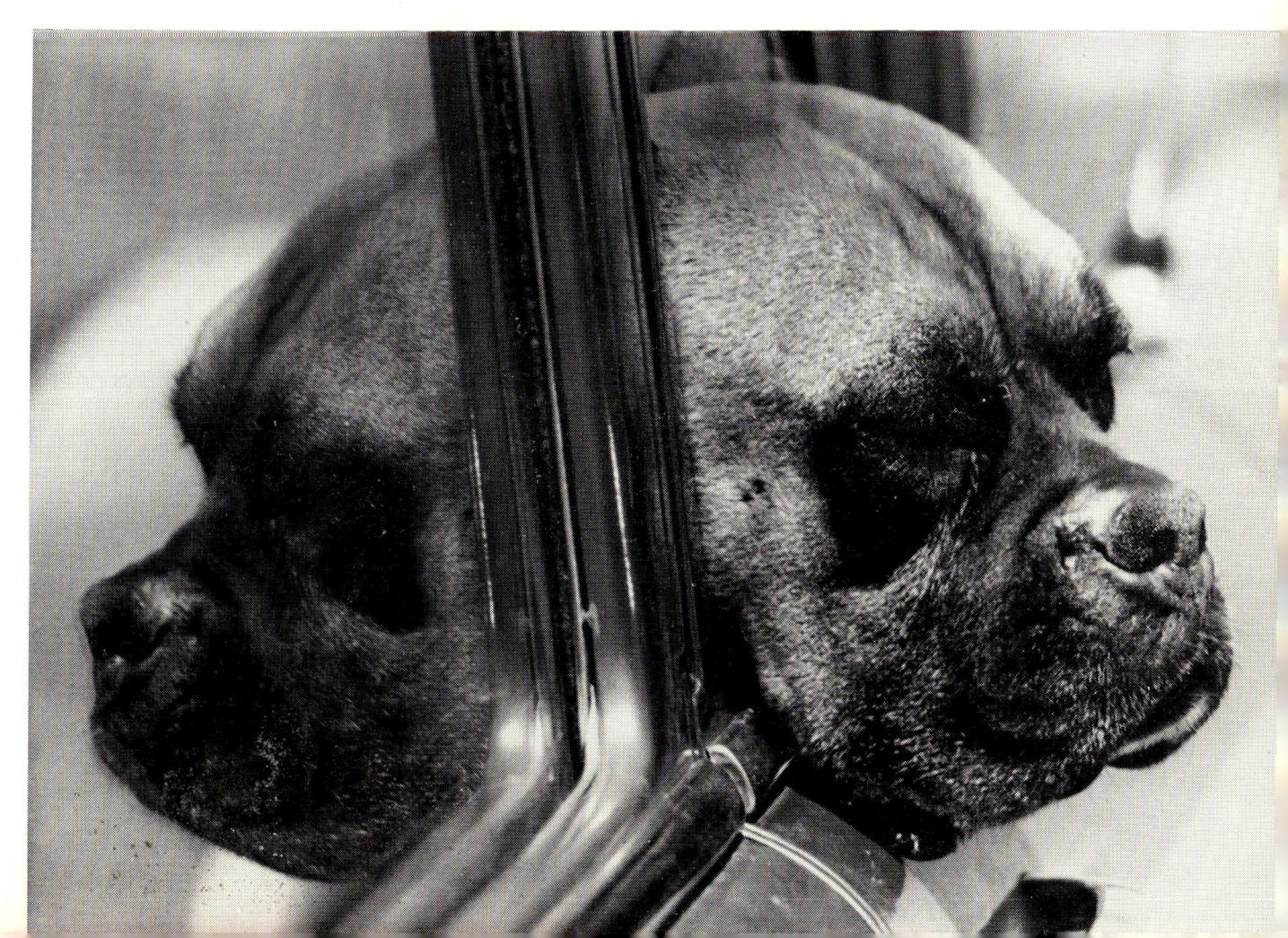

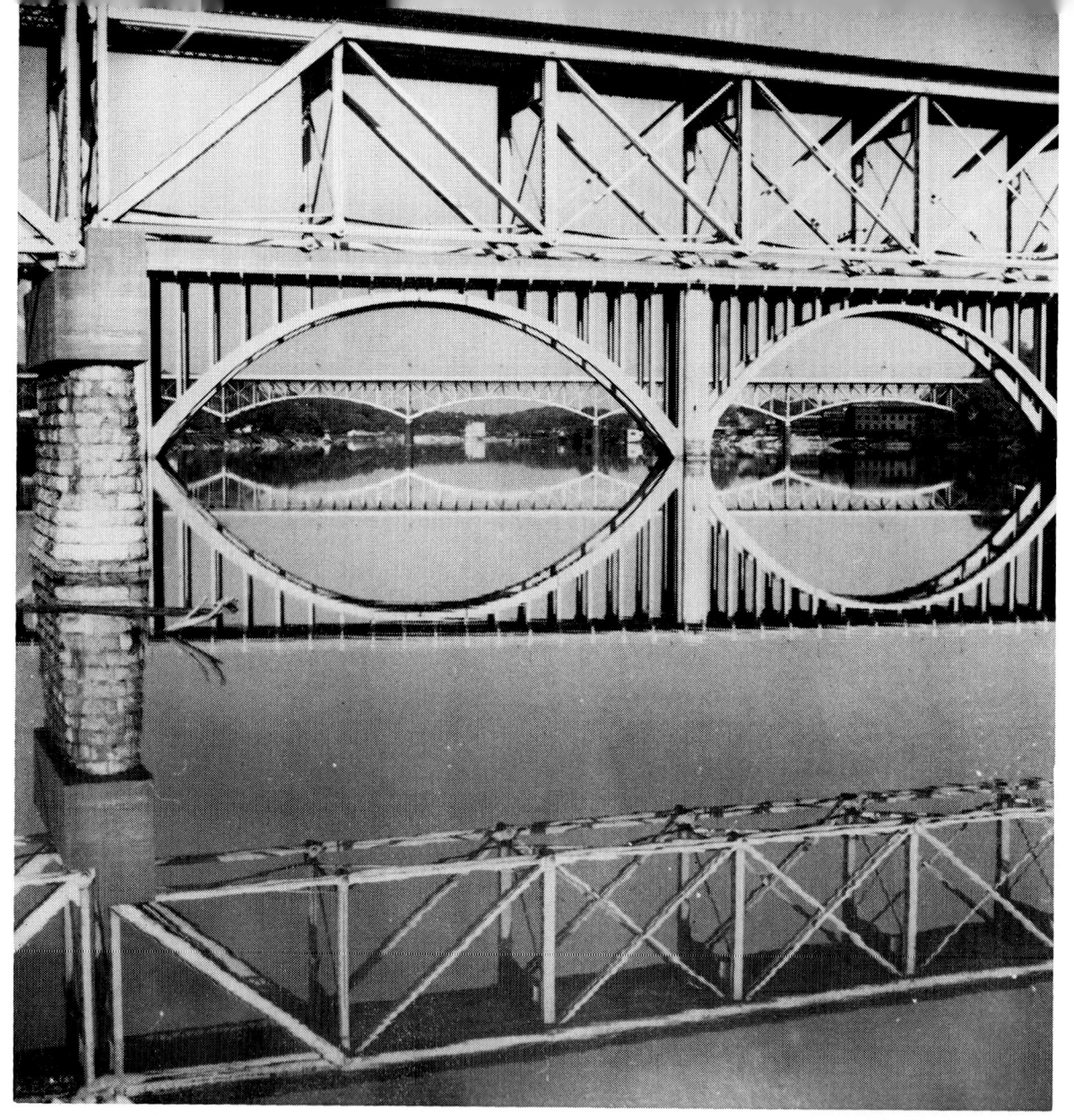

131    The fun of this picture lies in the series of repetitions with variations in the bridges, their reflections, their parts. The longer you look, the more repeats you see.

*Knoxville* News-Sentinel *photo by Bill Dye*

132    Helmets and head shapes are repeated many times and are varied in color and size. Full length figures in the background carry on the feeling of repetition.

*Fritz Shellman, Oconto County (Wis.)* Times-Herald

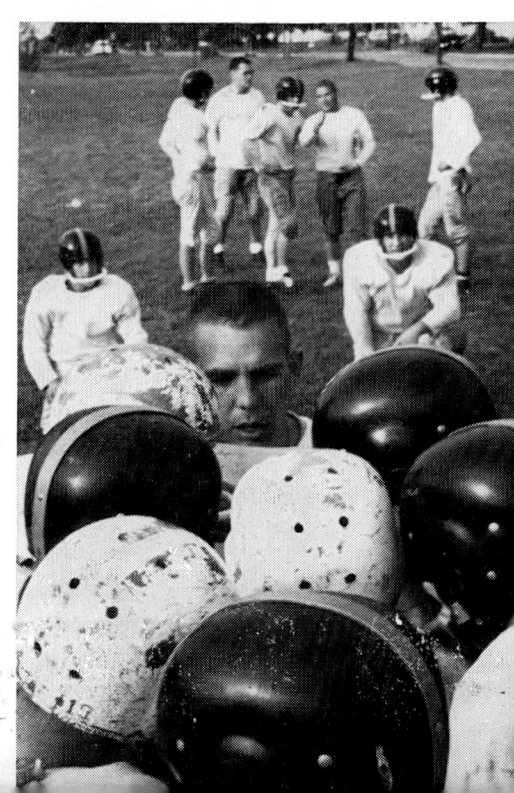

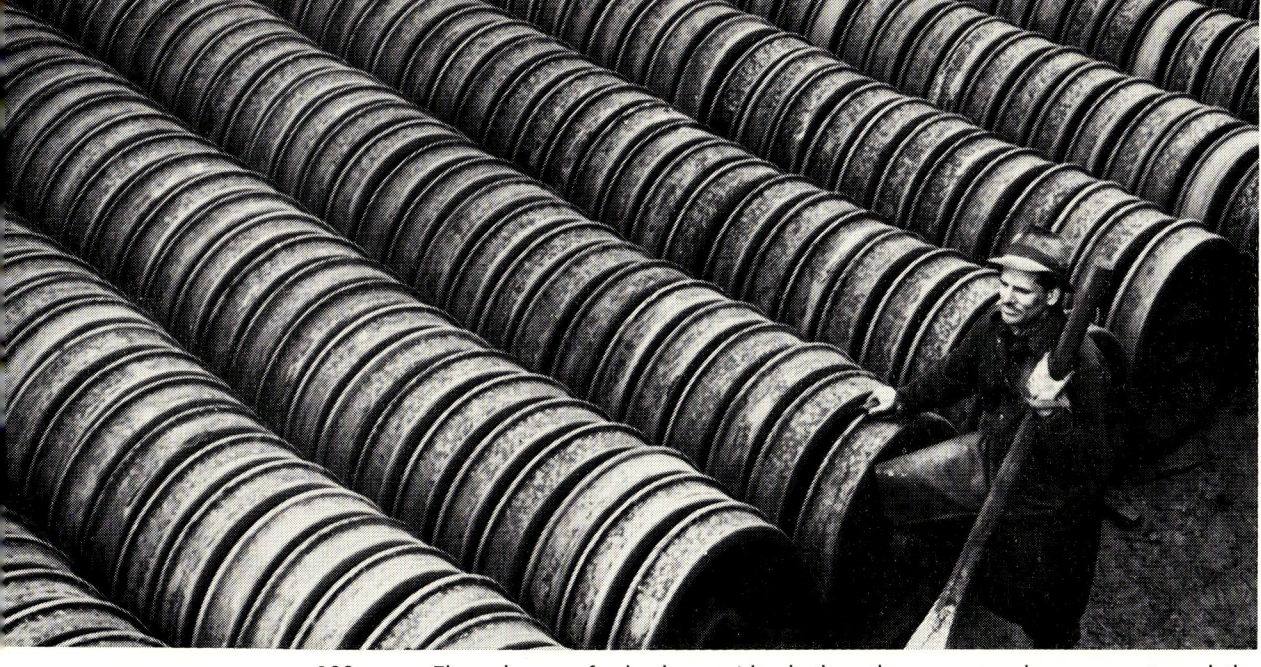

133 The columns of wheels provide rhythm, the man a welcome accent, and the diagonal lines a feeling of movement.
The Conductor & Brakeman, The Roadman's Magazine and Authenticated News, New York.

he notices a strong triangle, for instance, in your picture, discovery of other triangles can provide him with the fun that comes from finding the familiar. He can enjoy finding repetitions of certain kinds of curves, or lines, or shapes, or colors if you are working with colored film. He may not be aware that he enjoys your picture more if it contains repetitions, but it is well established that repetition can provide pictorial pleasure.

But too much of the familiar can easily become tiresome. "Oh, Ma, not eggs for breakfast again!" Just as a boy can quickly tire of one food if served too often, viewers of a picture can become bored if it has too many exact repetitions.

So the clever photographer looks for ways to obtain repeated elements in his pictures, but he doesn't want many elements exactly alike. A picture that has repetition with variation provides its viewer with the fun of discovering the familiar, but he is saved from boredom resulting from too much of the familiar because repetition is accompanied by variation. Finding changes and differences arouses new interests.

The principle of repetition with variation is found throughout art. In music, whether in a sonata or a popular piece, certain themes, sounds, elements are repeated, but with variation. In architecture, certain masses, forms, decorations are repeated but, to avoid monotony, repeated with variations. In an art more closely related to photography — painting — repetition with variation is of great importance.

There is no reason why this principle so important in art can't often be applied in news photography. A photographer with his eyes open will be amazed at how often he can use it.

**Rhythm in Pictures Pleasurable**

Certain kinds of repetitions can result in rhythm which in pictures — as in music, dancing, marching, poetry — provides pleasure.

The 1 2 3; 1 2 3; 1 2 3 of the waltz; or the 1 2 3 4; 1 2 3 4; 1 2 3 4 of marching provide pleasure.

So does the red, blue, blue, yellow, red; red, blue, blue, yellow, red; red, blue, blue, yellow, red of a design in a rug or woven basket.

In poetry rhythm delights, whether a nursery rhyme repeated again and again by children, or a highly sophisticated sonnet.

— 101

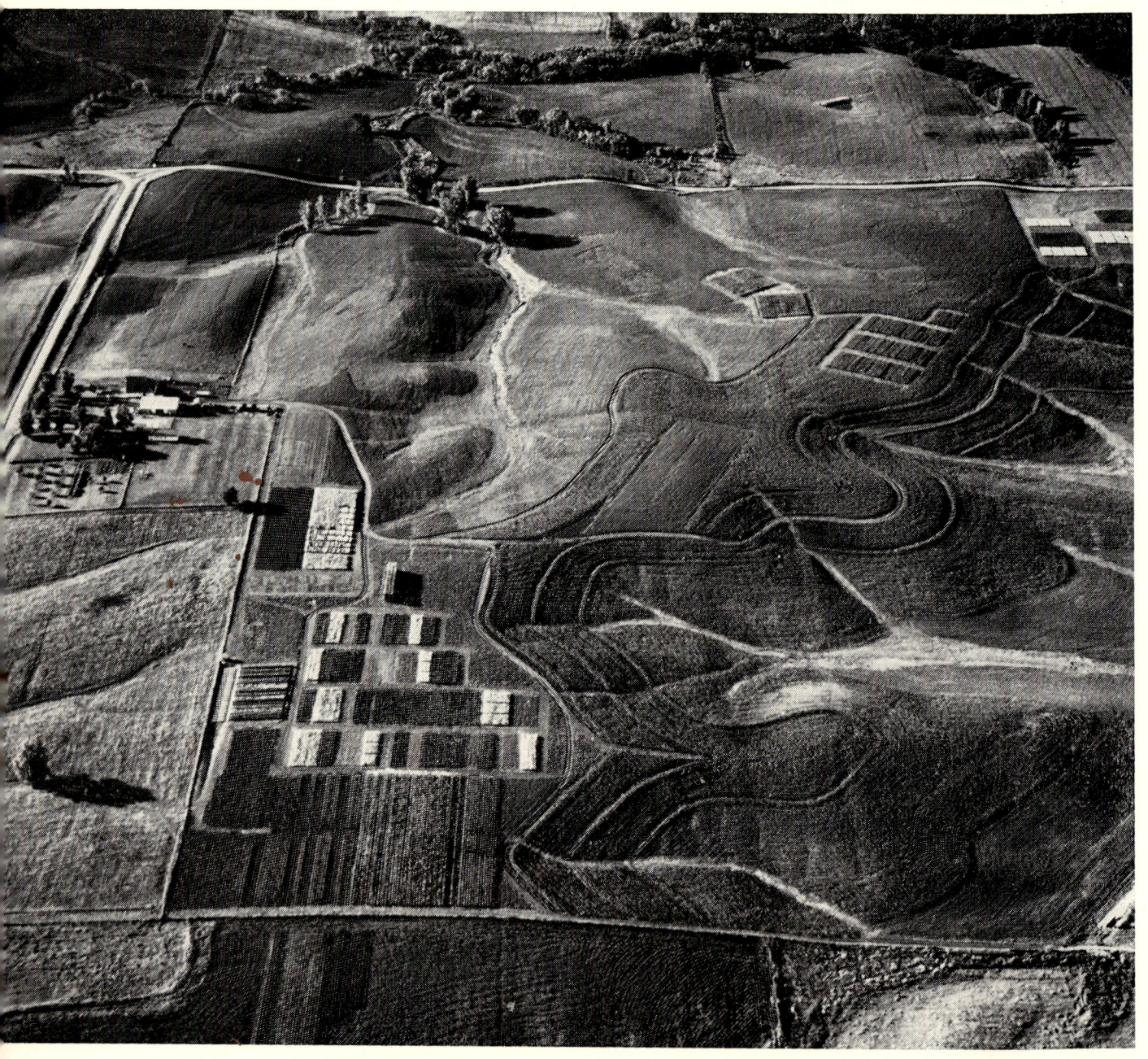

134 - Viewed from the air, fields form a pattern as in this photo by Charles Benn.
*Iowa State University Photo*

**Rhythm Important in Pictures**

Rhythm can be an important factor in the pleasure that pictures are capable of delivering. Rhythm in pictures is achieved by alternating or repeating certain shapes, lines or other elements in certain orders. Curves lend themselves nicely to rhythm because they relate to each other gracefully, but rhythm can be achieved by the use of shades, shapes, colors and other pictorial elements. A too constant rhythm can become monotonous and some variation is helpful.

Rhythm can be used by news photographers to enhance the pleasure their pictures can give.

**Patterns Can Enhance Pictures Too**

When lines, shapes, colors occur within a picture in an ordered way, somewhat as they do in wallpaper or rug designs, they create patterns which often enhance the attractiveness of pictures. Patterns often are geometric, but not always. Free rhythm patterns are possible.

Pictures that are purely pattern are monotonous and seldom are used. Some variation or the superimposition of a point of interest creates interest and kills monotony.

The delight that comes from repetition with variation in a picture is illustrated not only in the photographs in this chapter but also in others scattered throughout the book. Especially good examples are Photo 2 in which the human figures repeat each other, the sacks repeat each other and shapes of sacks and of figures are somewhat similar, and Photos 126, 127, 128 and 129 where repetitions are easy to find.

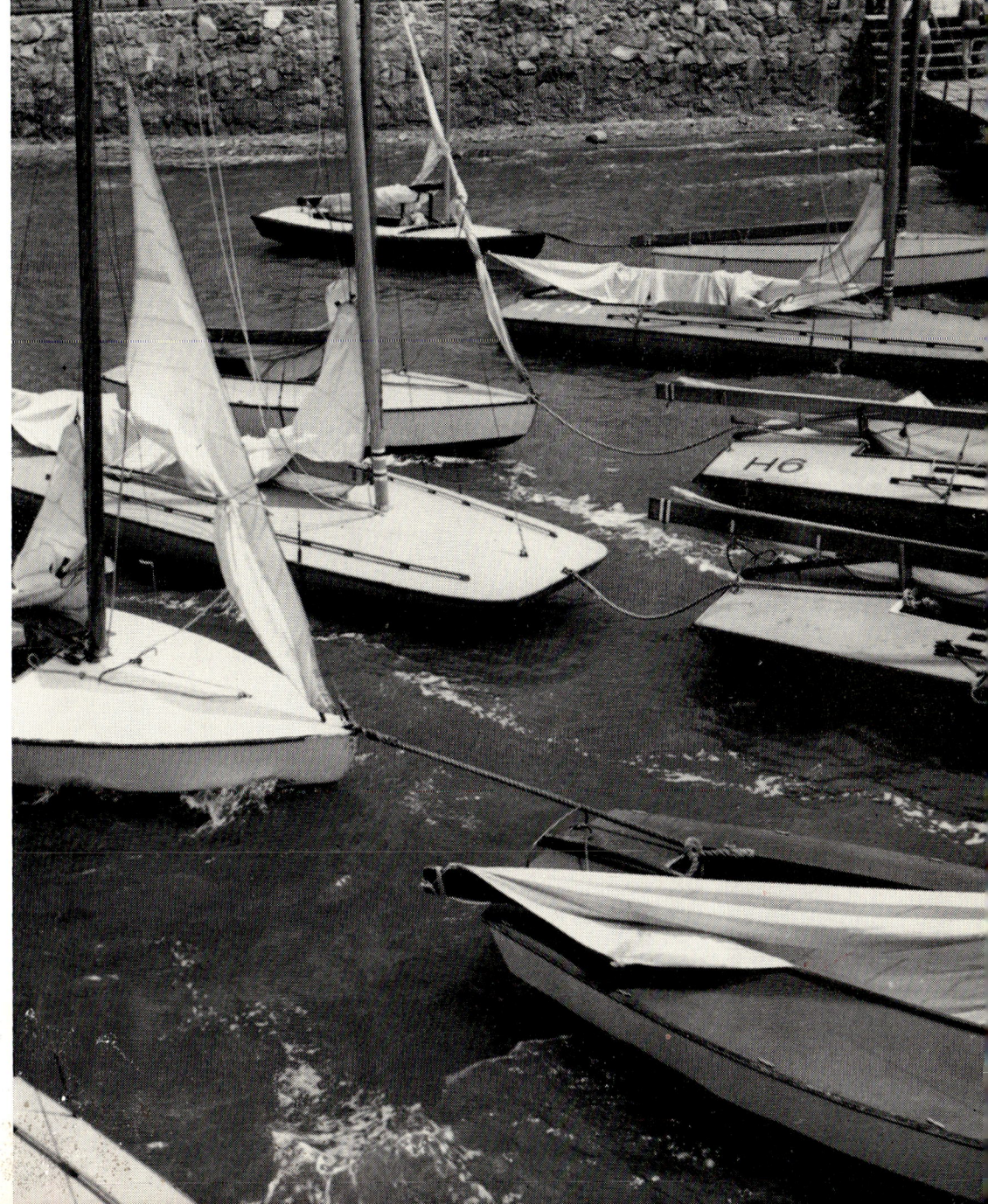

135 An orderly repetition of boat shapes creates rhythm.
*Elwin Musser, Mason City (Iowa) Globe-Gazette*

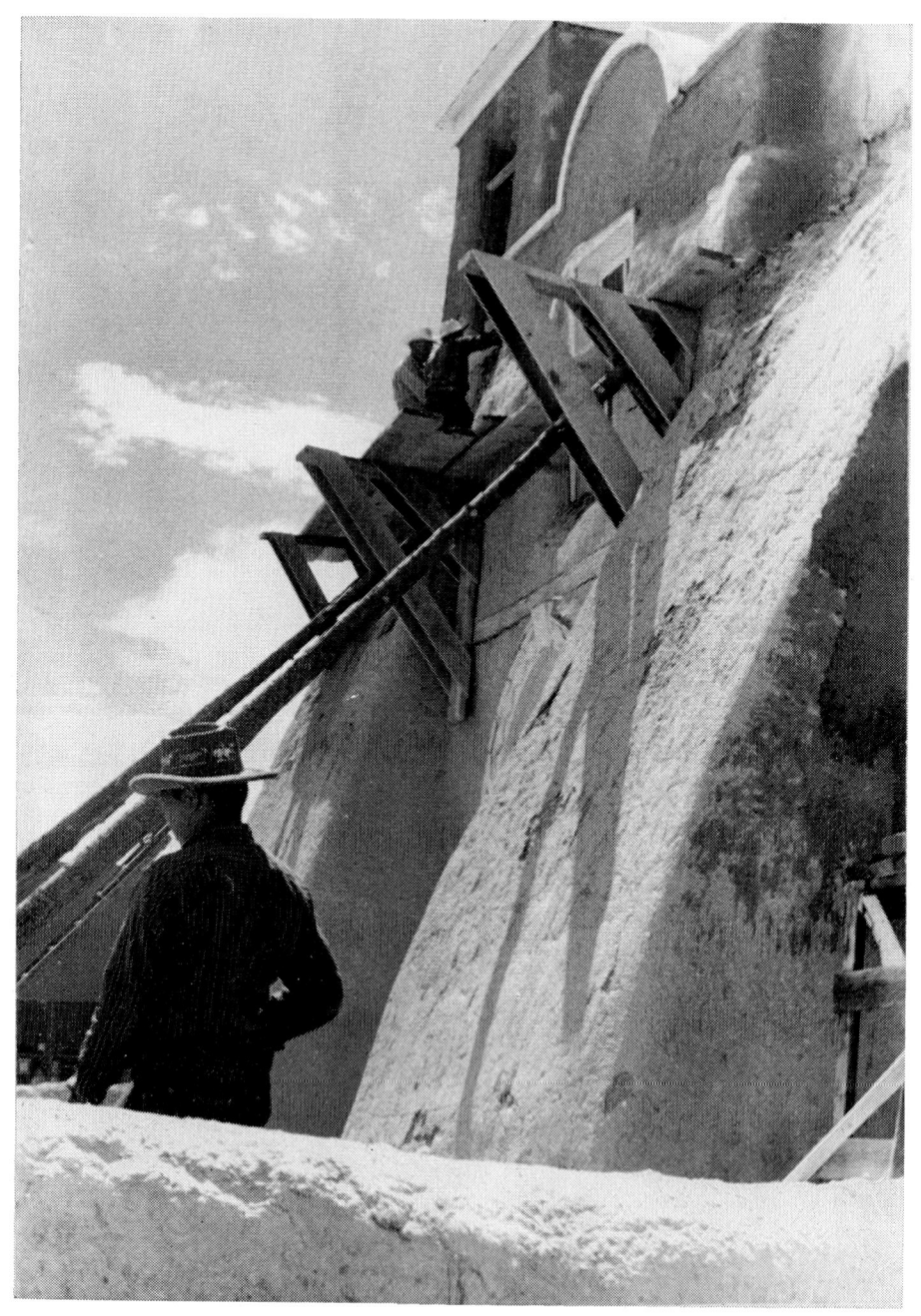

136   Good texture rendering enhances this construction picture.
*Mildred T. Crews for* El Crepusculo, *Taos, N. Mex.*

CHAPTER 13

# Texture Brings Fun of Touch to Pictures

WHEN YOU SEE a soft and woolly surface, usually you feel a strong urge to touch it. You have the same desire when you see a smooth and shining surface, or a rough and rugged one. Sometimes, when a sign commands, "Do not touch," you look both ways to see if anybody is watching and then steal a quick contact with your finger to satisfy your overwhelming desire to feel.

You can provide much of the delight people find in the feel of surfaces by a good rendering of texture in your photographs, for the word texture is used here as meaning a pictorial rendering of surfaces in such a way that the viewer gets much the same sensation he would if he rubbed his finger across the subject.

**Texture Enhances Reality**

Good rendering of texture in a photograph can greatly enhance the degree of reality it conveys. The viewer not only sees in the picture a representation of the subject matter but also gains the sensation of feeling it.

Not only can the rendering of textures give the illusion of touching the surface of the subject, but also sometimes can create the illusion of qualities internal to the surface. For instance, texture in the picture of a piece of cake might suggest whiteness and lightness of the whole cake.

In some advertising pictures the rendering of textures can be the most important purpose of the picture. Pictures of a loaf of bread sliced open, of rugs, of upholstery, of fabrics used in advertising rely heavily on the depiction of surface textures.

Often the story, or an important part of the story, to be conveyed in a picture in a newspaper or magazine concerns textures. Textures of clothing, wall surfaces in architectural studies, skin, plowed fields are essential to telling the desired story. Without good textures, pictures often do not tell either accurate or adequate stories.

If painters and sculptors spend much time and effort rendering interesting surfaces to delight the viewers of their works, why isn't it worthwhile for news photographers to give thought and effort to render texture to please the viewers of photographs too? Usually it takes just a little different lighting, a slight change in camera angle to improve the rendering of the texture of an important part of the subject matter in a picture. To do so may please hundreds of viewers.

When an area in a photograph shows rich texture, the textured area usually forms a shape and should be so considered in planning the photograph.

— 105

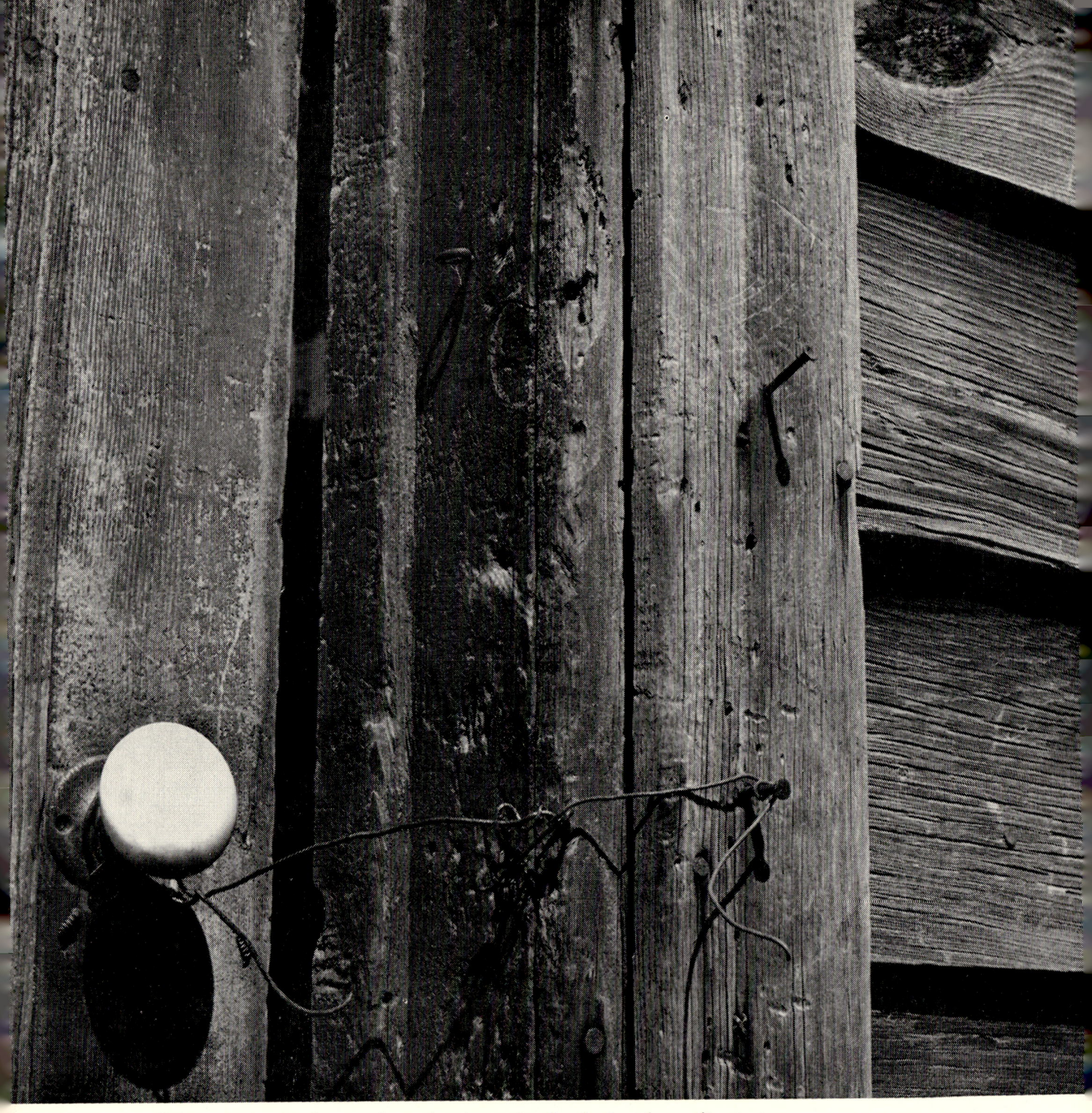

137   If some photographers take pictures just for the joy of recording texture. . . .

138   Why shouldn't news photographers seek good texture rendering more often, as in this picture made as part of a series about construction activities. Notice how lines are made to run diagonally across picture, and that this photograph has pattern, too.

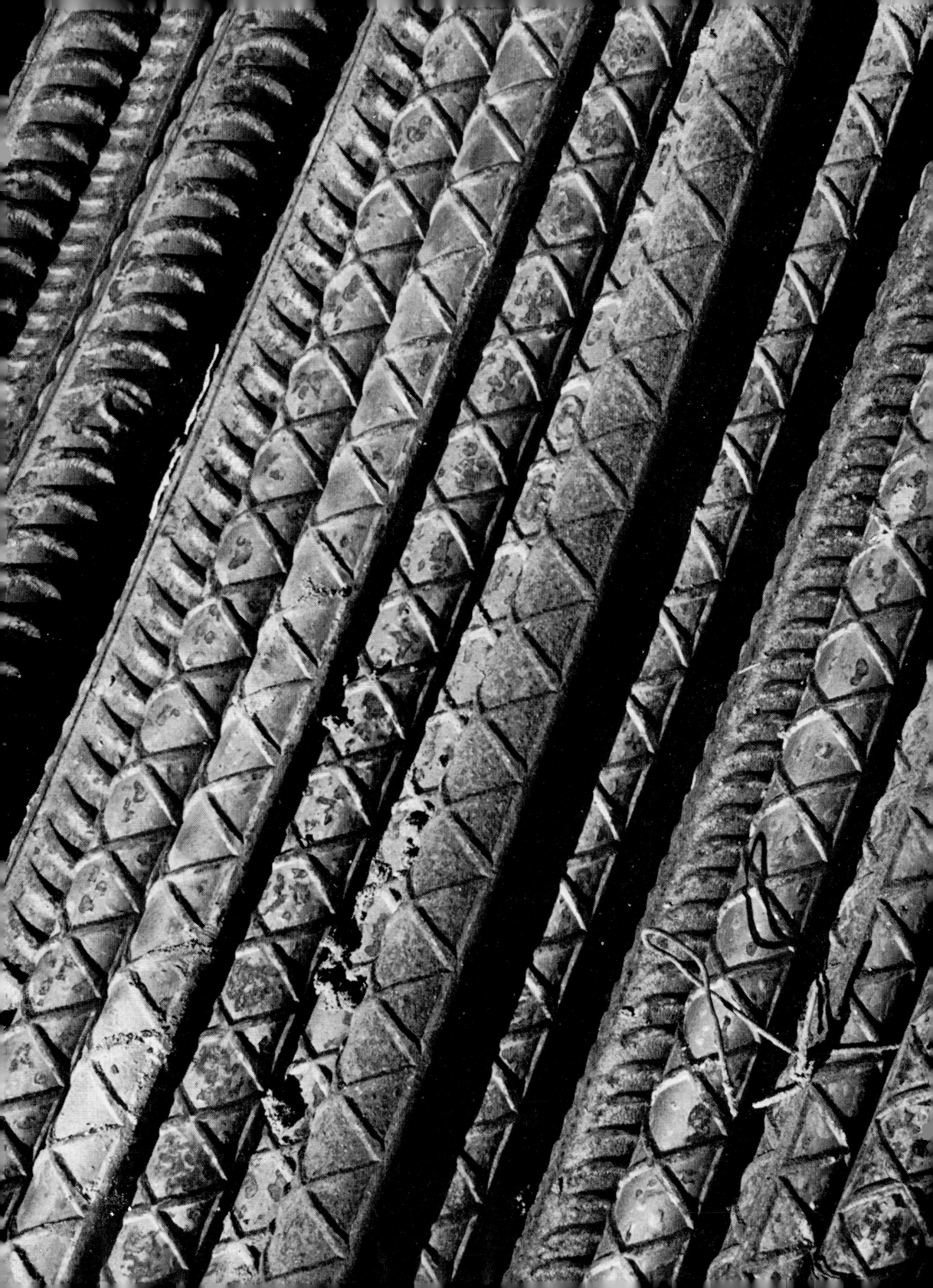

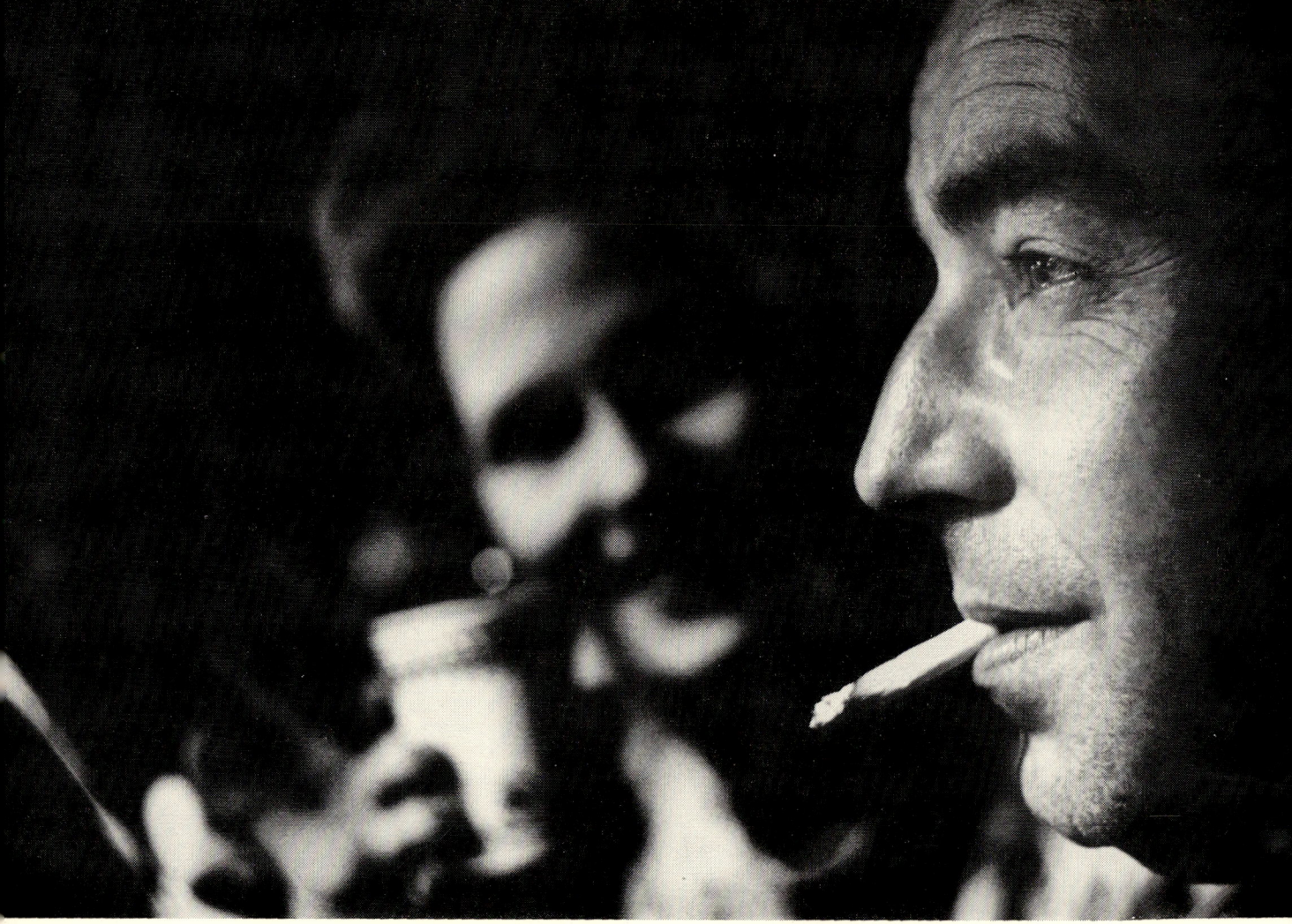

139   Skin texture becomes an important factor in a picture.
Home & Highway Magazine, *published by Allstate Insurance Companies.*

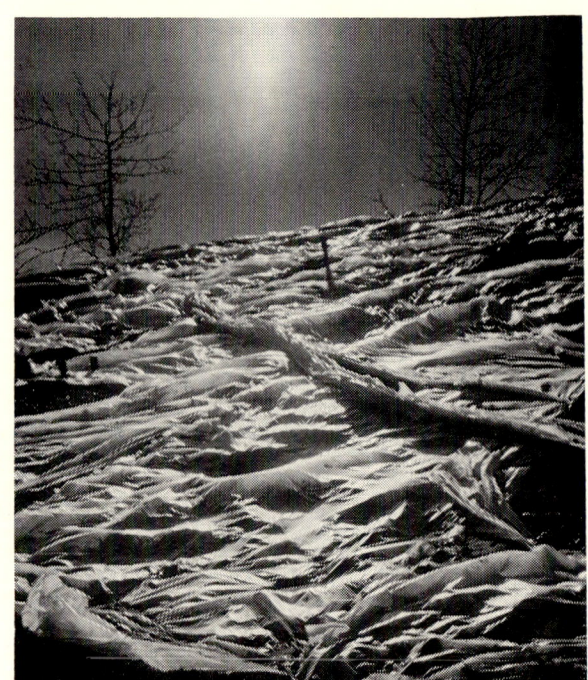

140   Knowing how to photograph texture produced this striking picture of plastic used in a hillside soil experiment.

108 —

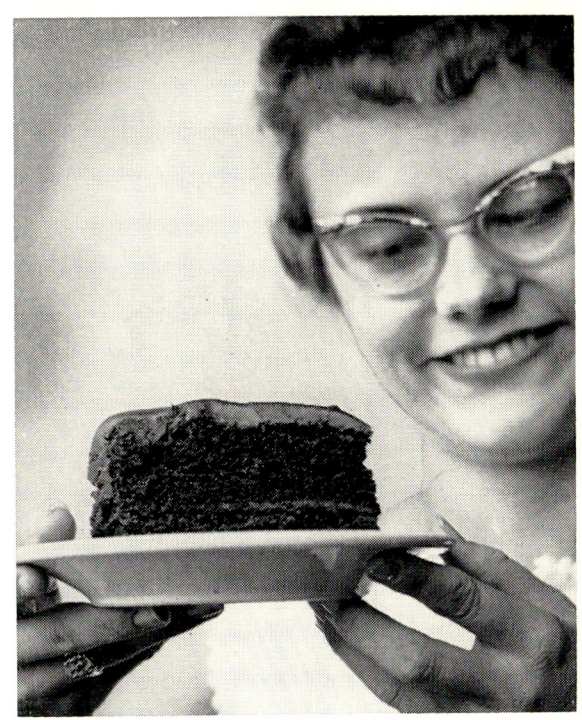

141   Foods photography can be greatly enhanced by good rendering of texture.

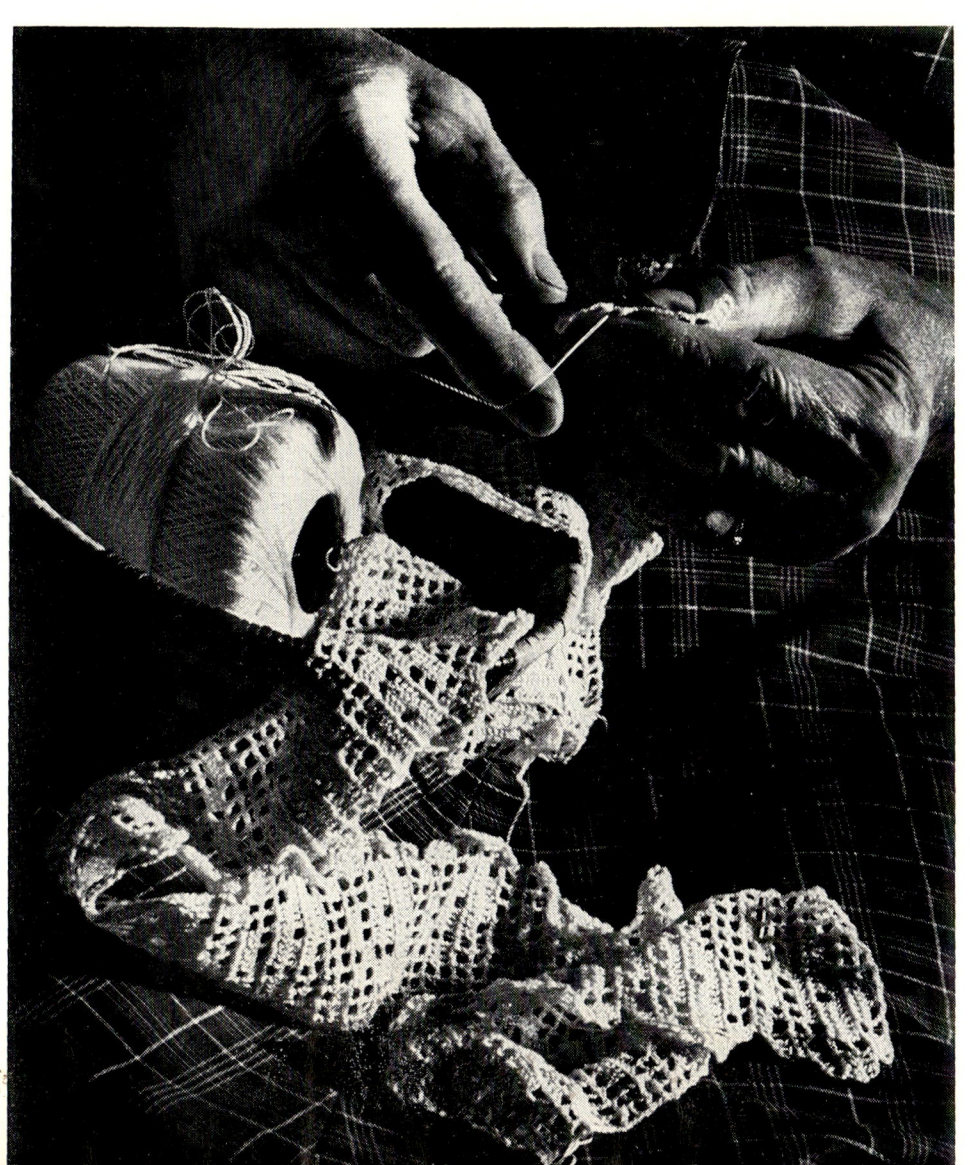

142   Fabrics reflect an almost infinite range of textures.

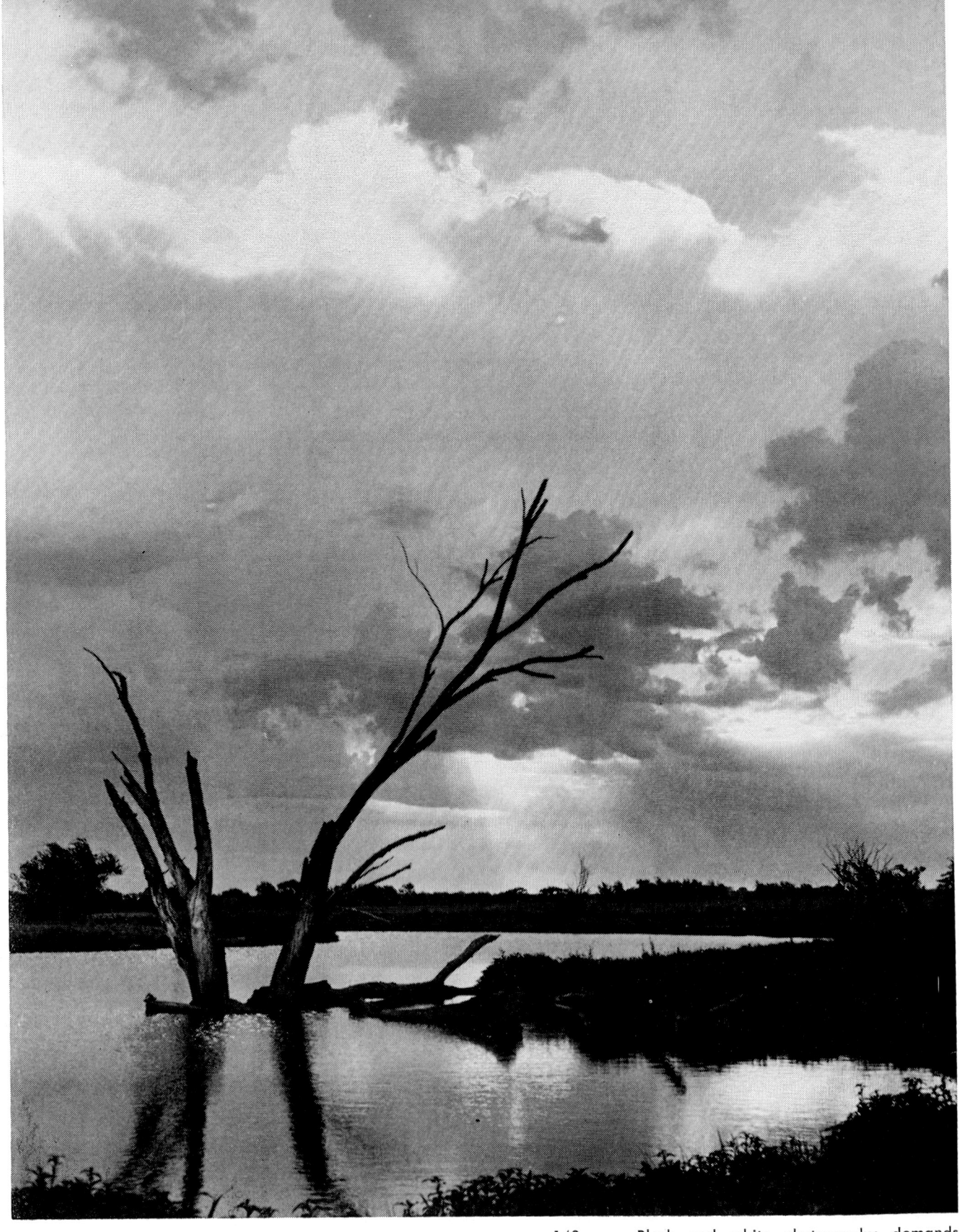

143  Black and white photography demands skillful handling of darks, lights and middle tones.
*Leonard Bacon, Lawrence, Kansas, Journal-World*

CHAPTER **14**

# Tone Values and the Magic of Light

THE DARKS AND LIGHTS and middle tones are important factors in black and white photography. Their relative values have much to do with the quality of a picture, and to an extent such relationships are under the control of the photographer. He can to some degree select and arrange subject matter and to some extent can control the value of tones through exposure, development, printing.

Here are a few of many facts about the *relationships* of tone values that could be of value to a photographer in helping to create desired results:

1. The value of a given tone is changed by its relationship with adjacent and surrounding tones. For instance, when a gray area is surrounded by black, the gray looks much lighter than it would if viewed without its dark surroundings. Likewise, when gray is surrounded by white, the gray looks darker than it would if looked at alone.
2. A light tone area in a picture looks larger than does a dark area that covers the same amount of space.

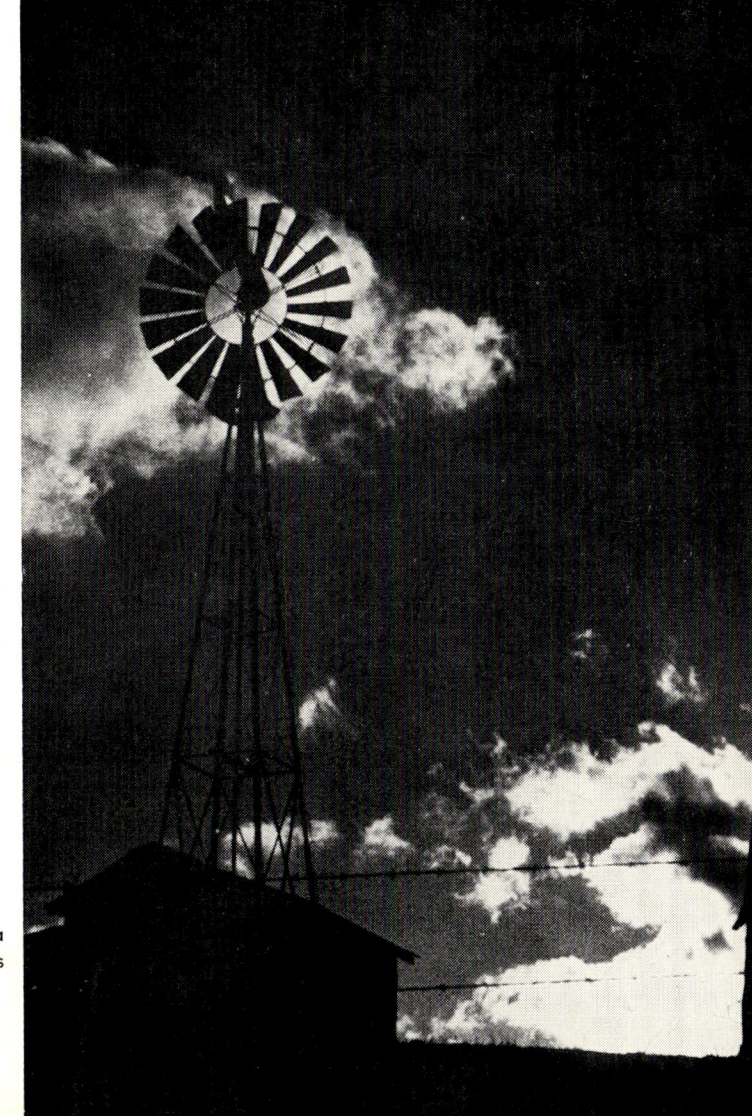

144   A light object against a dark background, or the reverse, is dramatized.
*By Larry Mulvehill, Middletown, New York,* Daily Record

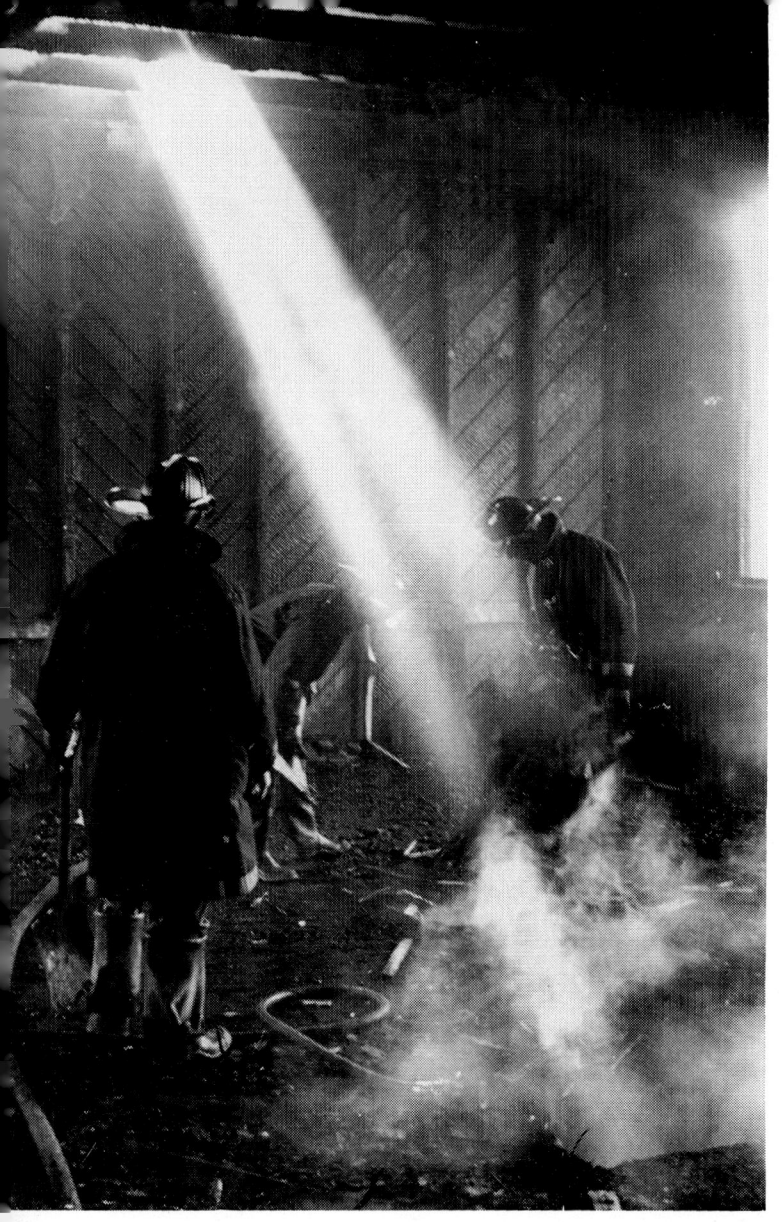

**145** A streak of light can become a line compositionally.
*Photo by Hugh M. Gillespie for Montgomery County (Md.) Sentinel*

3. The darkest dark contrasted against the lightest light will attract attention to that point of a picture. Such a point becomes the center of interest if it is the only one in the picture. The reverse of this is true, too. The lightest light against the darkest dark will attract attention to that point in a picture.

**Some Practical Applications**

Some of the practical applications that can be made of this information include:

1. A light object against a dark background, or the reverse, is dramatized. An example is Photo 144.

2. The apparent size of a white or comparatively light object in a photograph is greater than the apparent size of a dark object that occupies the same amount of picture surface. Knowing this can help in planning balance.

3. Knowing that the lightest light against the darkest dark (and vice versa) creates a center of interest helps the photographer play up or down such centers of interest in accordance with his plan. It also helps him work out balance.

In Photo 144, two centers of interest develop with the windmill, probably because of its more interesting shape, emerging as the real center. These two centers are important in establishing the balance of that picture.

**Magic of Light**

After all, light is photography. How it is controlled by means of the lens to cause chemical reactions results in pictures. How lights and darks are distributed has much to do with the attractiveness or the effect of the picture.

A streak of light can become a line compositionally; the patches of darks and lights become shapes; the relationships of these designs of lights, darks and intermediates become part of a picture's design. Notice how dark and light masses become abstract shapes and part of the composition in Photo 143.

Backlighting creates a certain feeling in a picture, light from above seems natural while light from a low source creates a sense of drama, as do theater footlights. The harshness or softness of light, the qualities of contrasts created by light, reflections and shadows, glares and highlights all are elements used in designing good photographs.

**146** Backlighting creates a certain feeling in a picture.
*Bruce Roberts, staff photographer, Charlotte Observer*

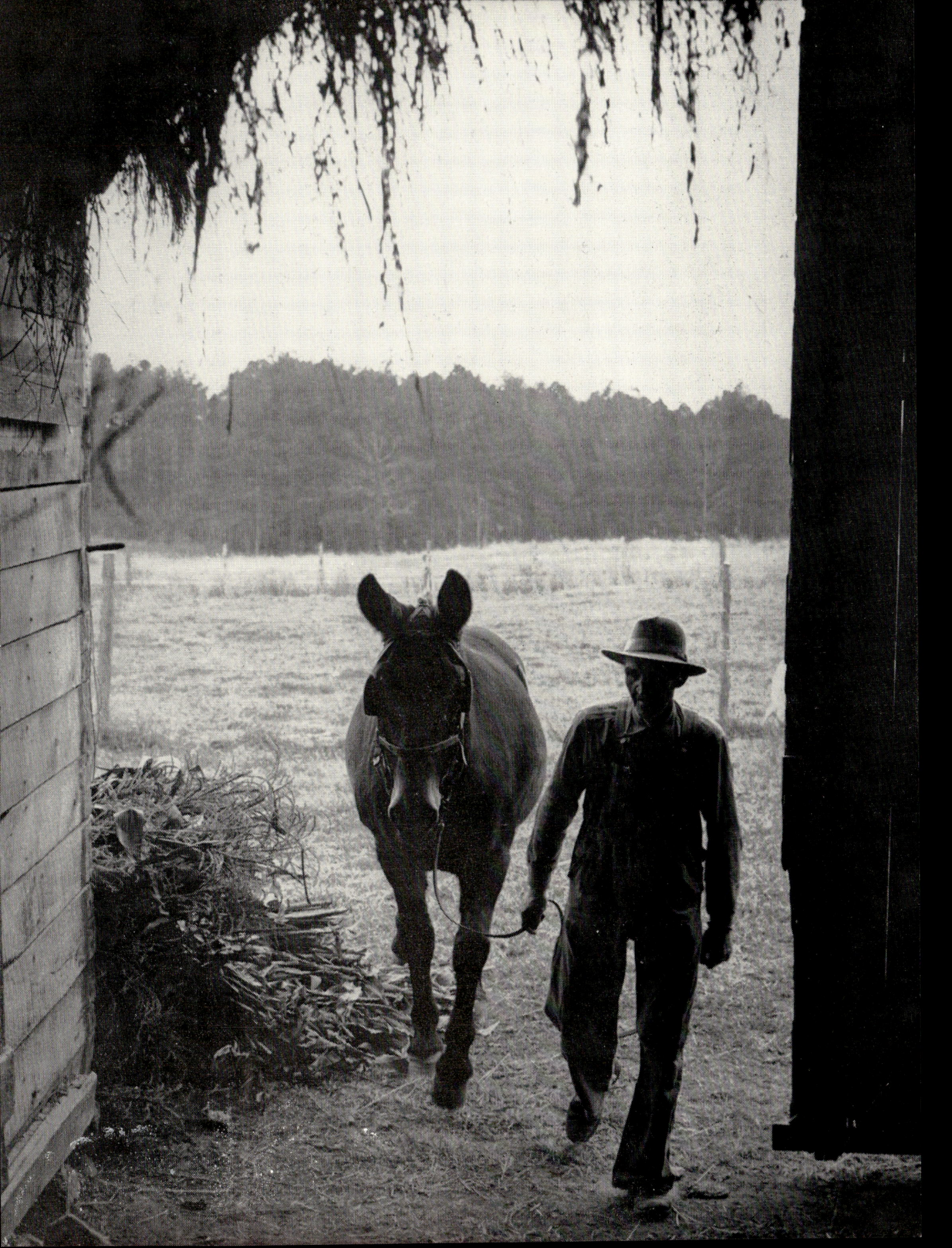

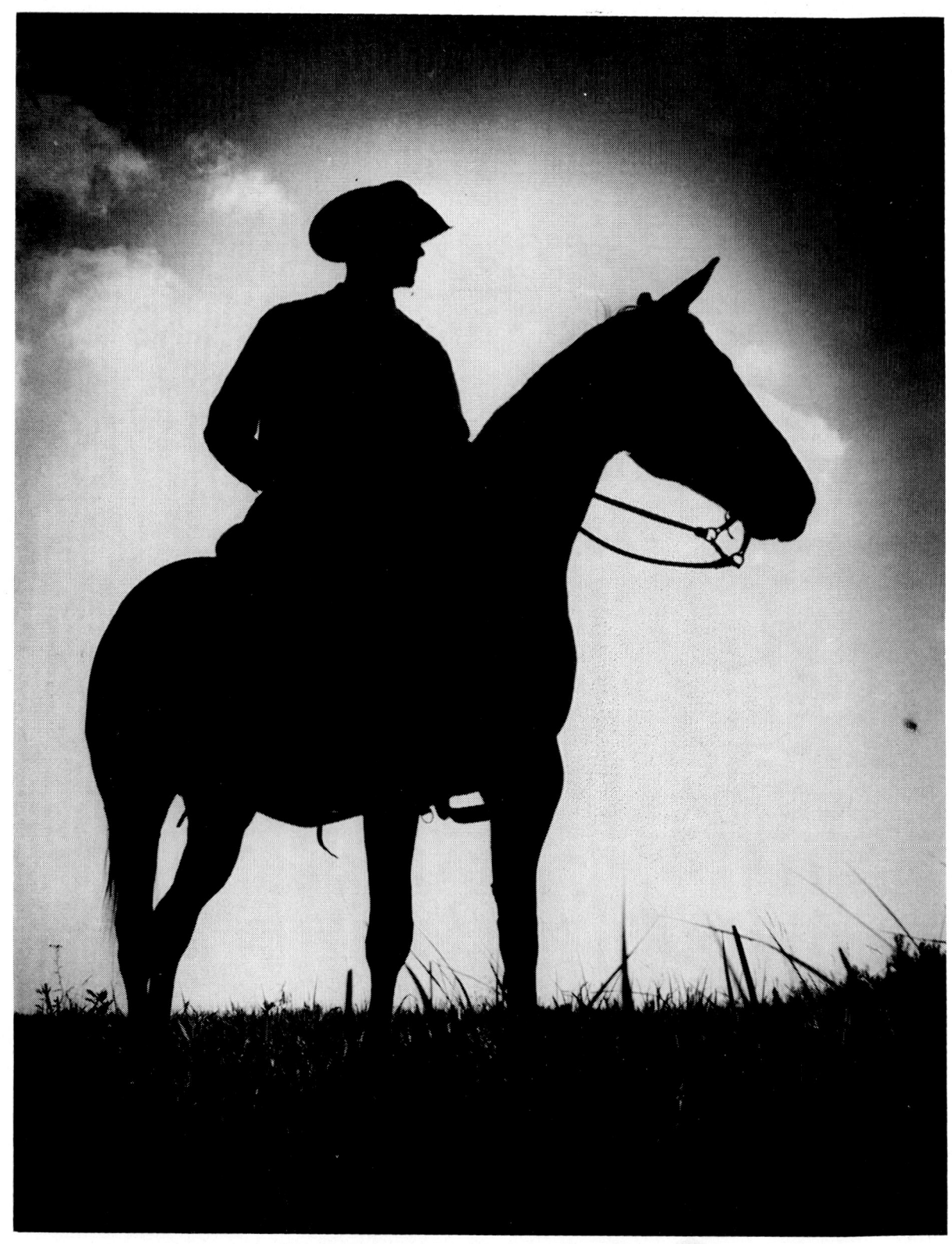

147   Once in awhile, a complete silhouette produces an arresting picture.

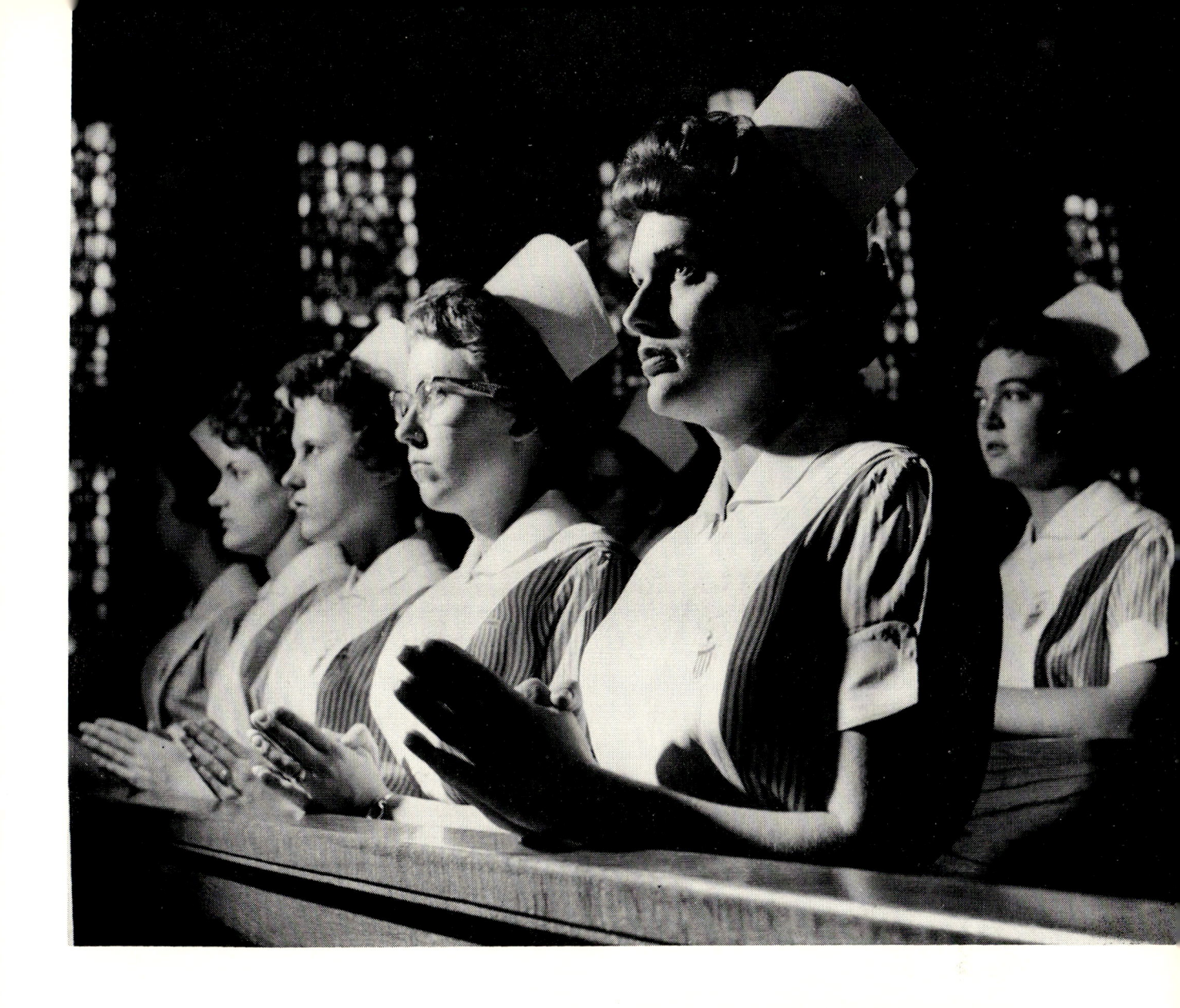

148–149
These two pictures illustrate how the photographer can dramatize his subject by thoughtful manipulation of the light source. In the picture above, the resulting dark background and softening shadows give an emotional impact lacking in the more conventionally lighted news picture at the right.

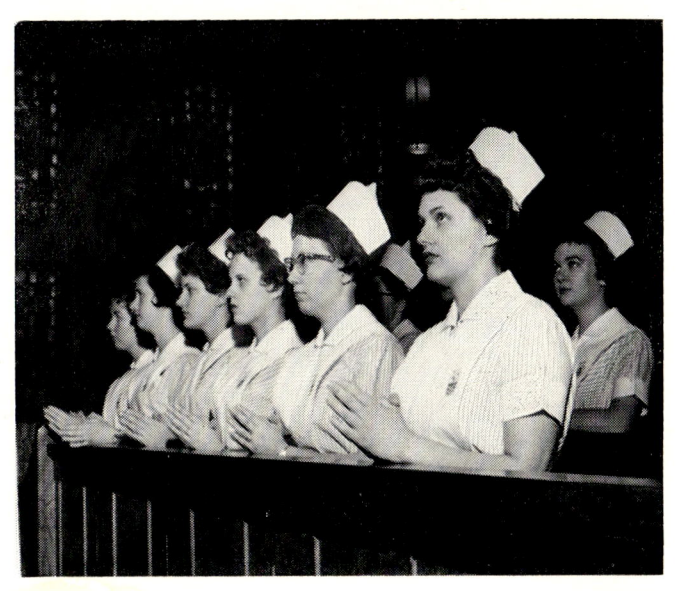

— 115

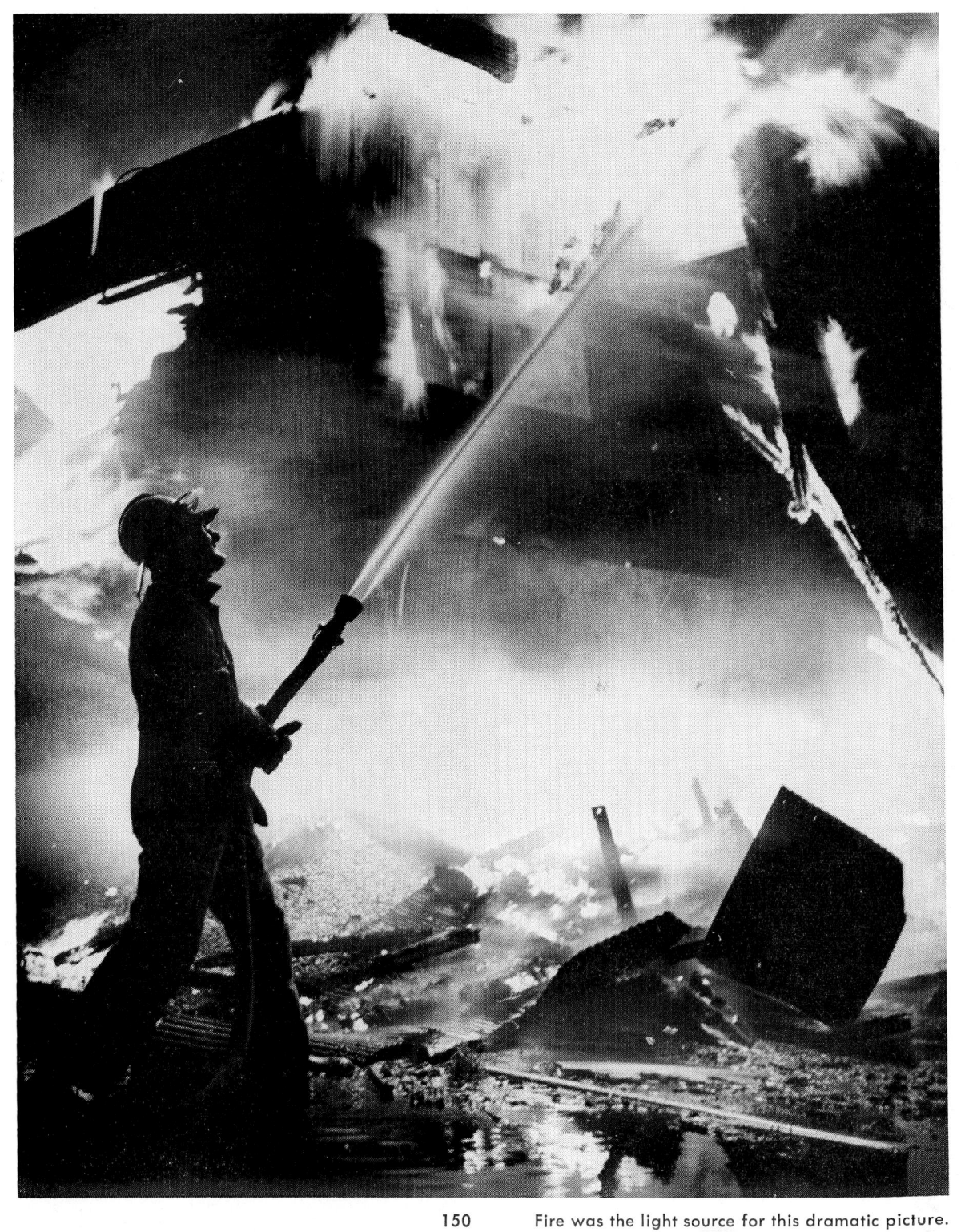

150  Fire was the light source for this dramatic picture.

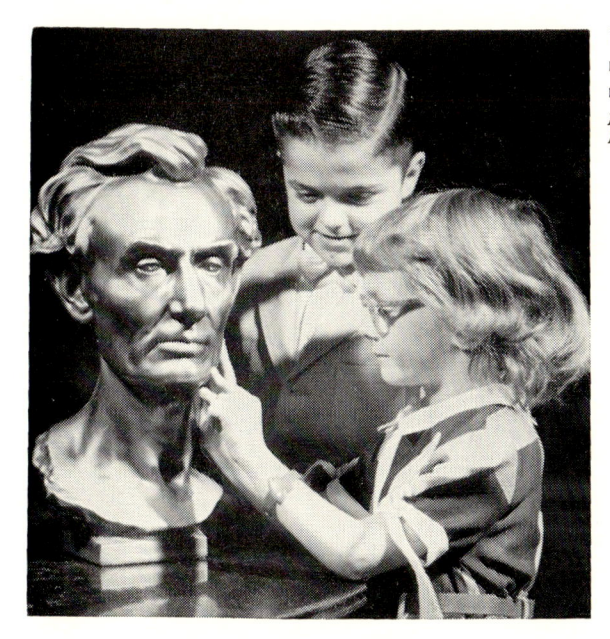

151   An extraordinarily good use of light made this picture sparkle.
*Elwin Musser,*
*Mason City (Iowa)* Globe-Gazette

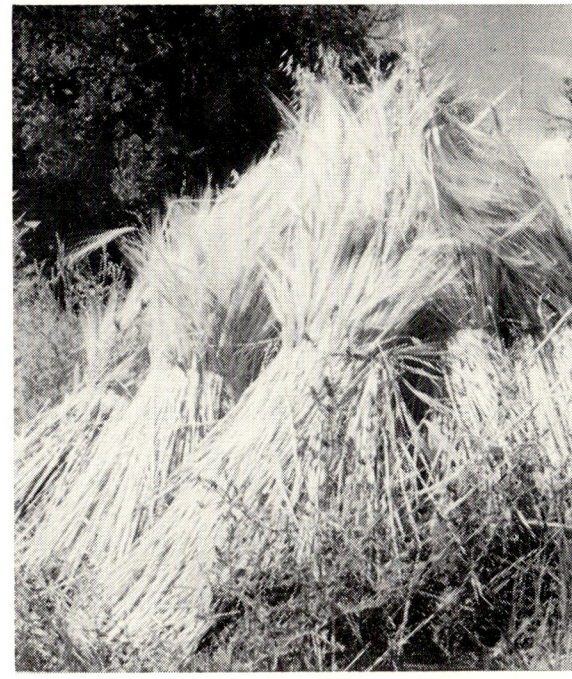

152   An appreciation of outdoor light accounts for much of the quality of this picture of grain.
*Mildred T. Crews for*
*El Crepusculo, Taos, N. Mex.*

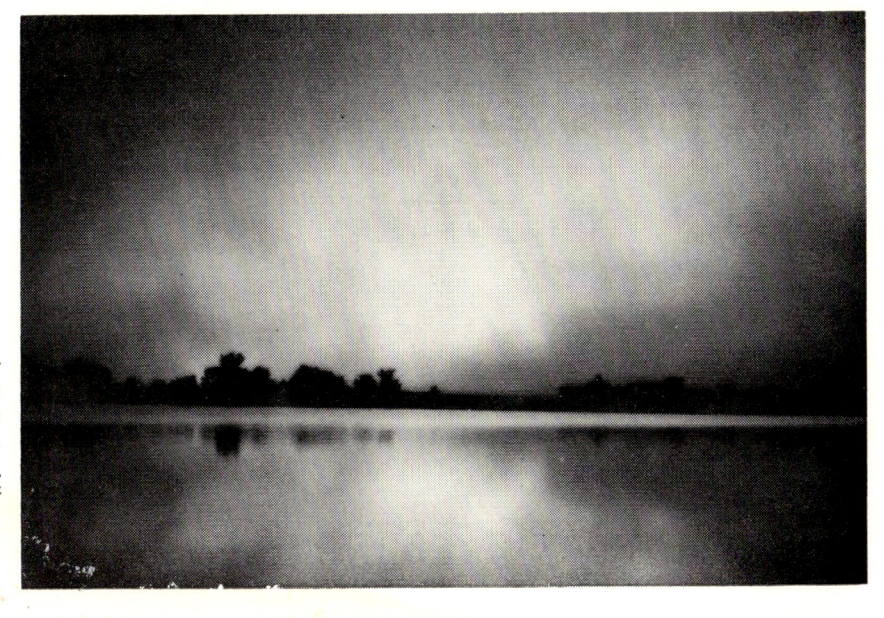

153   Sometimes curious sources of light can be utilized — in this case the aurora borealis.
*Rockwell City (Iowa) Advocate,*
*Photo by Karl F. Schwartz*

— 117

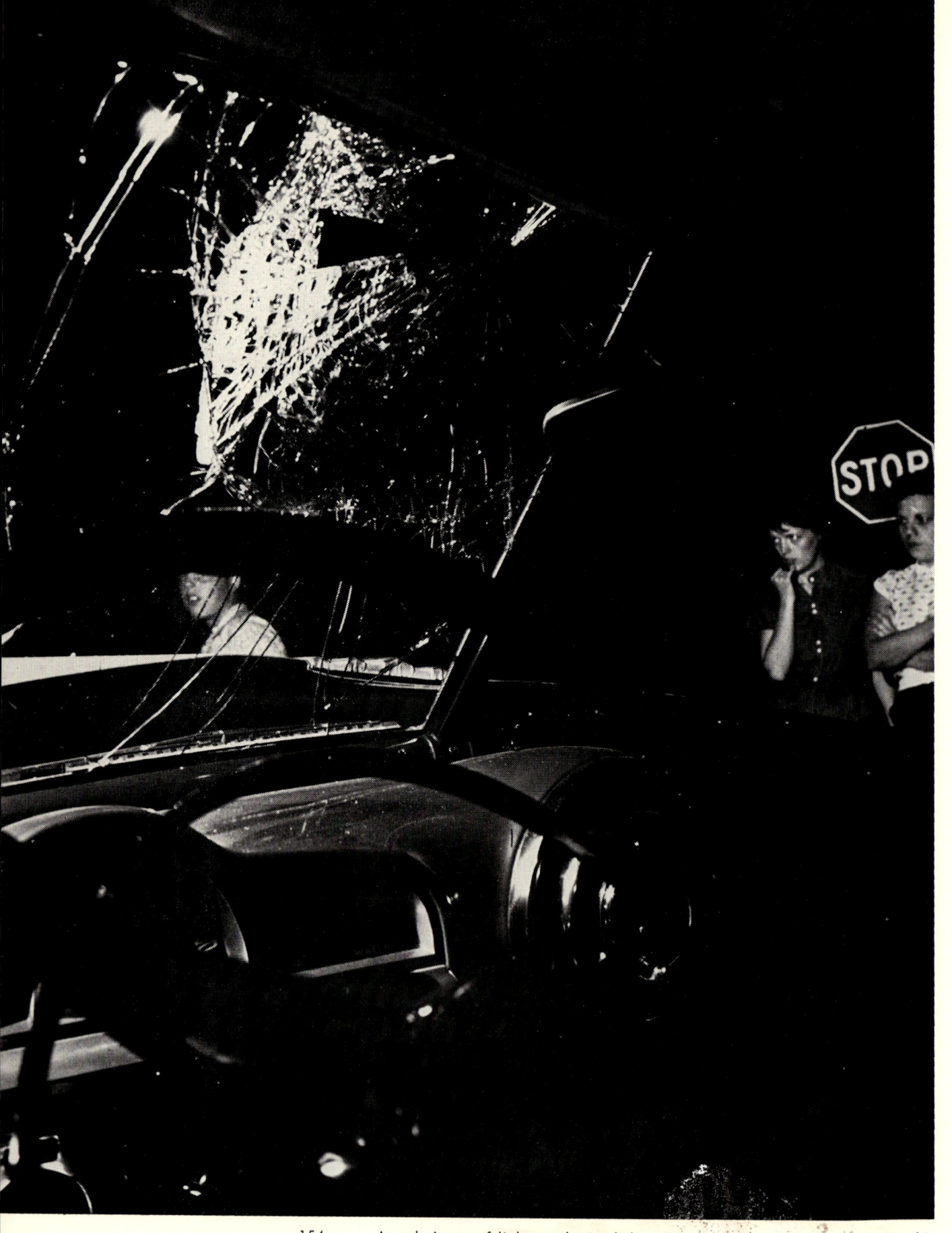

154   An adroit use of light emphasized the two important points of interest in this picture titled "Somebody Didn't."
*Lowell Georgia, Green Bay (Wis.) Press-Gazette, staff photographer*

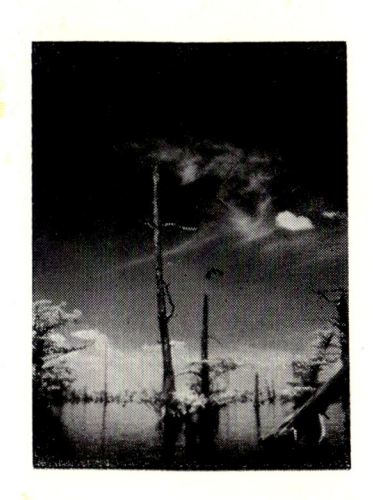

**PART 3**

Practical Photo Problems
Require Practical Solutions

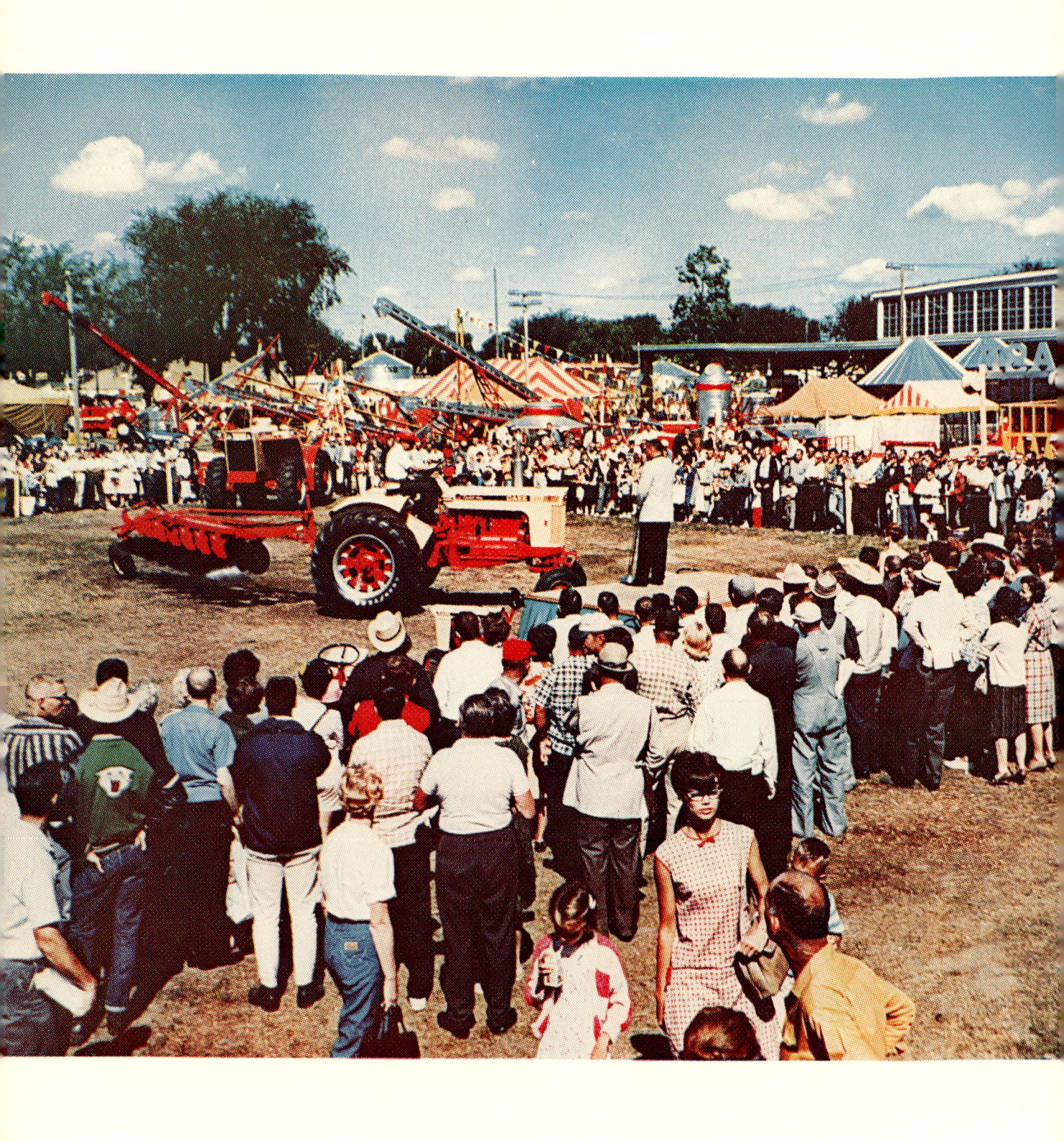

CHAPTER 15

# ROP Brightens America's Newspapers

THE WORLD around us is an endless variety of colors. These colors add to our enjoyment of life, help us to identify the objects we see, and give us information that we would find difficult or impossible to interpret in any other form. The same advantages exist when objects are reproduced in color, as is evidenced by the unqualified success of color illustrations in national magazines and commercial advertising, of color motion pictures, and of color snapshots.

Recognizing these advantages, more newspaper publishers every day are using editorial color for local scenes and events. Many of these newspapers — especially those enjoying large circulation — use color daily in the coverage of spot news as well as features. Color advertising in the press can be seen every day of the week.

The use of color illustrations need not be (and is not) restricted to the large metropolitan dailies. A considerable number of smaller-circulation newspapers, and even some weeklies, include editorial color in their editions. And practically all of these publishers — large and small — have found that the *use* of editorial color stimulates the *sale* of color advertising. This, of course, results in increased revenue per page.

In newspaper work, ROP (meaning "run of paper") color usually is printed in three colors only; that is, with no black printer. It begins with a picture which can be made in one of three ways:

### One-Shot Color
A special camera exposes three separation negatives simultaneously.

### Reversal Color
Almost any camera exposes reversal color film such as Kodachrome or Kodak Ektachrome Film. A color transparency results.

### Negative Color
Almost any camera exposes negative color film such as Kodacolor or Kodak Ektacolor Film. A color negative is produced.

Since the negative color method is used in most newspaper work, it will be described in detail.[1] Its advantages are: (a) lightweight,

OP brings even more impact to the news pages.
ourtesy Des Moines (Iowa) Sunday Register

---
[1] Technical details of this method are in a pamphlet, *Three-Color Separation Prints from Color Negatives* E-47, available free from the Photo Press Sales Division, Eastman Kodak Company, Rochester 4, New York.

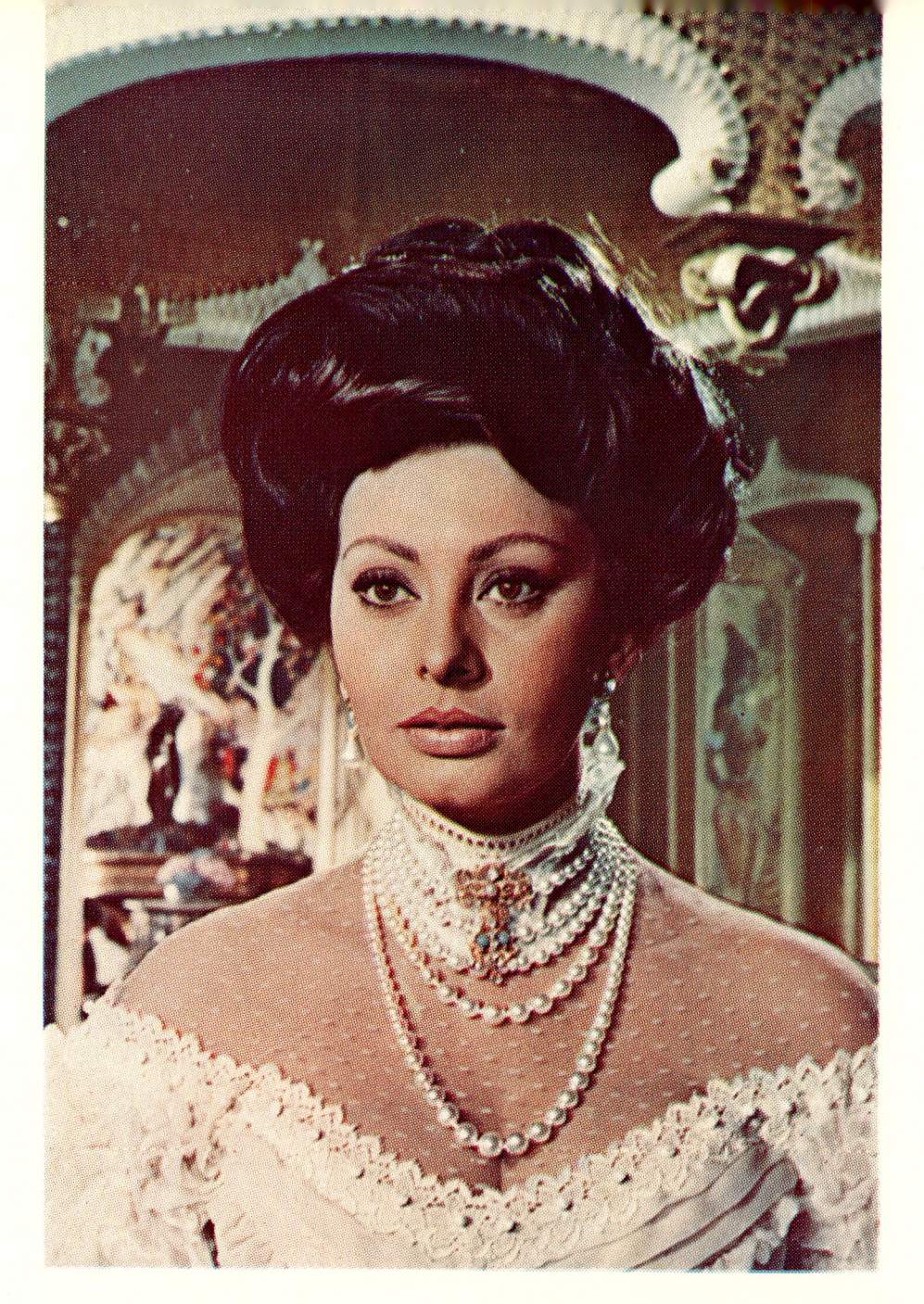

155    ROP color brings added glamor and life to all parts of the newspaper. This shot appeared in the entertainment section.
*Courtesy Des Moines (Iowa)* Sunday Register

high-speed cameras can be used, (b) the film has adequate speed for most situations, (c) full-color "proof" prints can be made directly from the color negative (on Kodak Ektacolor Paper), (d) film processing is not difficult, although it does require careful attention to details, and (e) no black-and-white separation negatives are needed because the separation prints are made directly from the color negative.

Whatever camera or film is used, the picture subjects selected for newspaper reproduction should preferably be bold and should contain bright colors. Subjects composed of fine detail and pastel colors are less desirable.

**Separation Print Quality**

Good halftone cuts start with separation prints which are properly balanced in density and contrast. Such prints *can* be made on a trial-and-error basis, but this may be costly and time consuming, as the need for correction in any of the prints may not become apparent until after the cuts and color proofs have been made. To avoid this, most publishers use instruments such as the Kodak Reflection-Transmission Color Densitometer, Model RT, and the Curtis Color Analyst (see illustration, page 127).

The densitometer is used to measure selected gray-scale steps as well as white or light-gray picture areas on the prints. By this means, the density and contrast relationships of the prints can be evaluated.

With the Color Analyst the three separation prints are viewed as a color picture. If the result is unsatisfactory, the Analyst indicates what corrections should be made in the prints. The Analyst can also be used to evaluate engraver's proofs.

**Separation Prints to Halftone Cuts**

Starting with well-balanced separation prints, the objective should be to faithfully reproduce their tonal ranges. Usually, no matter how a print may appear, no attempt should be made to distort, lighten, or darken the image during its reproduction.

The halftone cuts can be made by photoengraving or on an electronic engraving device. Both methods produce good results and are being used generally. In making the cuts, each print must be screened at a different angle to avoid a moiré pattern during printing. This can be accomplished on an electronic machine only by placing each print on the machine at the appropriate angle.

The size of the halftone cut is optional, but experience has shown that large cuts are easier to register than are small ones.

156  Story-telling quality can be enhanced by use of color. This picture acted as a drawing card to its related news story.
*Courtesy Des Moines (Iowa) Sunday Register.*

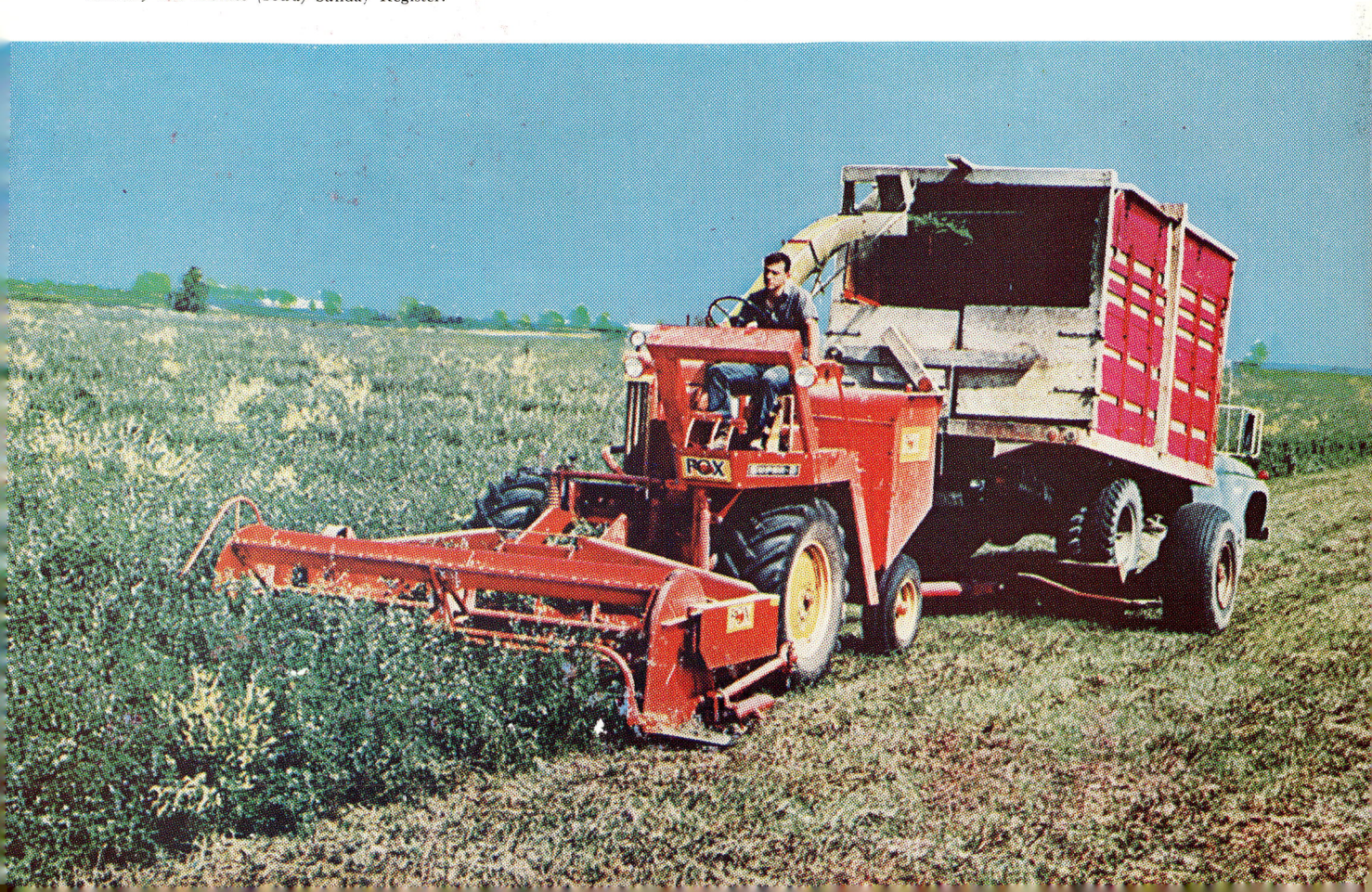

124

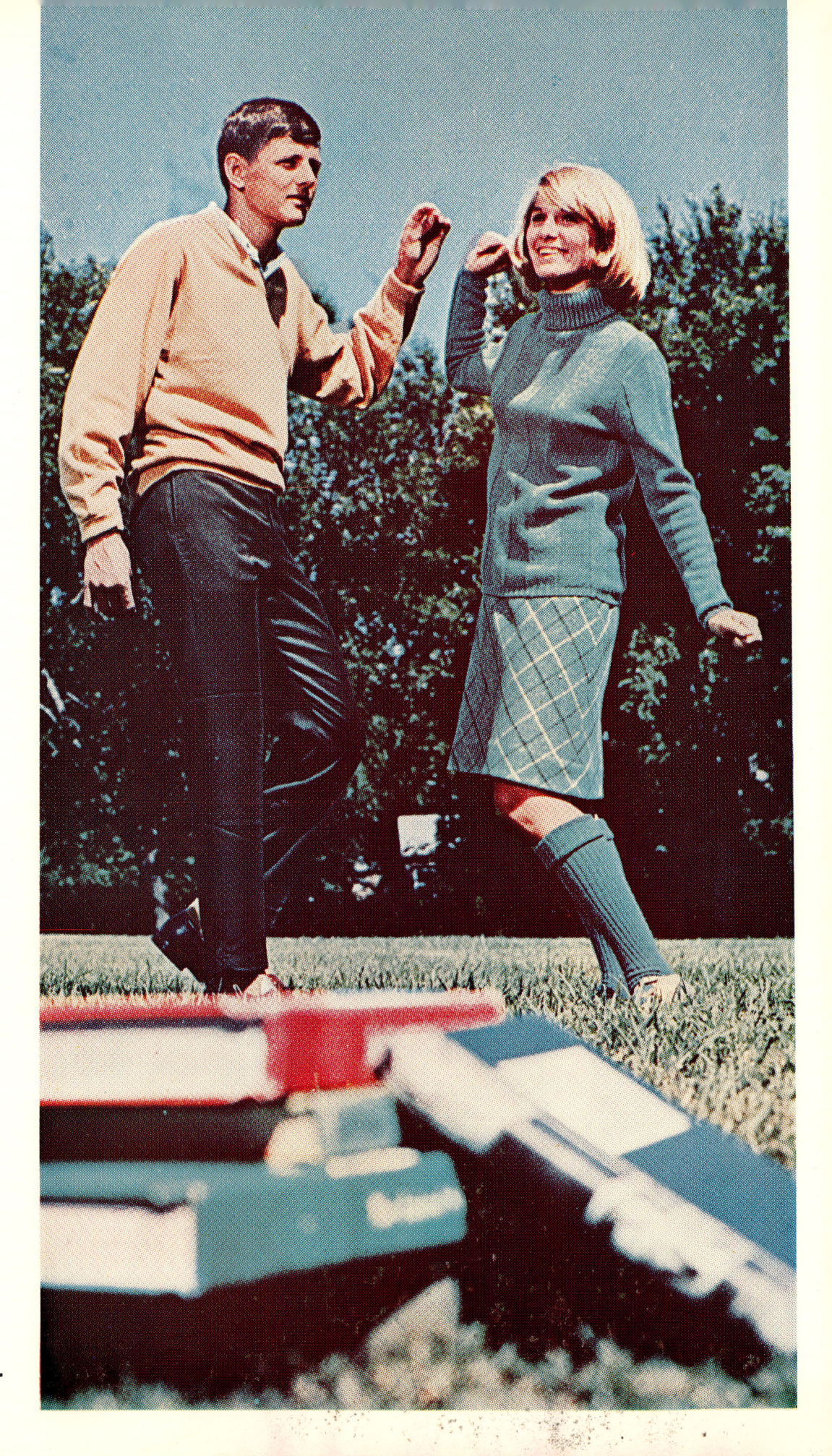

**Teen-age fashions with a back-to-school theme set the pace for this colorful picture, designed to catch the eye of all youthful readers.**
*Courtesy Des Moines (Iowa)* Sunday Register

After the cuts are made, they should be proofed in color. Then, if one color is too strong or too weak, correction can be made by re-etching, by remarking the cut, or by making a corrected separation print and a new cut. However, no correction should be necessary if the cuts were made correctly from properly balanced prints.

157   The three-color ROP separations made from a color negative on panchromatic enlarging paper. These black-and-white separations for photomechanical reproduction are made by either the press photographer or engraver. The three separation prints are given to the engraver to make color plates.

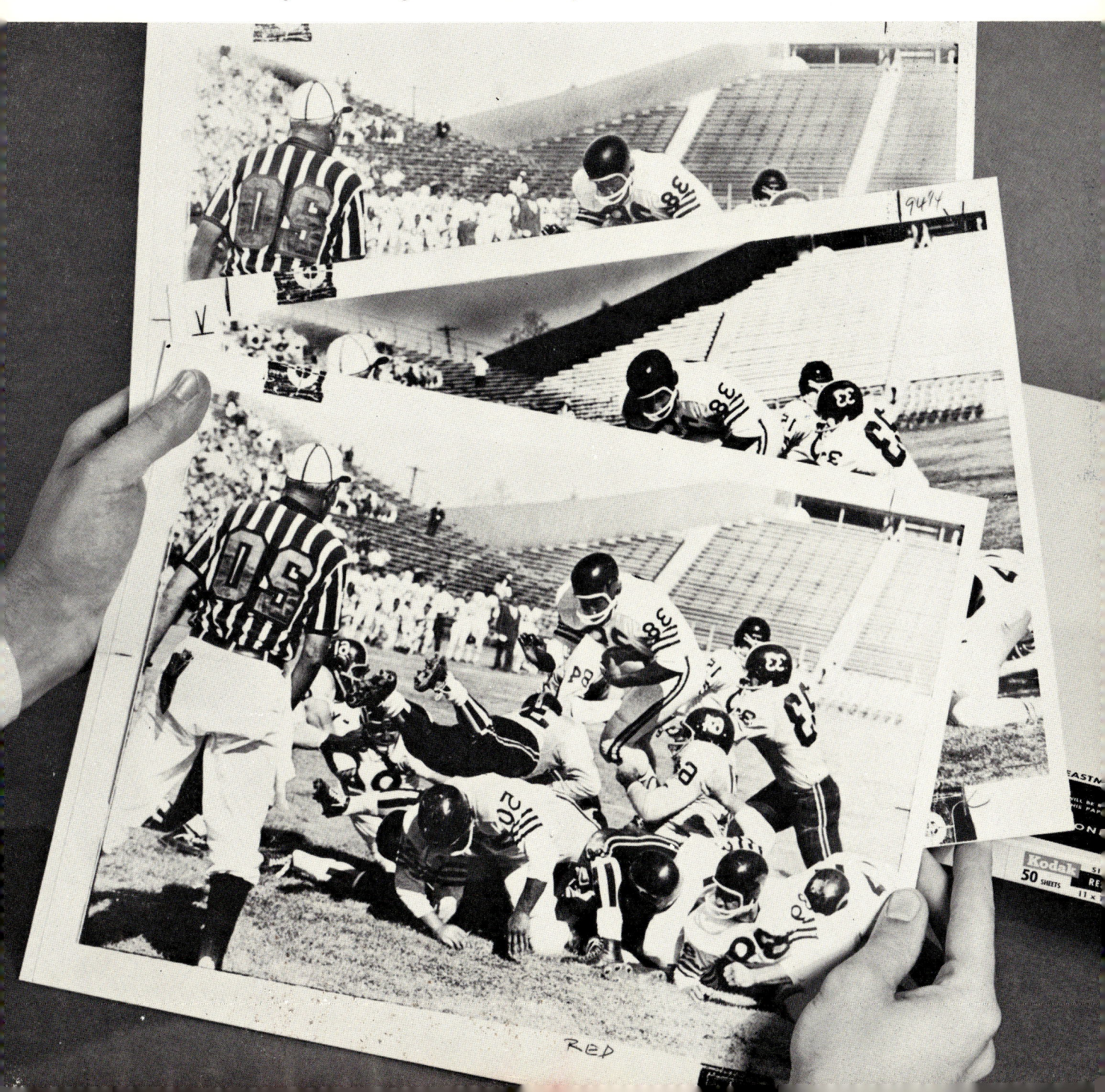

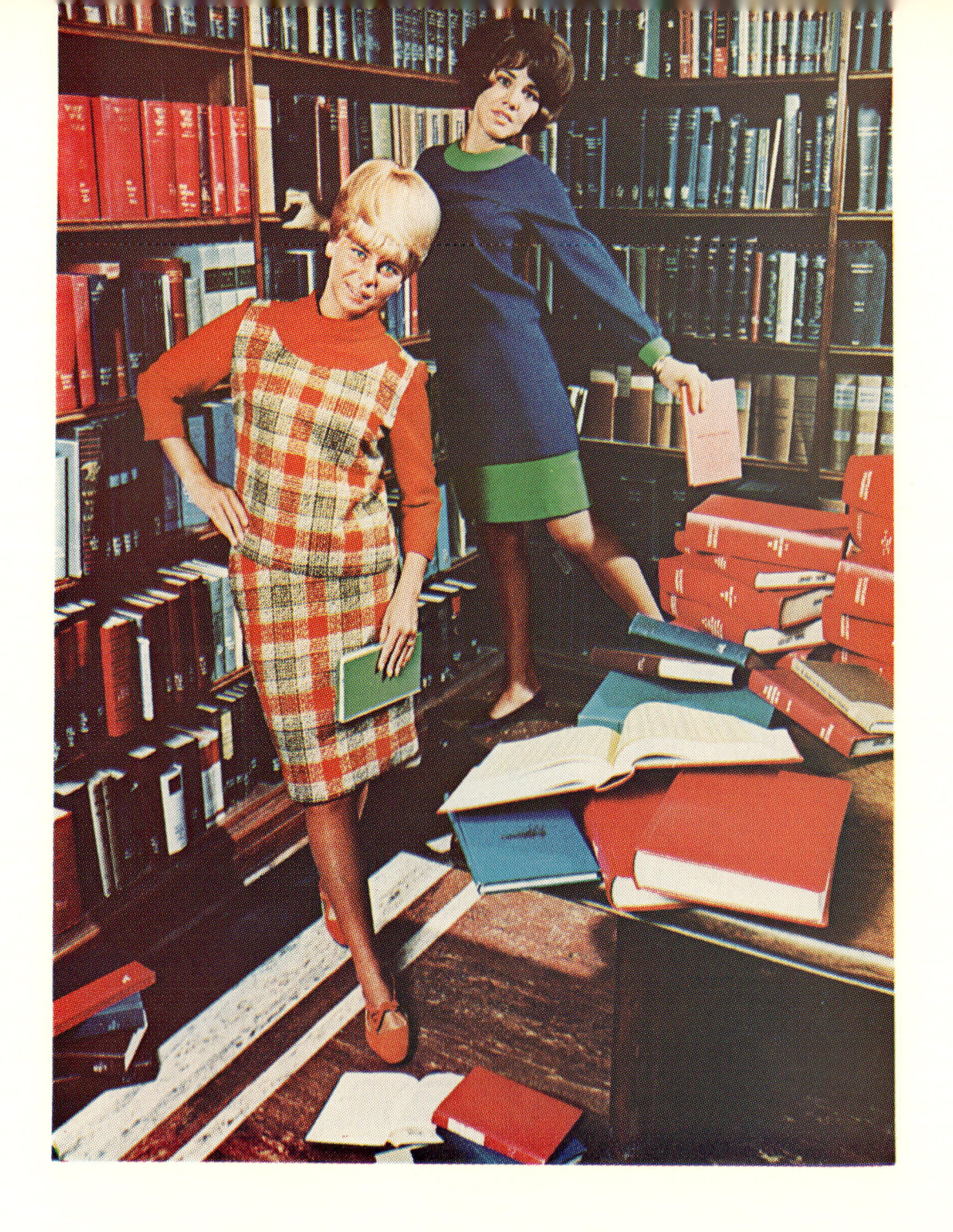

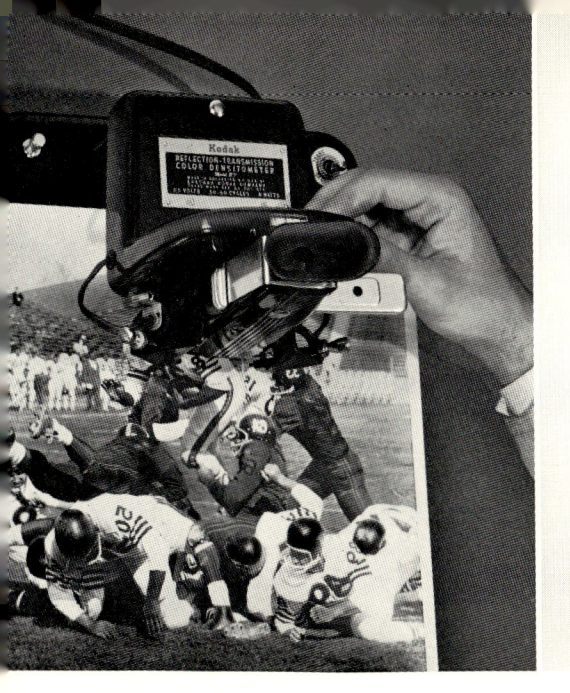

**158a** A reflection transmission densitometer used by the photographer or engraver to accurately measure densities of the original color negative and reflection densities of the separation prints (the latter as shown here).

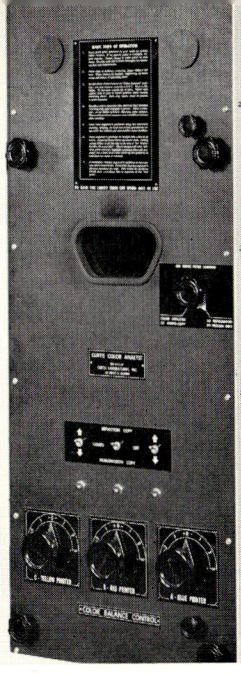

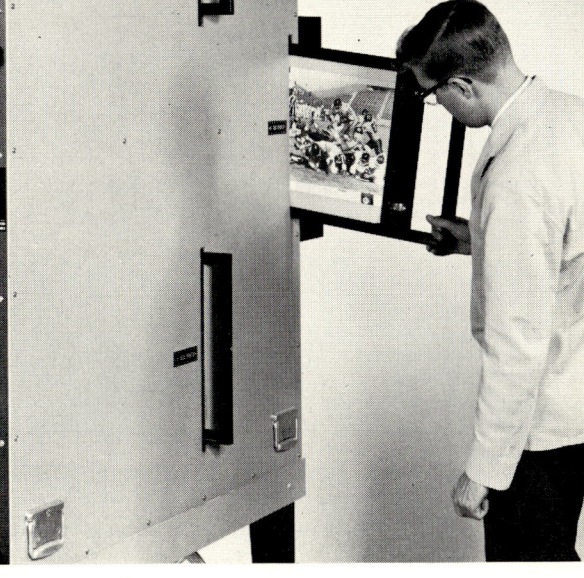

**158b** The Curtis Color Analyst. The technician is viewing the red printer. The yellow printer is above and to his left, and below that is the blue printer. The three black-and-white separation prints may be positioned and registered with knobs on the front of the Analyst and, when lighted inside the Analyst through the appropriate filters for the three colors, allows the operator to see a close approximation of the color picture as it will be reproduced from the three ROP separations.

### To the Press

Color cuts can be stereotyped in the usual manner to make the press plates. Or, when only a single press unit is to be used, it may be practical to use the original halftone cuts on the press. With this alternate method, an area of proper base-height for the cuts is provided for in the page form, which is then stereotyped. The original cuts are attached to the press plates by means of double-coated tape. The use of flexible plastic cuts simplifies this operation, but zinc cuts can be curved to fit the press plates and attached in the same way.

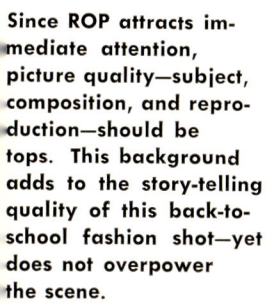

With either method, special care is needed to assure exact register of the three-color images. This requires precise positioning of the images at all stages of production; in the page forms, the press plates, and the press.

Many newspapers use direct-pressure molding equipment. With this equipment the mats are baked on the page forms, and register problems caused by non-uniform shrinkage of the mats are eliminated. However, other molding equipment and regular high-shrink mats or low-shrink glass-fiber mats are being used successfully by many newspapers. Press plates intended for long runs should be nickel plated. This hardens the plates and makes them stand up better during the run.

### Printing

The American News Publishers Association (ANPA) has standards for the cyan, magenta, and yellow inks used in three-color

**Since ROP attracts immediate attention, picture quality—subject, composition, and reproduction—should be tops. This background adds to the story-telling quality of this back-to-school fashion shot—yet does not overpower the scene.**
*Courtesy Des Moines (Iowa) Sunday Register.*

— 127

ROP printing. (In the trade, these colors are referred to as blue, red, and yellow.) The normal printing sequence is yellow — red — blue, but other sequences are sometimes used.

Printing is done as usual, except that the press must be adjusted carefully to maintain good register and color-ink balance. Register is controlled by orientation of the three-color plates. Poor results will be obtained, even with plates which are near-perfect in balance, if they are not printed in register or if too much or too little of one color is being laid down on the paper.

**Cost of ROP Color**

The cost of setting-up for color must be estimated on an individual basis because of the many variables involved. For a modern shop, an absolute minimum of extra equipment in the photographic department would be filters and a register board and punch (for making separation prints), plus an inexpensive densitometer. These items would cost approximately $250. The investment would increase to $3000 or more with the purchase of an electronic densitometer and a Color Analyst, but these instruments are well worth the cost because of the convenience and assurance they provide.

The stereotype and engraving departments probably would require little or no additional equipment.

The press room may already be equipped to run color. Even so, extra color-decks for frequent color runs or portable ink fountains for less frequent runs may be required. Most regular presses can be used to print color by using three press cylinders for color only. However, this will reduce the maximum number of pages which can be printed.

**Value of Color**

The printing of good ROP color presents challenges to the photographic and mechanical departments of a newspaper. It requires special cooperative efforts and a will to succeed. It may be frustrating and discouraging — especially on the first few attempts. On the other hand, successful color printing gives the pleasure of accomplishment, improves the appearance of the paper, identifies the paper as being progressive, and gives the readers and advertisers more for their money.

Is ROP color worth the effort and cost? Perhaps the answer to this is the fact that at the present time about 300 newspapers are printing editorial color and several hundred more are planning to do so in the foreseeable future. The trend is to color. And the colorless newspaper very likely will be in the minority much sooner than we think.

Color can be photographed in black and white, too. The warm brilliance of yellow sunlight filtering through this maple will loom large in the memory and recall of one who has walked in an autumn wood.

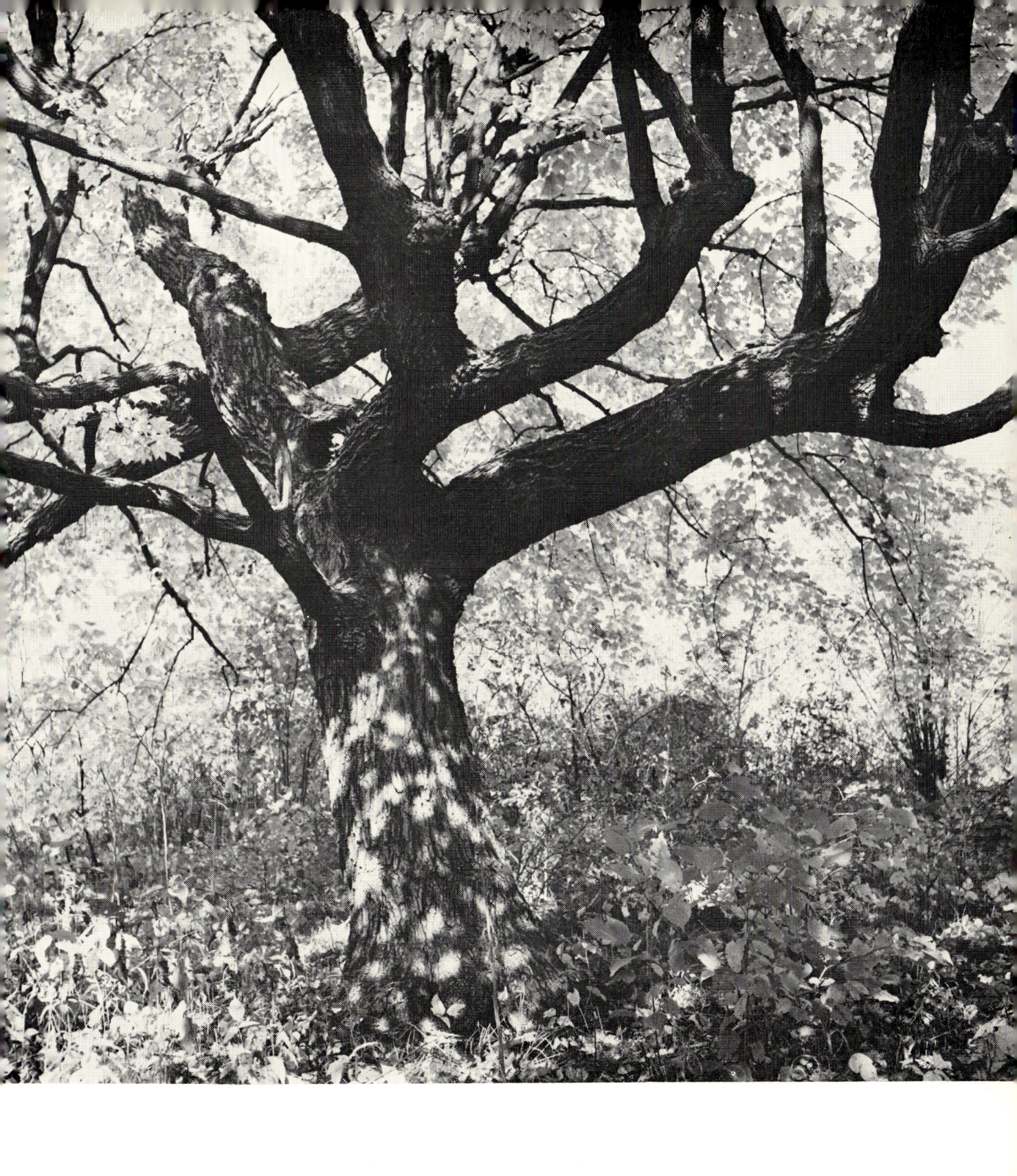

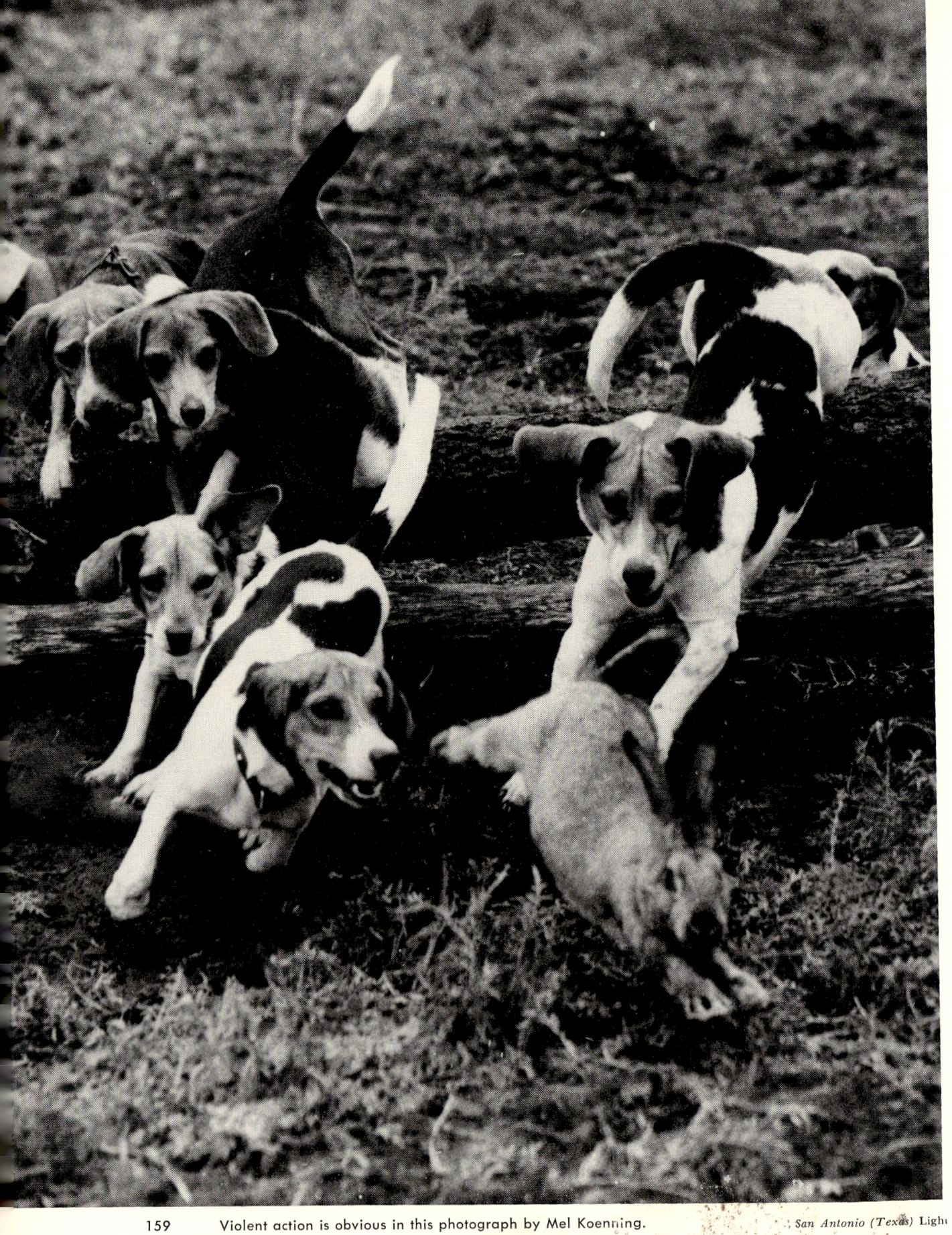

159   Violent action is obvious in this photograph by Mel Koenning. *San Antonio (Texas) Light*

CHAPTER 16

# How To Load Pictures With Action

When a picture conveys a strong impression of movement, it usually gives somebody looking at it a feeling that he has participated in the action, at least that he saw it happen.

Because a reader can be expected to have a deeper interest in the picture of an event in which he feels he has taken part, it seems smart to load most news pictures with as much feeling of movement as possible. The problem is how to convey as convincingly as possible the maximum impression of action in a picture that, after all, ends as only a pattern of ink on paper.

Just to point a camera at people or things in violent action and snap a picture doesn't always produce completely satisfactory results. A frozen bit of action may look static, or the picture of one instant cut from an action that extended over some time may look nonsensical and ridiculous and not convey the impression of movement.

**Several Solutions Available**

There are several things that can be done to intensify the feeling of movement communicated by a still photograph.

1. One commonly used device is to blur the subject, a part of it, the background or in some cases the whole picture. Some rather extremely blurred pictures have been published and for many persons, at least, seem to have conveyed an intense feeling of motion. In some pictures both figures and background were blurred, in others only the figures were blurred and in some—as the result of panning—most of the blur was in the background. Sometimes extremely effective results are obtained by a more restrained technique in which only a part of the figure or thing shown is blurred, such as the club in the hands of a golfer.

2. Action is suggested when the subject pictured is in a position impossible to hold, such as a pole vaulter high in the air (Photo 167) or a dynamited chimney in the midst of its fall to the ground.

3. Facial expression is a form of movement. Smiles, snarls, laughs, contortions—all convey the feeling of movement.

4. The way lines and other elements behave inside a picture can convey a feeling of movement. Restless, uneasy lines, strong diagonals, opposing diagonals are among ways to achieve a feeling of motion through pictorial means rather than by dependence on what the subject is doing.

5. Action can be indicated by a succession of pictures showing progression of movement as in Photo 47.

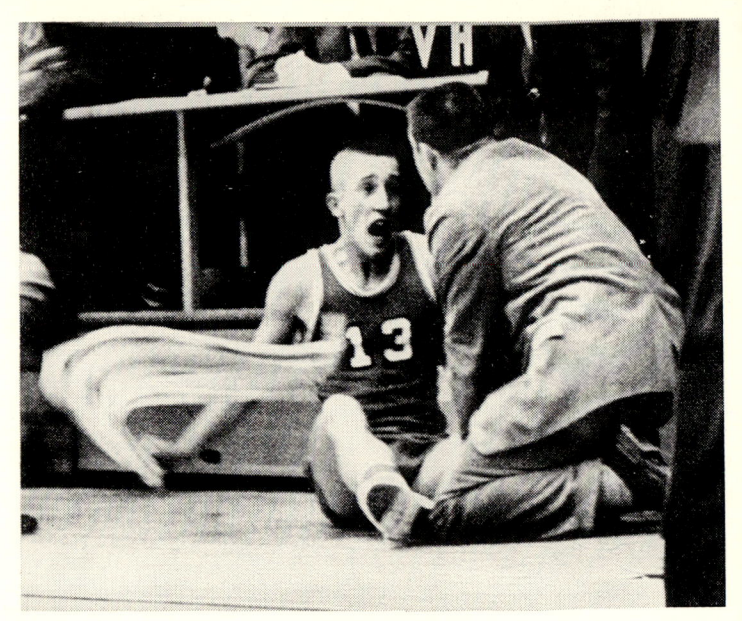

161     Taking a picture at a speed to blur a subject or part of it creates an impression of action.
*Dale Stierman, Dubuque (Iowa)* Telegraph-Herald

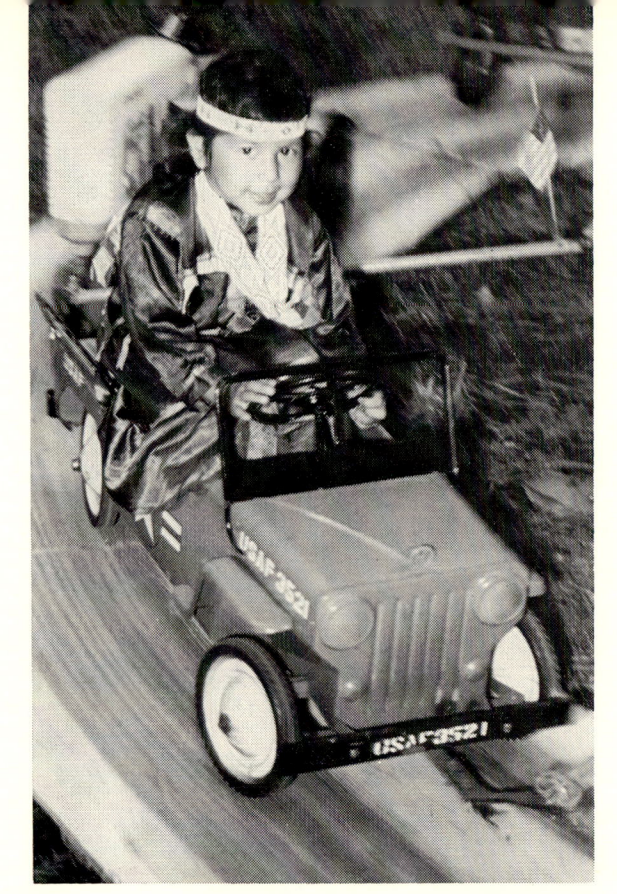

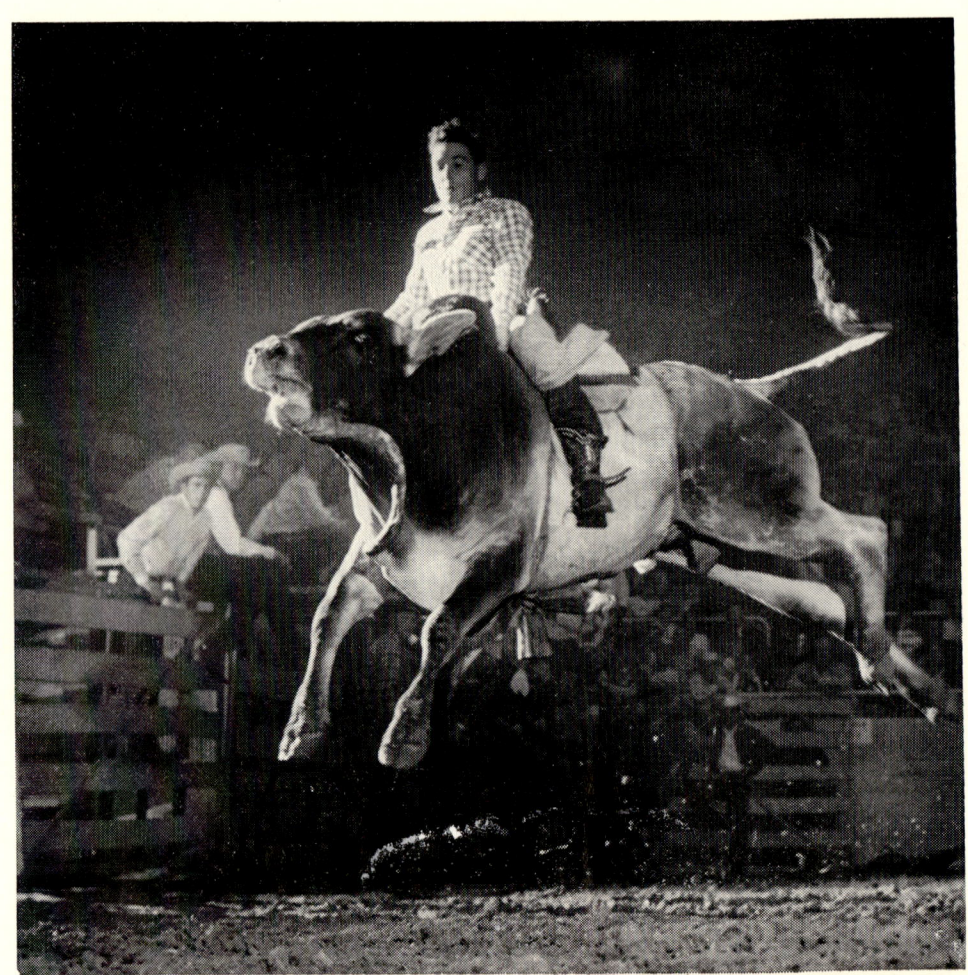

160     Moving a camera with an object results in a blurred background and a feeling of movement.
*Tom Merryman, Cedar Rapids (Iowa)* Gazette

162     Action is apparent in this shot since both animal and rider are in violent motion and in positions they can't hold.
*Bruce Roberts, staff photographer,*
*Charlotte* Observer

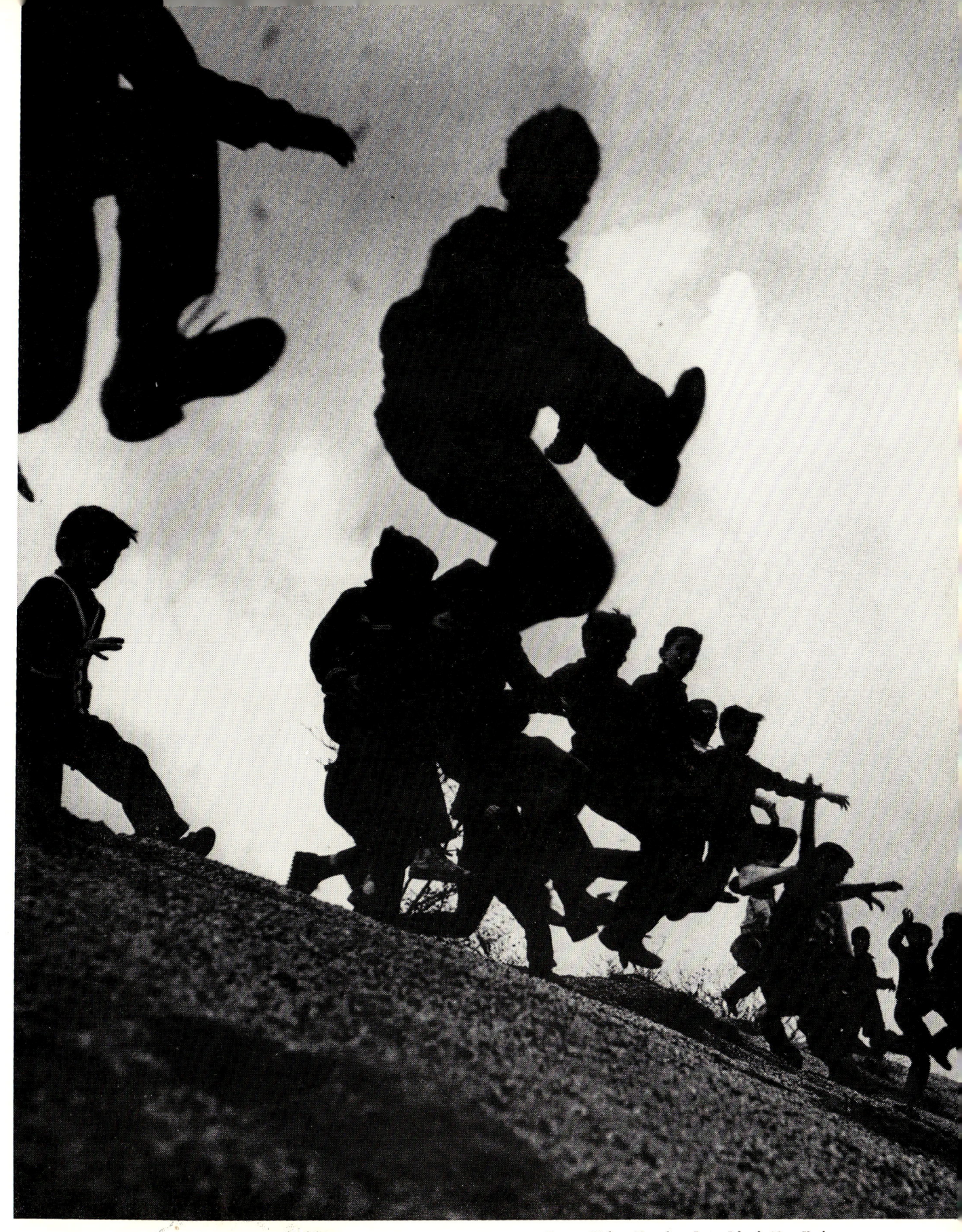

Harvey Weber, Newsday, Long Island, New York

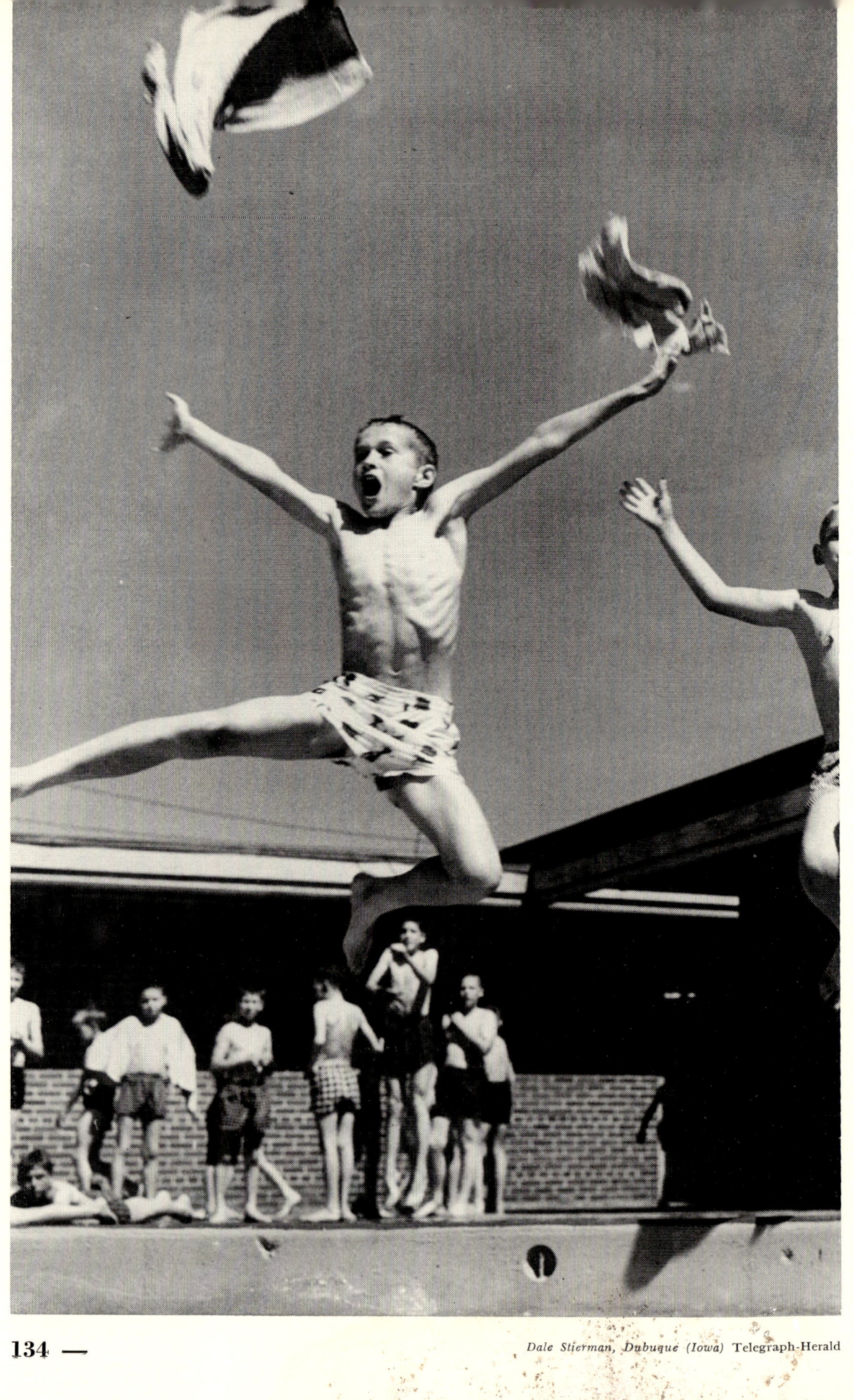

Dale Stierman, Dubuque (Iowa) Telegraph-Herald

164   In both this and the preceeding picture, the feeling of action created by boys in positions they can't hold is enhanced by diagonal lines. Blur in the towels increases the feeling of action.

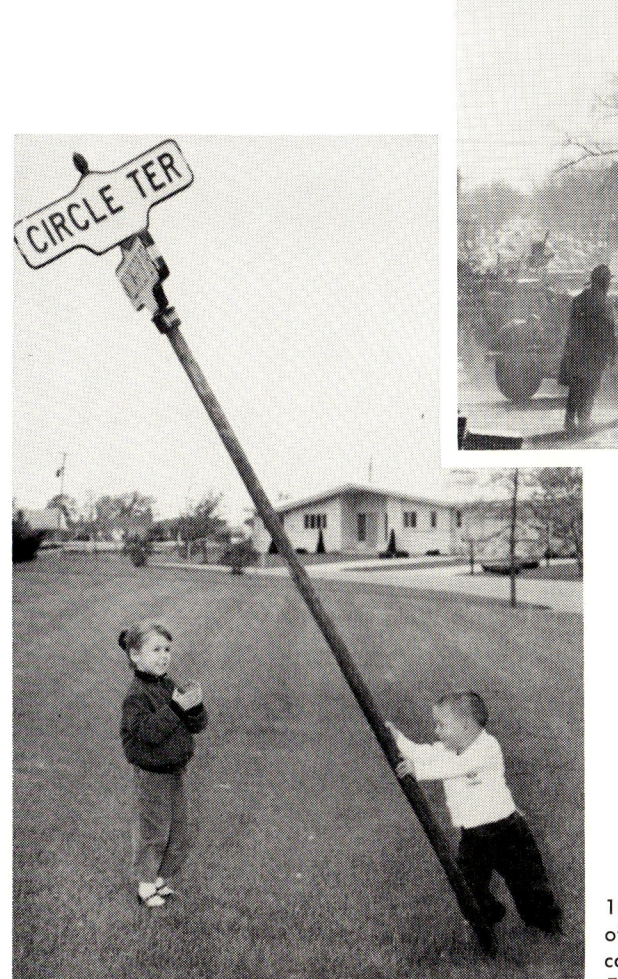

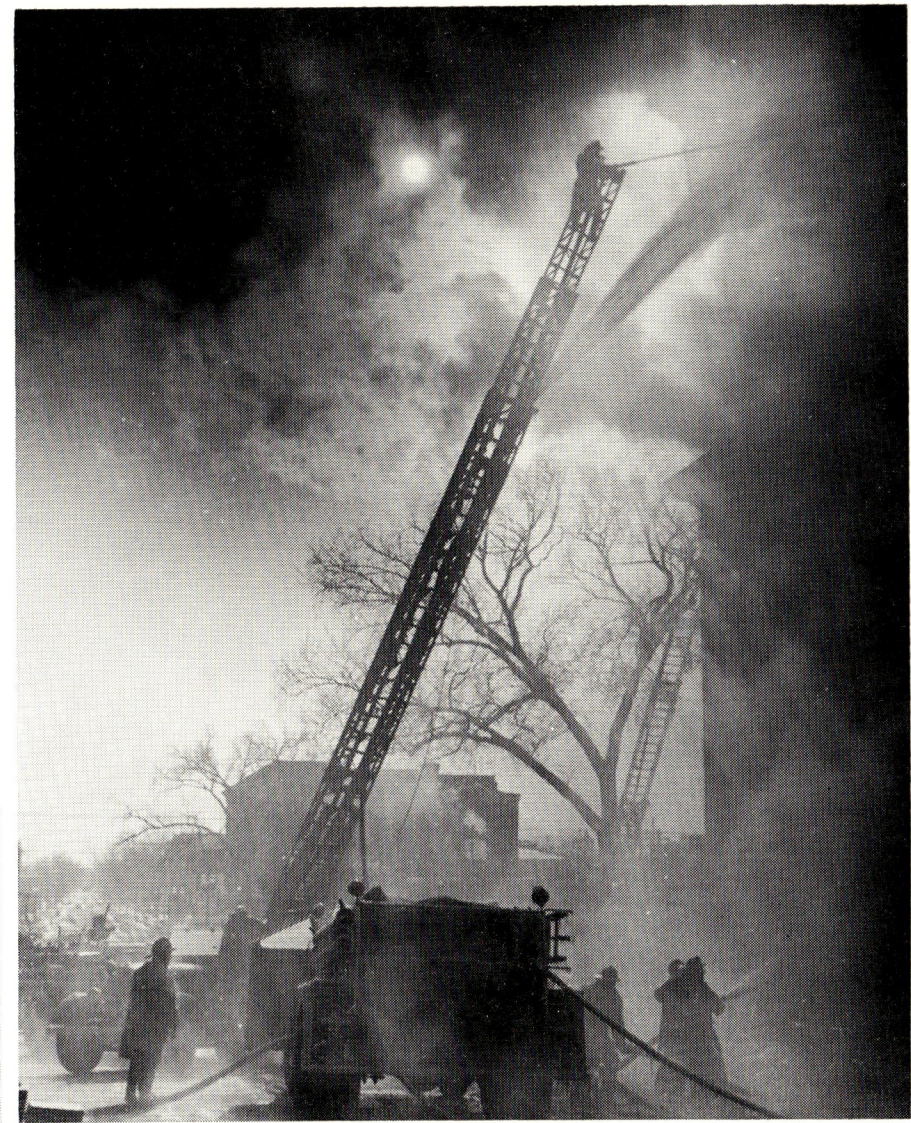

166   The strong diagonal lines of the ladder, repeated in the background, as well as the swirling smoke give this picture a strong feeling of movement.

165   A strong diagonal line provides a feeling of action for this picture, which otherwise is pretty calm.
Elwin Musser, Mason City (Iowa) Globe-Gazette

— 135

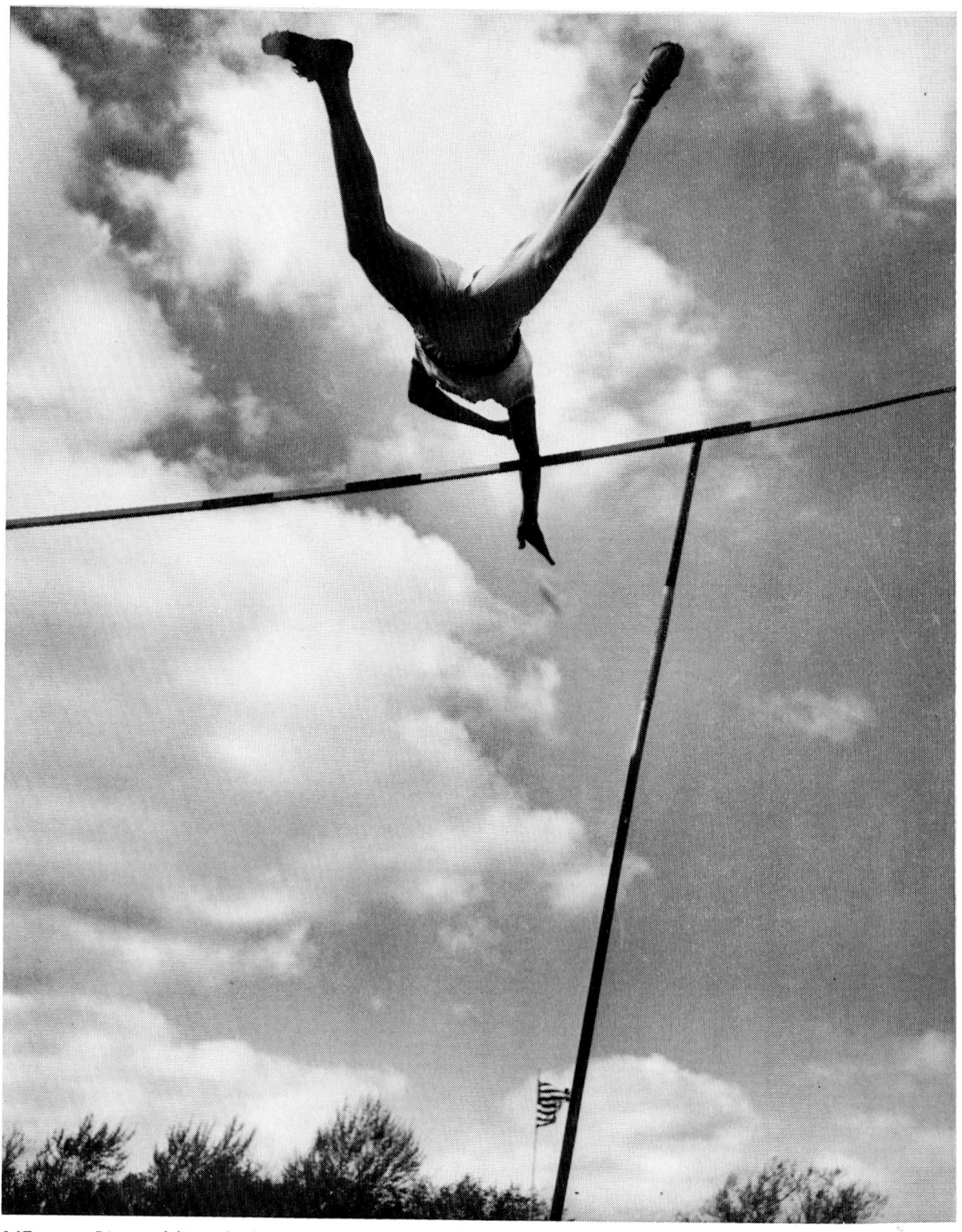

167   Diagonal lines, body in position it can't hold, low angle shot all combine to provide a sense of movement.

*Staff photo by Del Borer, Des Moines* Register

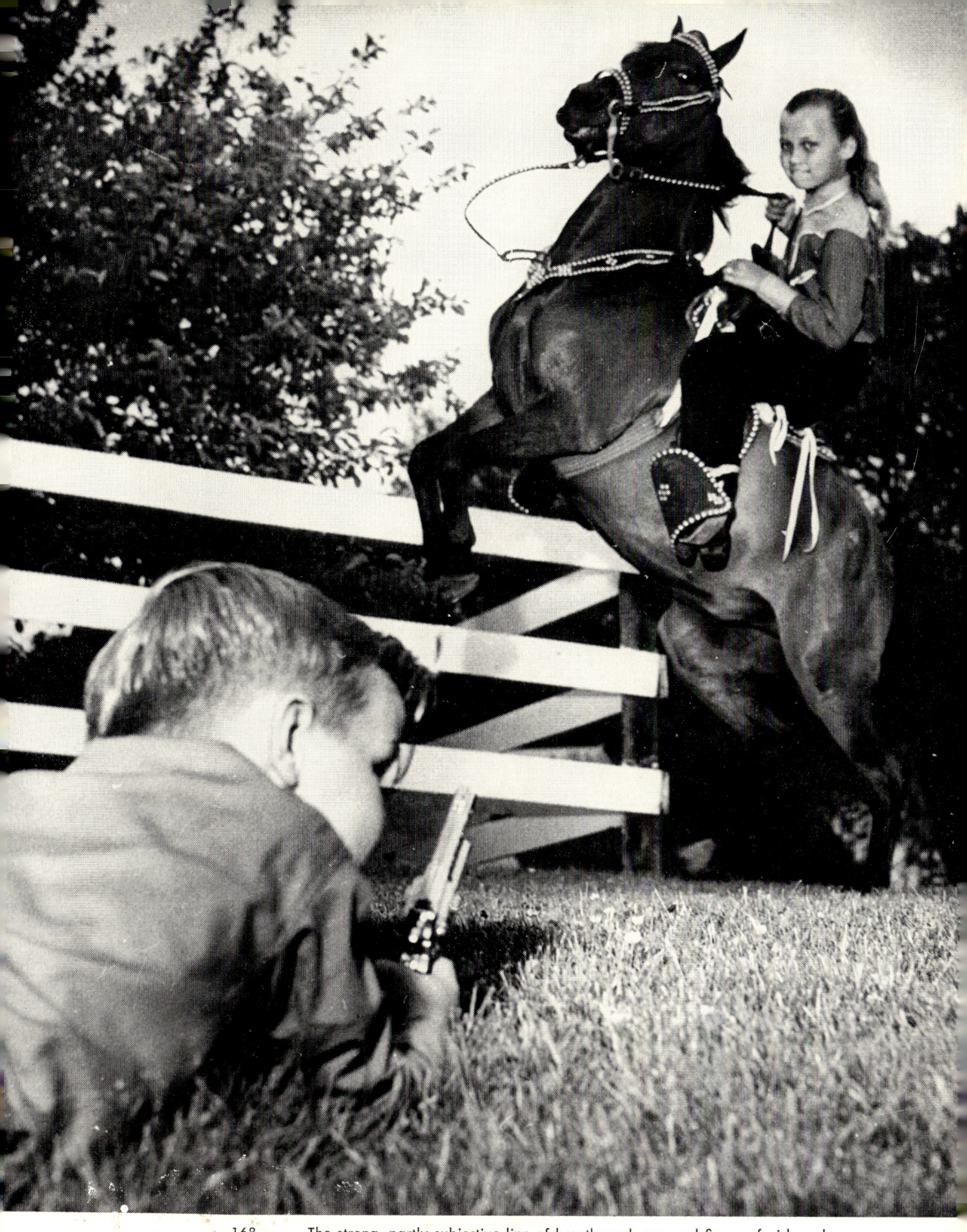

168     The strong, partly subjective line of boy through gun and figure of girl, and a cross diagonal formed by the horse combine to give an impression of action and conflict.

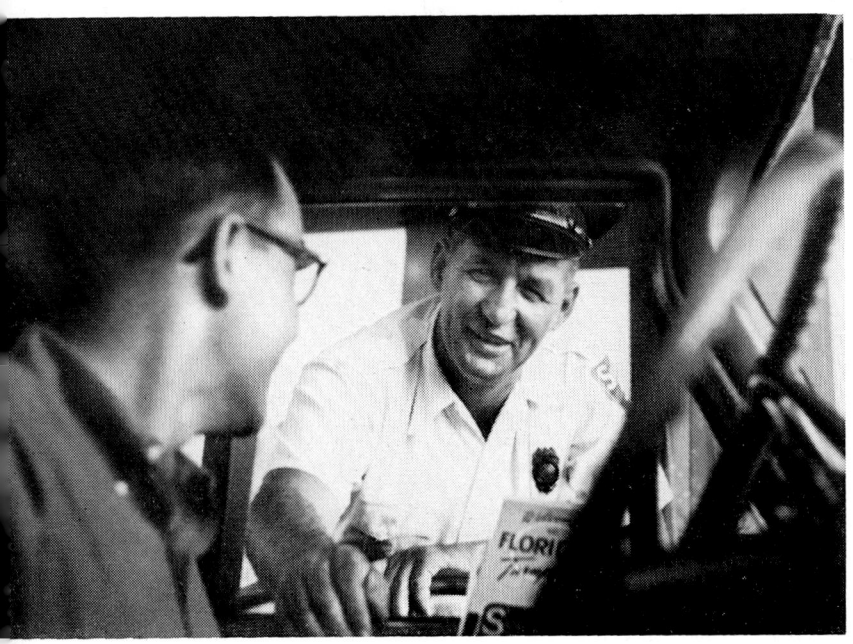

**169** Lively expression suggests movement.
*Home & Highway Magazine, published by Allstate Insurance Companies*

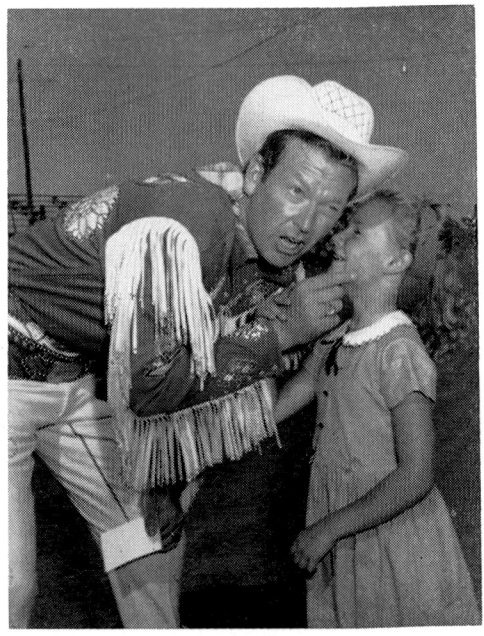

**170** Lively expression plus body in position it can't long hold suggest more movement.
*Elwin Musser, Mason City (Iowa) Globe-Gazette*

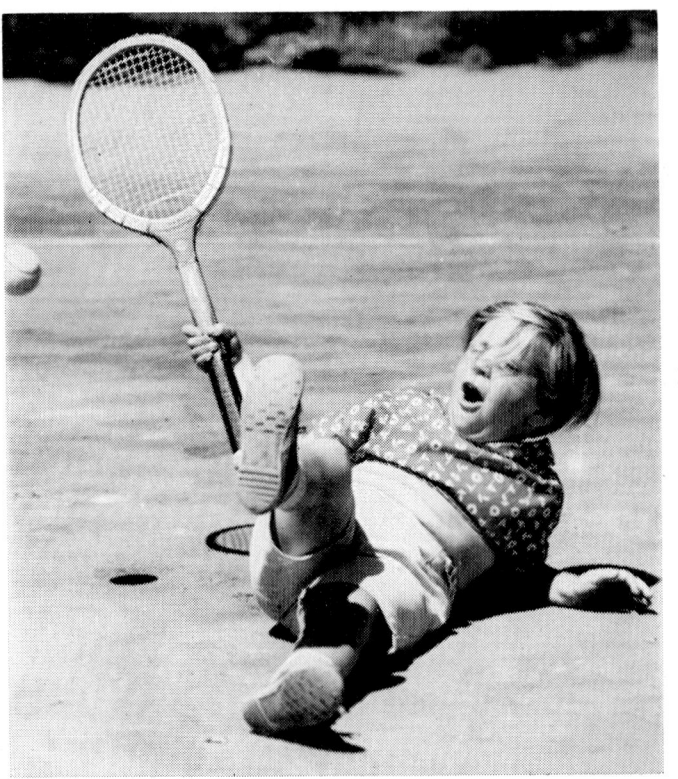

**171** Expression, lines, ball and foot in air all illustrate action.
*Staff photographer Arman G. Hatsian of the Hartford (Conn.) Courant*

**172** Again expression — this time on the face of a cautious cat, gave this otherwise static picture a feeling of action and saved this Groundhog's Day photograph from being an awful cliche.
*Davenport (Iowa) Morning Democrat*

— 138 —

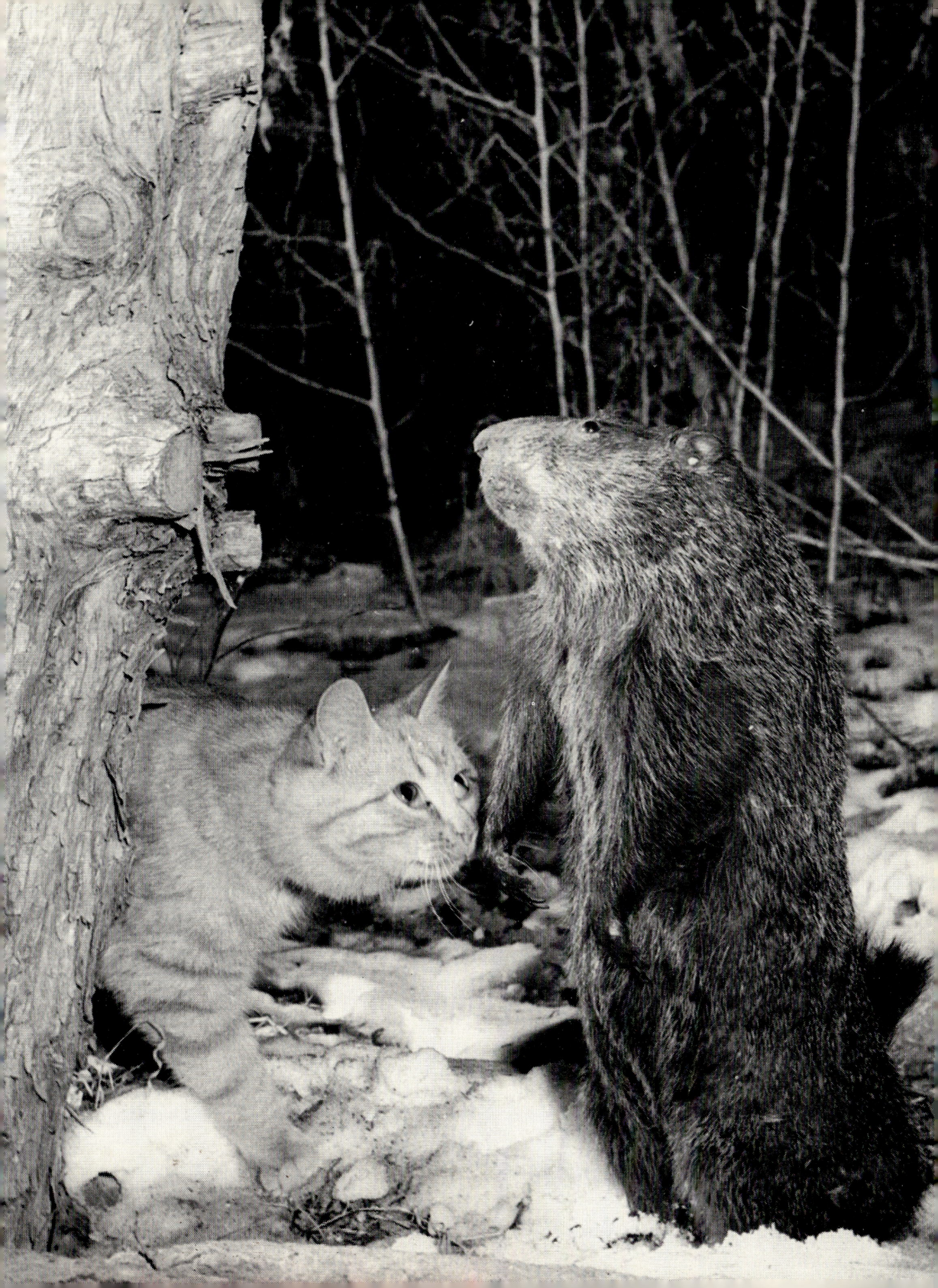

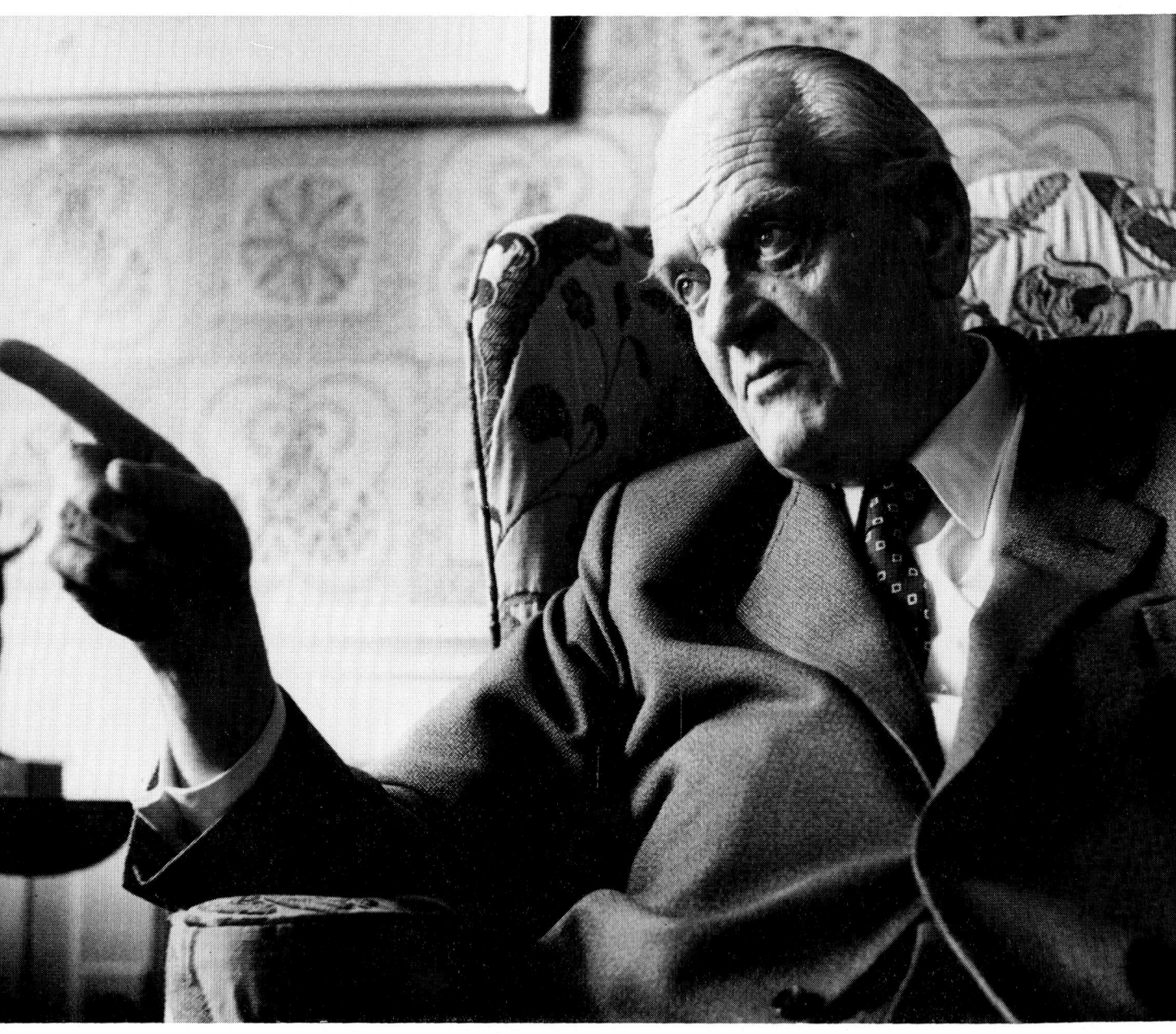

173   Good personality delineation makes a portrait interesting.
*Reprinted from* Nationwide World, *Magazine of Nationwide Insurance, photography by Gene Wells*

CHAPTER 17

# Good Portraits Tell a Story

BECAUSE OF THE INTENSE INTEREST of people in people, portraits make deeply appealing news pictures, whether they be of famous persons, loathsome criminals, pretty young hostesses, or of some fine old people with delightful hobbies to fill their waning years.

Almost any reasonably well-reproduced portrait is interesting, but the attention value of portraits can be greatly intensified if they are thoughtfully planned, given variety — and above all, tell a story. Portraits don't need to be stuffy, conventional, unimaginative. Ideas about news portraits no longer are dominated by the desire to make all of them rather formal so they can be filed and used again — probably with an obituary.

What are some of the devices that can be used to increase the appeal of news portraits?

**Try To Catch Individualism**

When a portrait tells a story obviously and well, it avoids that routine look that gives the readers the feeling that they've seen all this before. The most interesting story to be told, usually, concerns the personality and character of the subject. What are his features that give him individuality, make him different from others? A wry smile, a high forehead, a neat goatee? In the time you have to work, try to figure out such personality revealing traits and attempt to reveal them through emphasis in your picture. Better still, try to catch the evidences of kindliness, good nature or cruelty that characterize your subject.

**Expressions Indicate Action**

Action can be an extremely important story-telling element in a portrait. Sometimes it is difficult to catch the right smile, or grimace, or scowl, but when it is done successfully the expression makes the picture come to life. Some action can be injected into a picture by having the subject reaching for something, operating some instrument, painting, or doing some such slight activity. Such things as writing and holding open a book become obvious clichés. Some successful portraits show an individual while speaking, singing or in some such activity.

While many persons think of a portrait as a picture of a face only, or of head and shoulders at most, some closeup pictures of individuals are improved if they picture the sub-

*174    Try to catch the distinctive features of the individual — in this case poet Robert Frost*

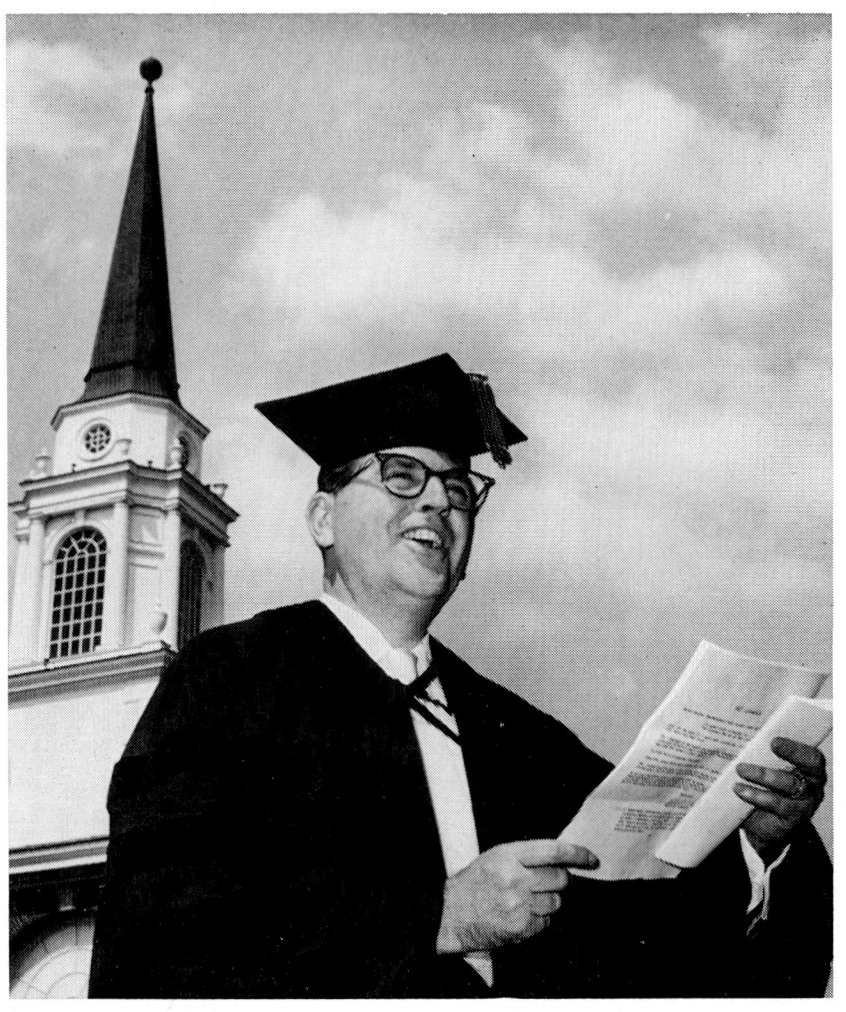

*175    Both background, such as this college chapel tower, and costume can enhance a portrait.*

ject from the waist up or are taken full length. Use of more than head and shoulders gives added opportunity to show clothing, action, background and frequently does a better job of story telling. But use of a full-length portrait requires more space, a factor to be considered.

**Composition Improves Portraits**

Portraits, like other photographs, are more pleasing when the elements within the frame of the picture are orderly and well planned. What has been said about composition needs to be applied to the making of portraits.

Intelligent cropping can help improve portraits by bettering such things as balance, by eliminating some unwanted material and by helping to emphasize points that should be played up. Tastes in cropping differ, but some rather extreme trimming of portraits until only parts of the features remained seem to have produced effective results in some cases. The trend seems to be toward a closer cropping of portraits when that seems desirable. But at any rate, cropping should be done at natural joints. Cropping should be deliberate, so that the intention is evident. No rules governing cropping seem to remain valid long.

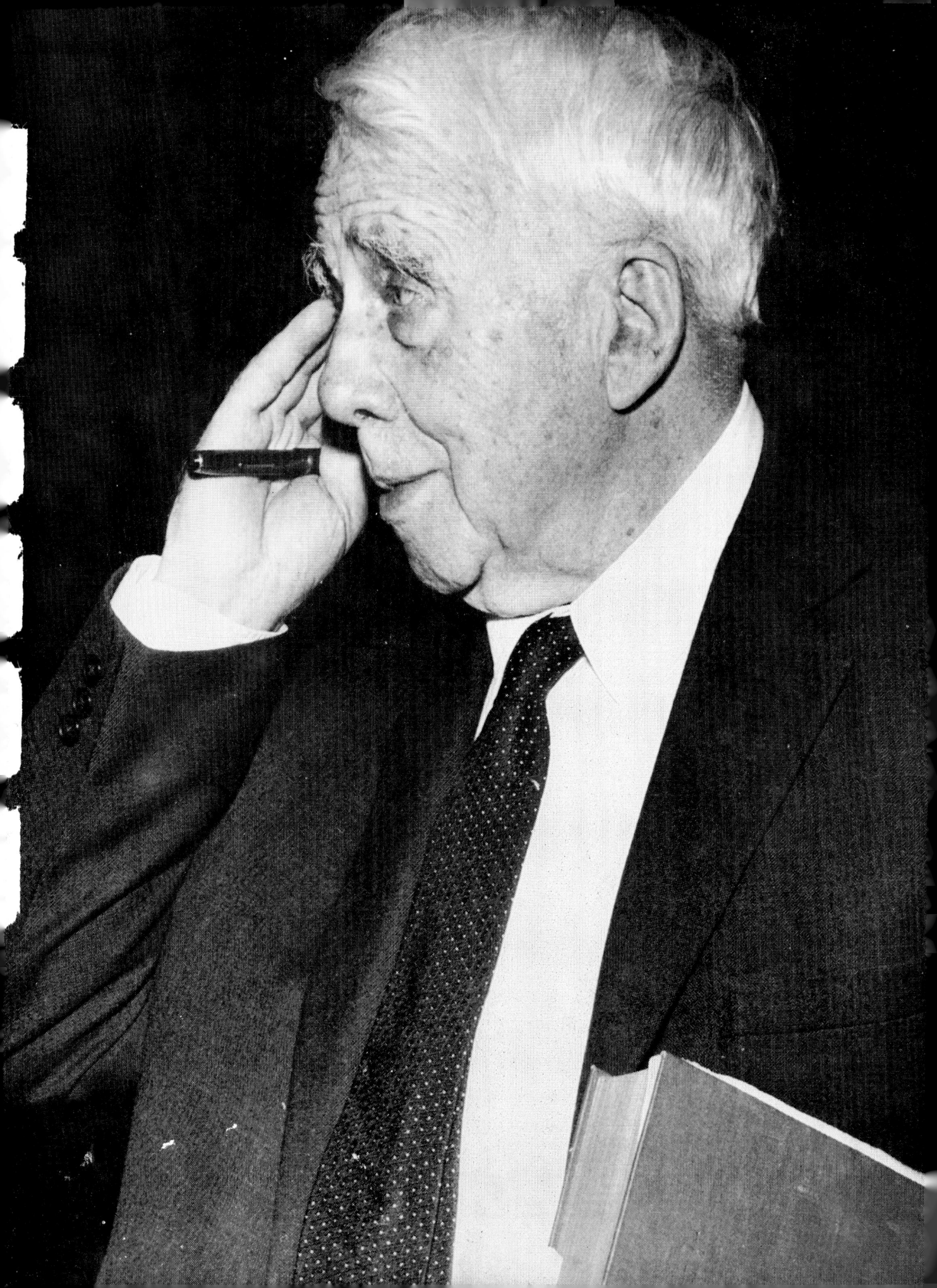

## Uniforms, Costumes an Aid

Uniforms and costumes can contribute much to the story-telling quality of a portrait, whether it be of a soldier, a chorus girl, a woman wearing an outrageous hat she has designed for a gag contest, a little girl with angel wings for a church pageant, or a lodge convention delegate in full regalia.

## Properties Help Tell Story

Some of the story-telling quality of a portrait can be obtained by use of simple "properties" — an object held in the hand of the subject or placed on a table near him. Such things as a compass held by a scoutmaster, a camera or exposure meter by a photographer, an interesting rock by a collector, or some other explanatory object can do much to break the formality of a picture and help explain why the person shown is newsworthy. But avoid like poison such clichés as a telephone held to an ear.

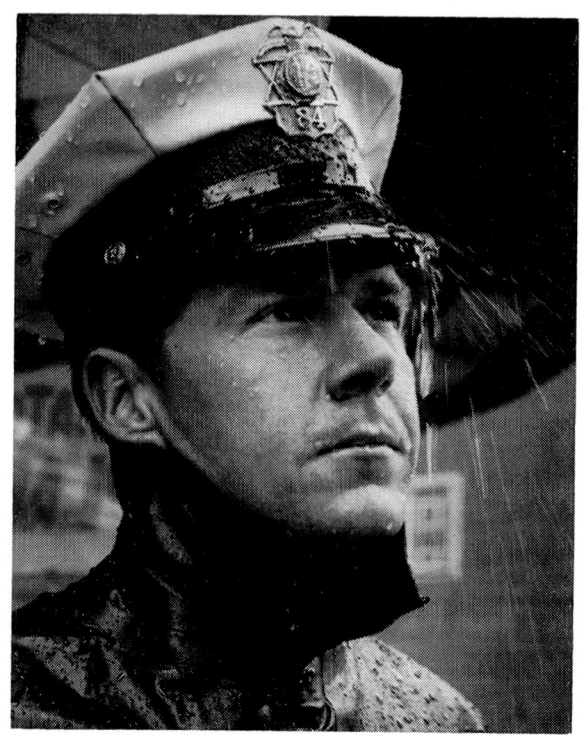

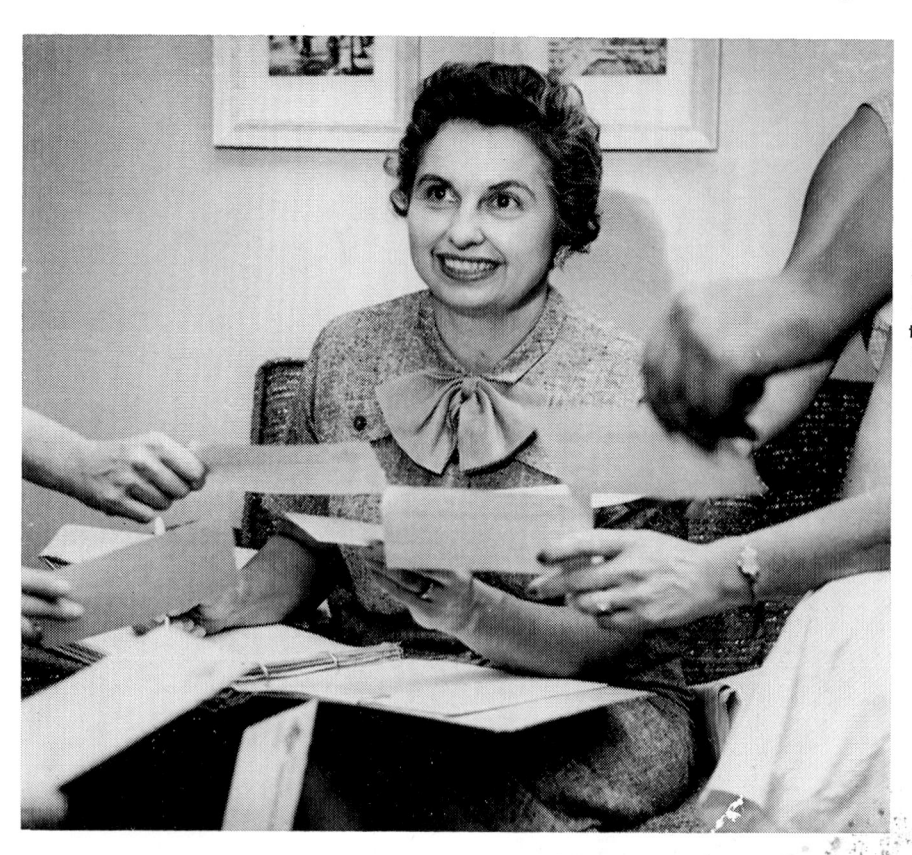

176   The uniform and the dripping rain combine to tell a story in this natural light picture of a policeman. *Bruce Roberts, staff photographer, Charlotte* Observer

177   Properties, in this case many checks, help tell the story about this secretary of an investment club.

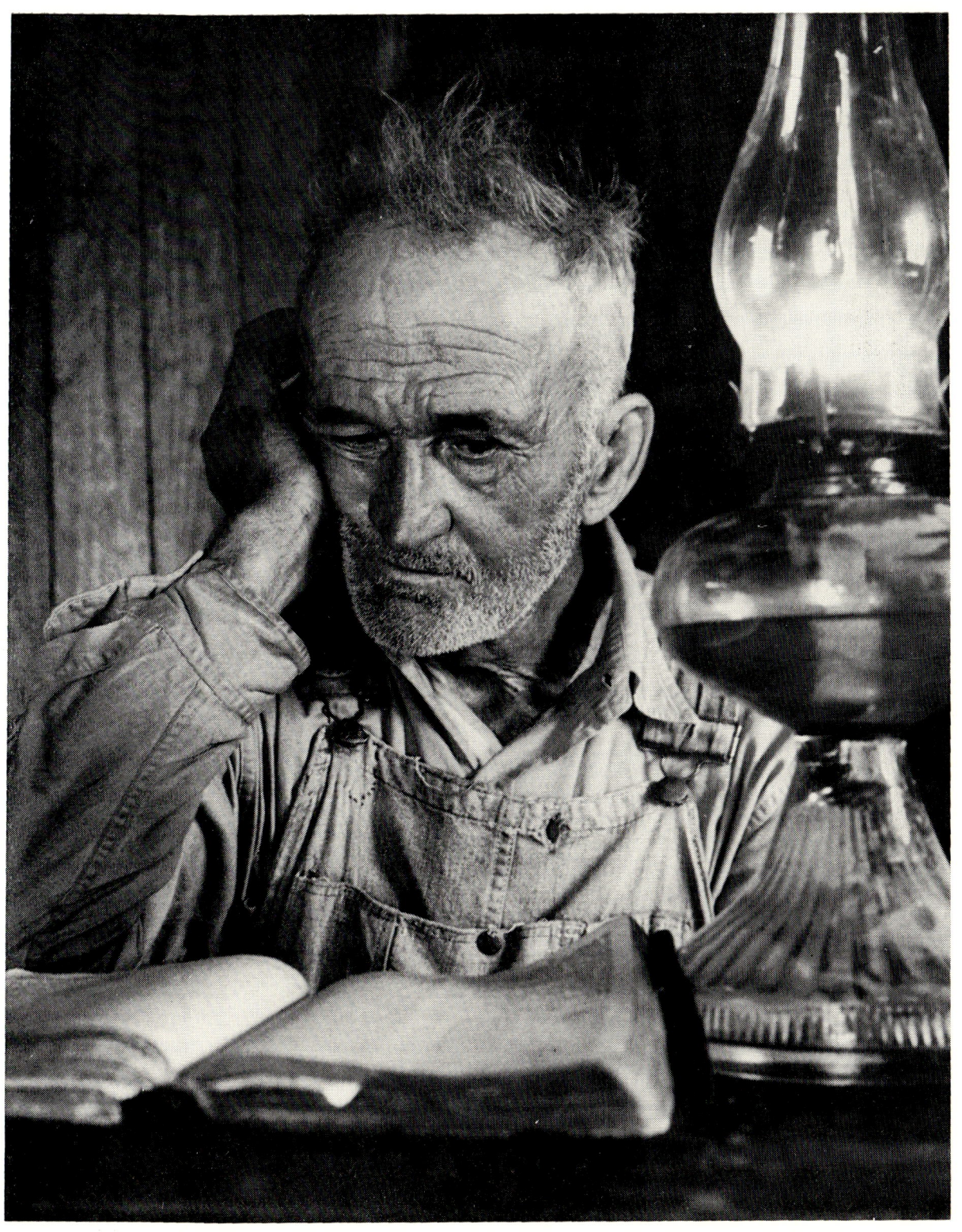

178  Notice how lamp, Bible, and arm combine to frame the face. These as well as clothing and beard help explain the personality of this man.
*Bruce Roberts, staff photographer, Charlotte* Observer

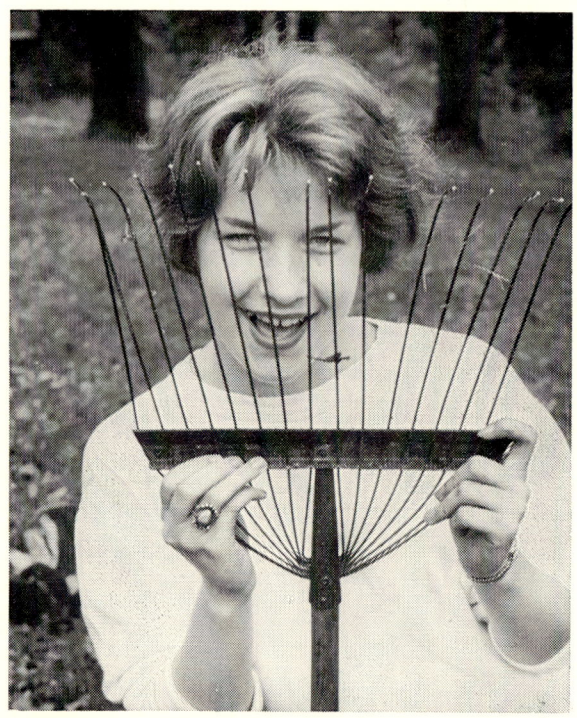

179    Use of a property that helps tell a story and frame an expressive face makes this portrait appealing.
L. W. Ward, Cedar Rapids (Iowa) Gazette

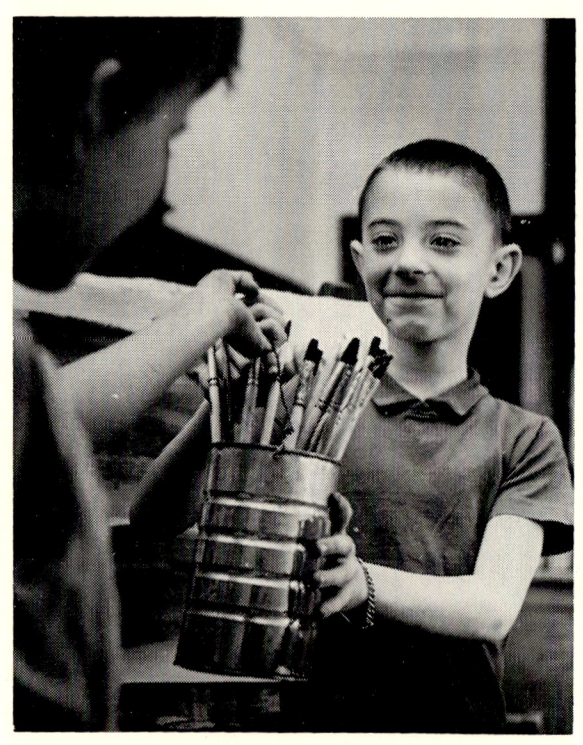

180    Good expression brings a portrait to life. Framing and the brushes help the composition.

### Good Lighting Vital

Good lighting is vital to successful portraiture, whether it be by flash, flood or natural light. Mercifully, gone are the days of the single flash on the camera. Bounce flash, use of more than one flash, use of fill-in flash for outdoor work are available when the situation indicates use of flash bulbs. More common use of small, candid-type cameras has increased the taking of natural-light portraits with their special qualities. Often floodlights are available when subjects can come to a studio or when time and situation permit the moving of floodlights to the place they are wanted.

The news photographer who feels unsure about portrait lighting might do well to borrow a bust of Plato or Bach to use as a model. It will stand quietly while the photographer practices and experiments until satisfied he has learned how to use light. Several books and publications are available concerning portrait lighting.

### Backgrounds Often Contribute

Sometimes background can be an important part of a portrait and can contribute to the proper telling of a story. Such things as a glimpse of a neat office behind an executive's face, a few flowers backgrounding the features of an enthusiastic gardener, a blackboard behind a teacher's face are important elements in a story. Such items must be kept simple, may be out of focus, certainly should not dominate the picture, should be integrated as a part of the composition. Such materials background both the picture and the personality of the subject.

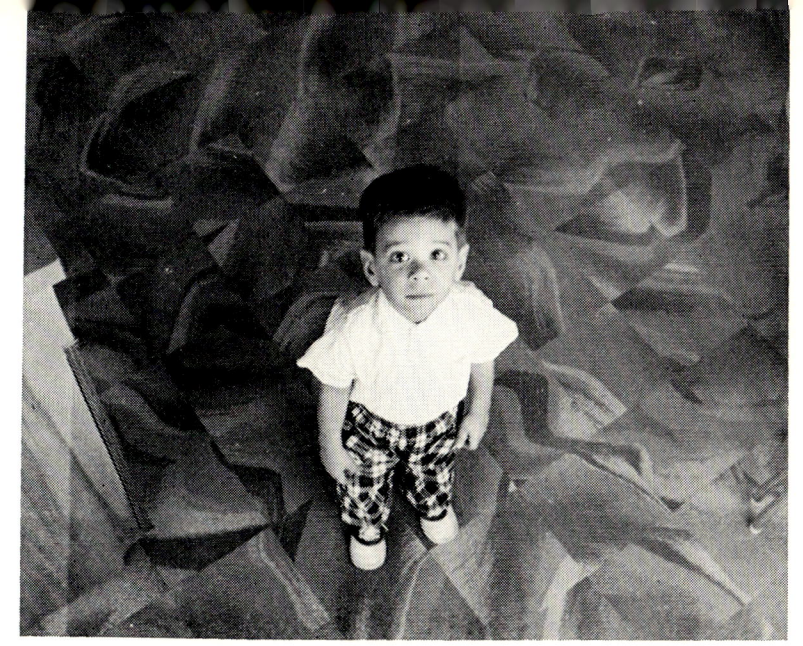

181    This picture of a little boy taken from a high angle and including a broad expanse of floor was part of a series that gave the impression of how BIG everything looks to a small child.

*Middletown (N.Y.)* Daily Record
*photo by Manny Fuchs*

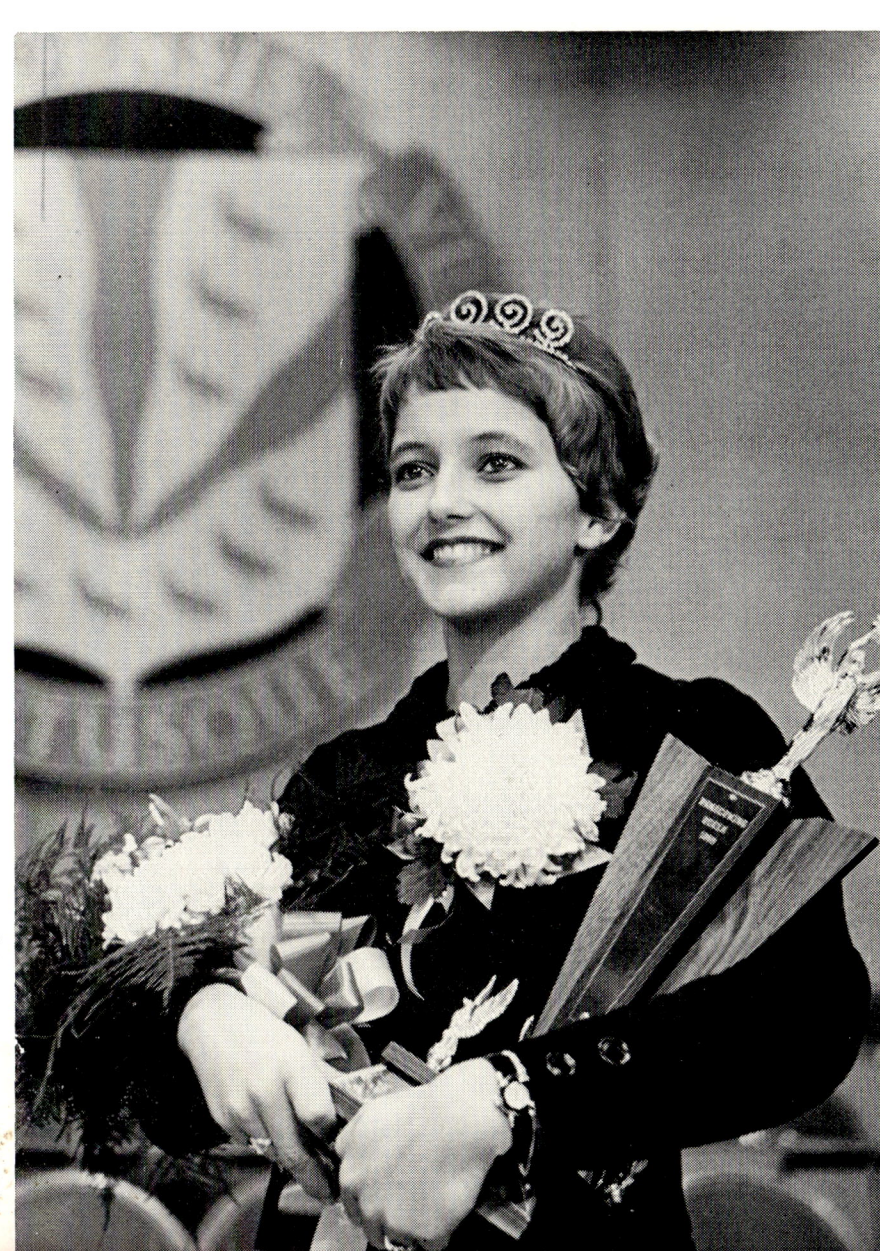

182    The ever-recurring assignment of photographing a "queen" can produce pictures that have dignity and good taste as well as beauty.

*L. W. Ward, Cedar Rapids (Iowa)* Gazette

CHAPTER 18

# Variety Is the Spice of Group Pictures

NEWSPAPERS, house organs and some magazines publish so many pictures of small groups that they are bound to start looking alike, routine and tiresome.

Yet pictures of from three to seven or eight persons are valuable, basically interesting and a vital part of news photography. Since the number of them printed isn't about to decrease, what can be done to relieve somewhat the feeling of monotony their frequency of publication tends to create?

Two suggestions should help: (1) Give them variety and (2) make them present a news story situation. Results from both suggestions often can be achieved from a single device.

The basic way to take the picture of a committee, newly elected officers or half a dozen honored persons is to line them up in a neat row or rows and shoot. That is the quickest, most efficient method, and it makes identification of individuals easy to obtain and easy for readers to follow. Long ago it was used because cameras had little depth of focus and the lineup was the only way to achieve a sharp image of all persons shown.

Today's splendid photographic equipment makes this reason invalid.

The lineup, with all its efficiency, if too often used, results in dreary monotony. Other methods of photographing small groups can result in interesting photographs.

### Nine Variations Proposed

Nine classifications of ways to vary small group pictures have emerged from a study of thousands of such pictures in newspapers, magazines and house organs. Undoubtedly, other classifications of variations could be devised on the basis of such a study. Each of these nine classifications can be varied in many ways. In addition, two or more of these variations can be combined in a single picture. Any news photographer with imagination, energy and perhaps a little extra time can give endless variety to small group pictures.

The nine suggestions for producing group picture variations are:

1. Emphasize one figure such as the president, the chairman, the oldest member or some-

body selected arbitrarily. Such emphasis can be given by placing the figure somewhat in advance of the others, by having him separated from others by spaces, by having him involved in action while others are not, by the fact that he is larger, or smaller or dressed differently than the others, or by several other means.
2. Distribute the figures interestingly rather than have them in a monotonously uniform line. The figures may be rather informally distributed, or may be arranged to create a geometric design.
3. Arrange the figures vertically rather than horizontally.
4. Use high or low camera angles. An almost too familiar version of this is the picture of basketball players taken down through the hoop. Although commonly used for sports and feature pictures, low and high angles can produce interesting but dignified pictures of groups. Low-angle shots involve certain problems and are less often used.

5. Direct the figures to look up, or down, or in some common direction to produce an effect.
6. When possible, use background to add information to the story. If the committee has to do with parks and playgrounds, let a fountain or some familiar park feature show; if a group of businessmen, background with a bit of Main Street architecture; if a church committee, show a fragment of their Gothic edifice.
7. Use properties when they create a good effect. Group the committee around an architect's model of the proposed hospital; add a dog as the center of interest for the group working on an animal rescue center; show the group planning a youth center looking at some athletic equipment. Let the properties describe part of the activities of the group pictured.

183  A simple way to vary a group picture is to place the emphasis on one figure in a group.

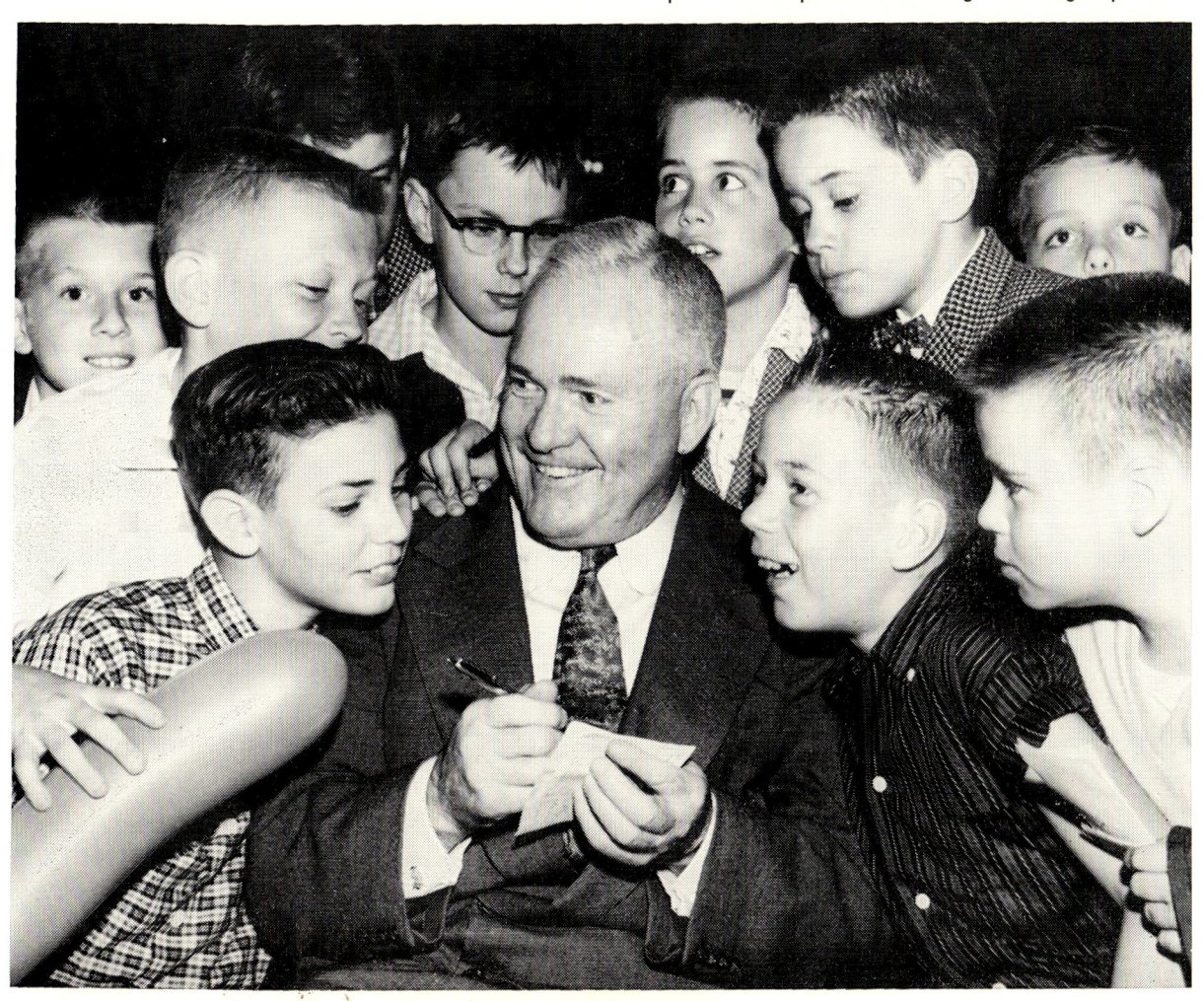

184   Distribute members of a group imaginatively — and informally.
Home & Highway Magazine, *published by Allstate Insurance Companies*

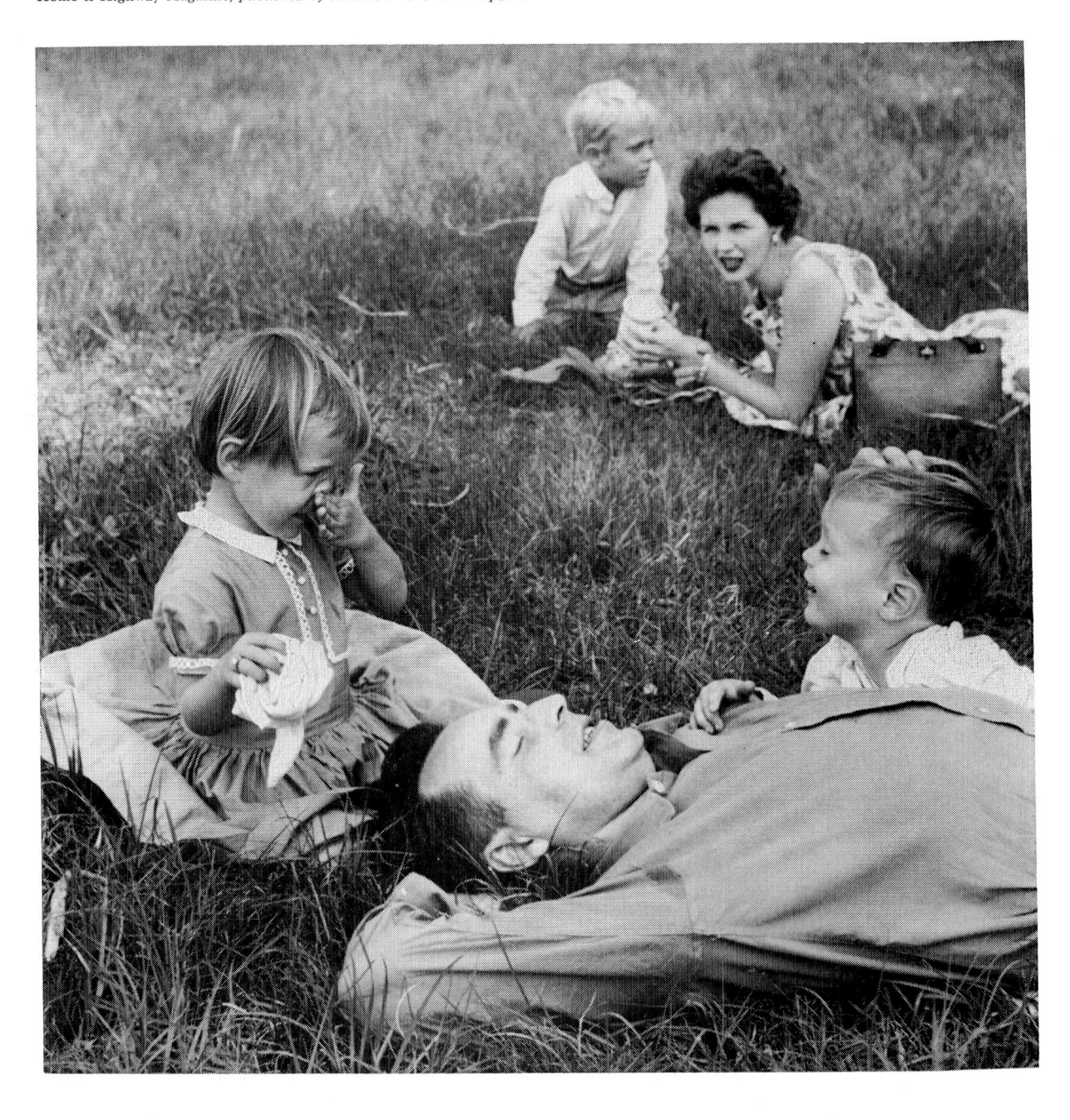

8. When appropriate, have members of the group in uniforms or costumes. Uniforms of nurses, American Legion members, Boy Scouts, National Guard units or lodge members add color to a photograph. Casts of amateur plays, people who plan to attend a charity costume ball, persons planning a centennial celebration are most interesting if photographed in costume.
9. Most important of all, make group pictures tell a news story, present a news situation. Have the group in action doing what it is supposed to do. Let the Arbor Day committee be busy planting a tree, the flower committee arranging bouquets, the cleanup committee cleaning up.

Some of the previous suggestions contribute toward making group pictures tell news stories. Good use of backgrounds, of properties, of dramatic arrangement of figures all add to the story-telling qualities of news pictures.

**Larger Groups Mean Bigger Problems**

Scout troops, classes, large committees, athletic squads and many other organizations containing more than seven or eight persons often have to be photographed. They make newsworthy pictures, especially in communities small enough that faces, like names, make news. But planning pictures of groups of that size presents additional problems.

The easiest and sometimes the only solution to this problem of photographing large groups is to stand the members in neat rows, especially if they are to be identified in cutlines.

But pictures of this sort can be improved by arranging members of the group in interesting patterns. This sometimes can be done on a stairway or the steps of a building or in an appropriate bit of landscape in a park or other open space.

Often it is desirable for the photographer to find a vantage point above the group so that he can shoot down. After sports writers called the football situation hopeless at one university, the squad was photographed from above in a formation that spelled "NUTS." At a 4-H Club convention, members were

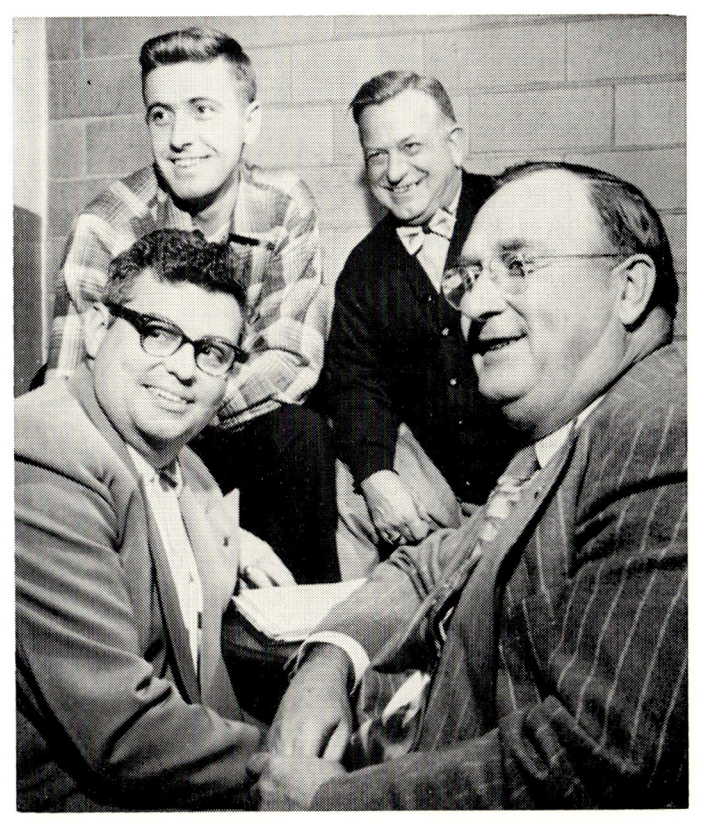

185    Ask everyone in the group to look in the same direction.
*Photo by Clifford R. Yeich, courtesy Reading (Pa.)* Times

grouped to form the insignia of their organization and photographed that way from the roof of a nearby building. At another convention, delegates were grouped to form a map of their state previously laid out on an open stretch of ground.

**Crowd Pictures Different**

The photography of a crowd presents problems somewhat different from those involved in picturing a large group. The picture of a sea of faces undoubtedly has some interest in spite of the monotony that occurs when the crowd is so big that interest in individual faces is lost. A crowd picture usually takes on added interest if it shows a center of interest such as a speaker or entertainer, a gate being besieged, the building around which the crowd clusters. A crowd picture should be more than a picture of a crowd. It must present a news situation clearly.

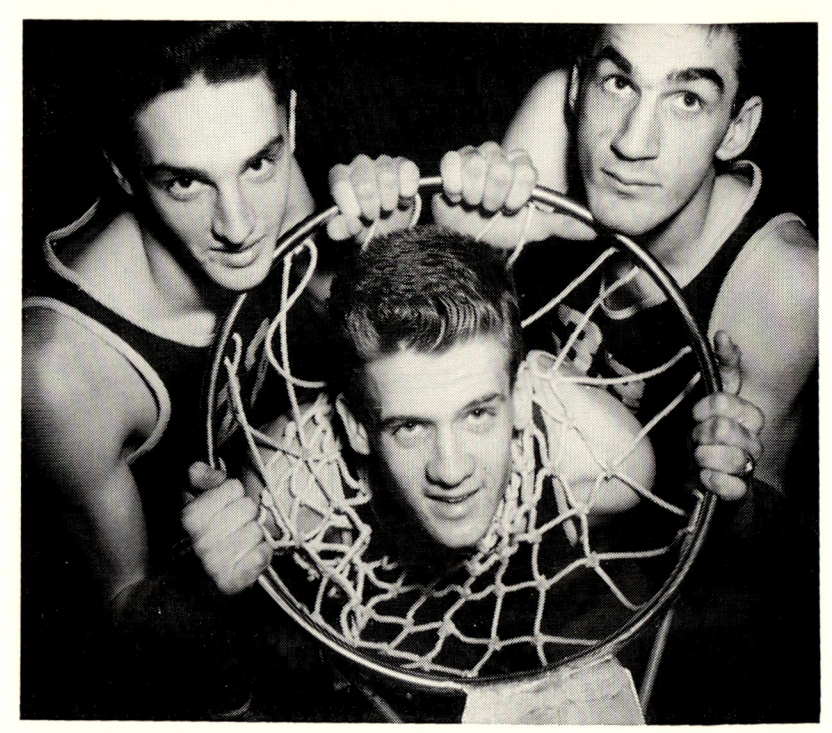

**187** Use high or low angles to photograph a group.
*Bob Weir, Malden (Mass.) Press*

**188** Formal arrangement of a group can be different and interesting.
*Fritz Shellman, Oconto County (Wis.) Times-Herald*

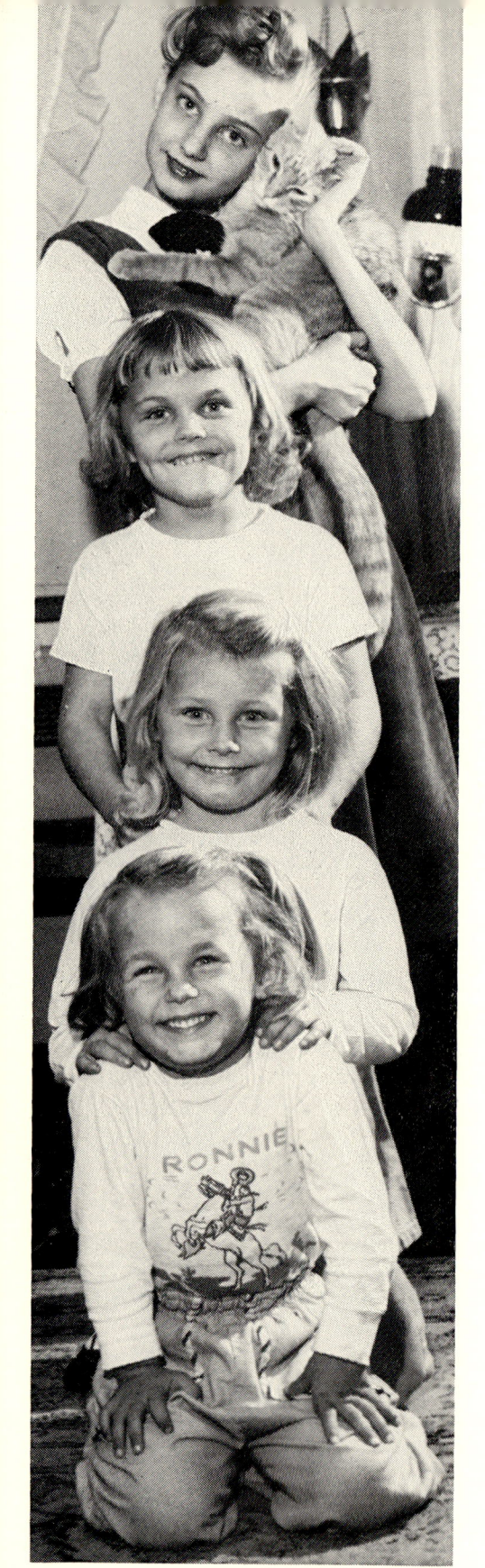

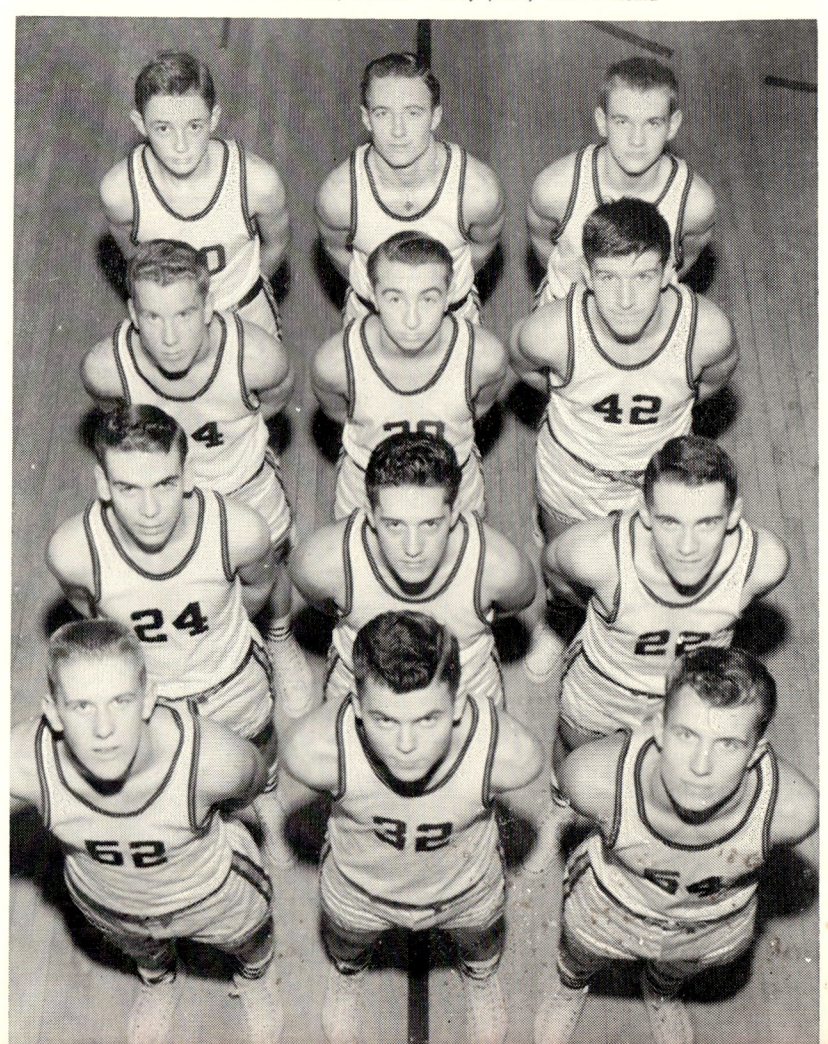

**186** Arrange the figures in a group vertically.

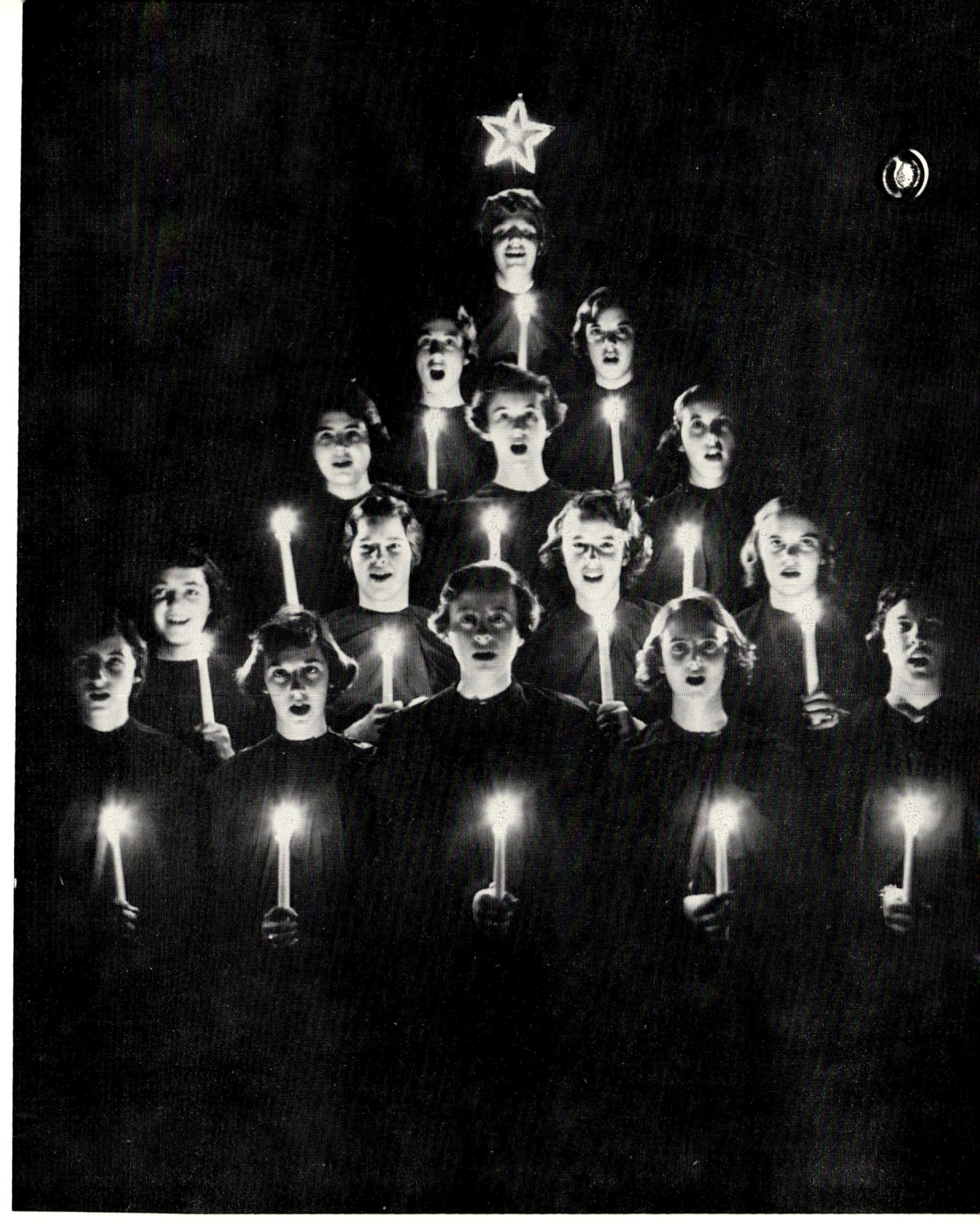

189  Triangular arrangement suggesting a Christmas tree covered with candles makes this group unique.
*Photo by Clifford R. Yeich, courtesy Reading (Pa.)* Times

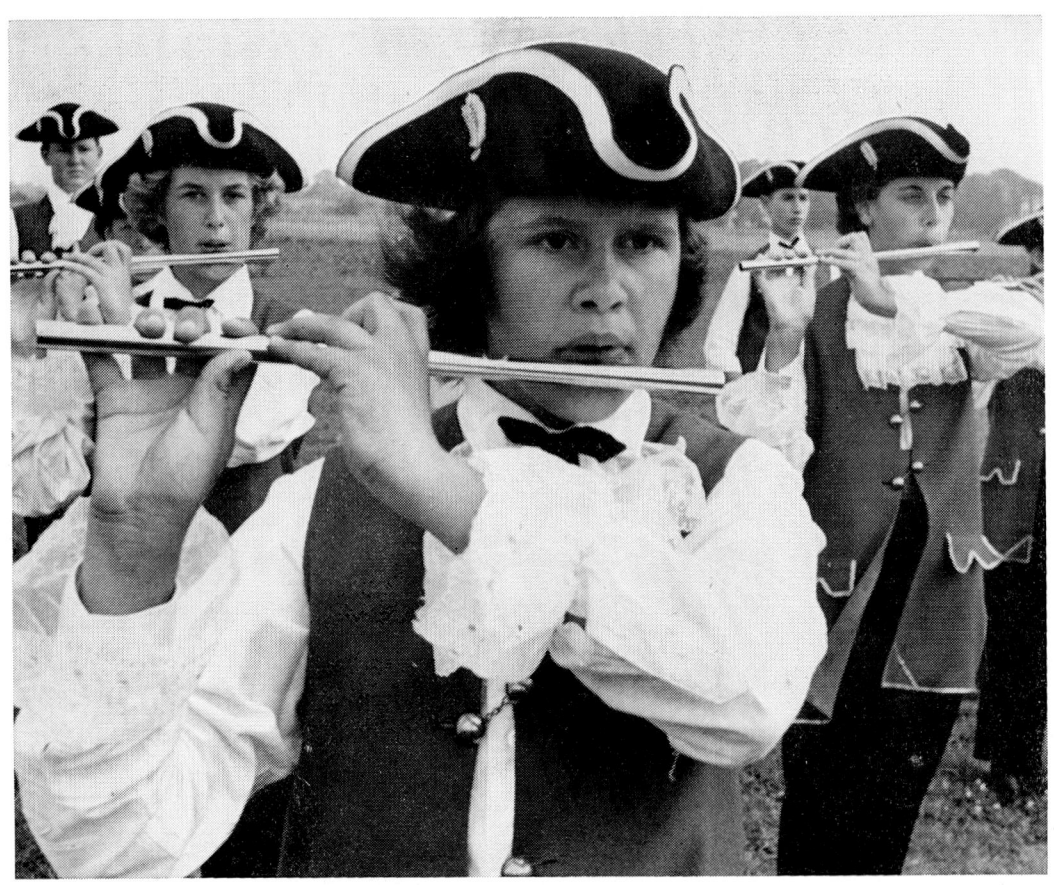

190     Uniforms or costumes add color to group pictures and tell part of the story.
*Marvin Sussman,* Newsday, Long Island, N.Y.

191     Background explains that this group has something to do with an art exhibit.

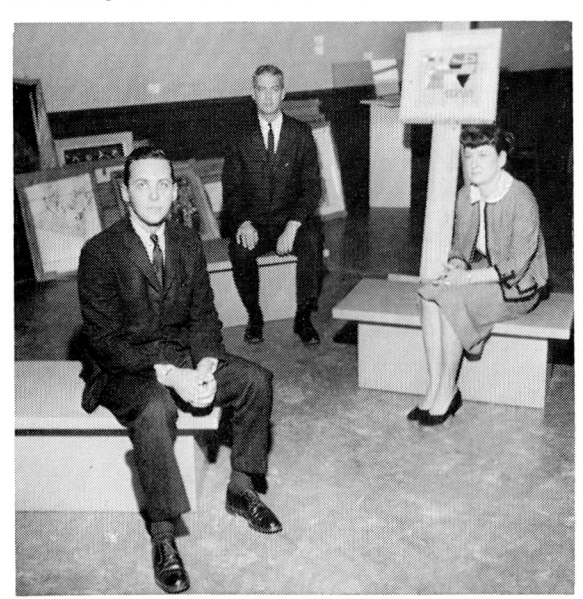

192     Properties and the arrangement of these 13 women give this picture story-telling quality.

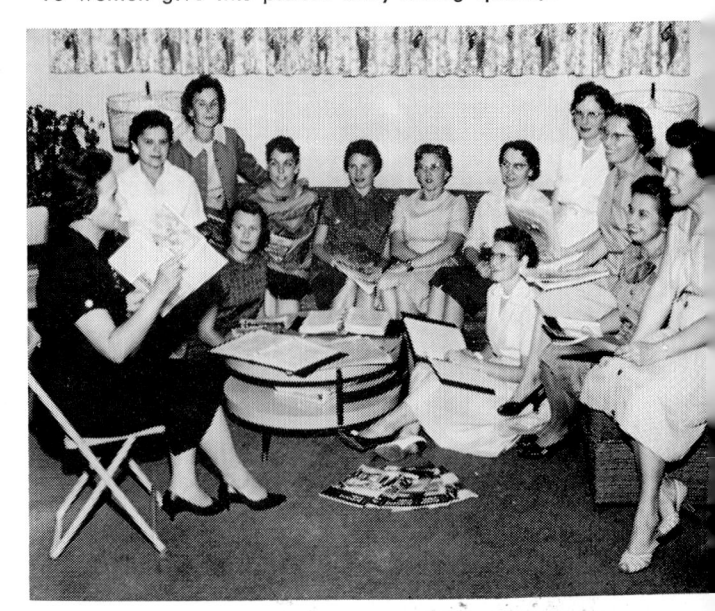

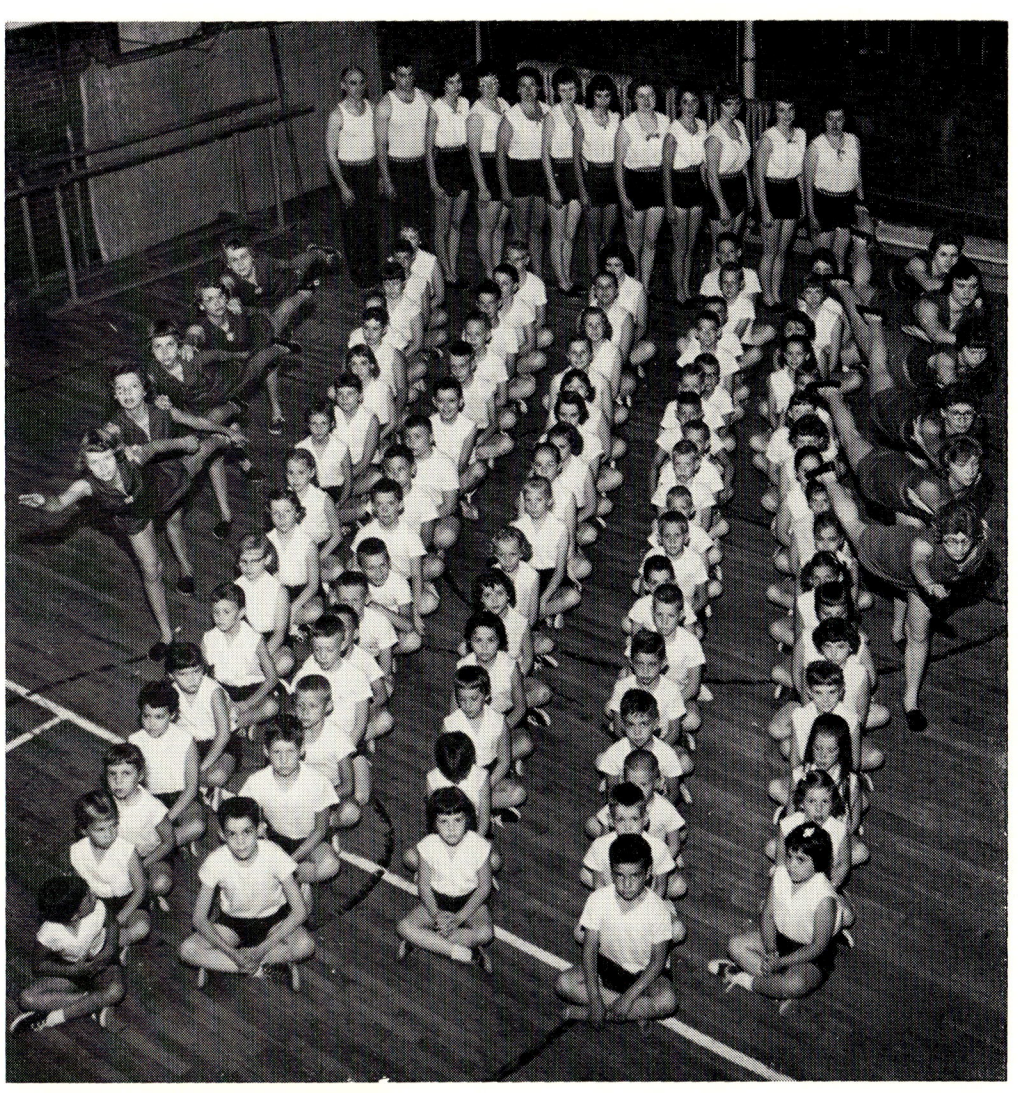

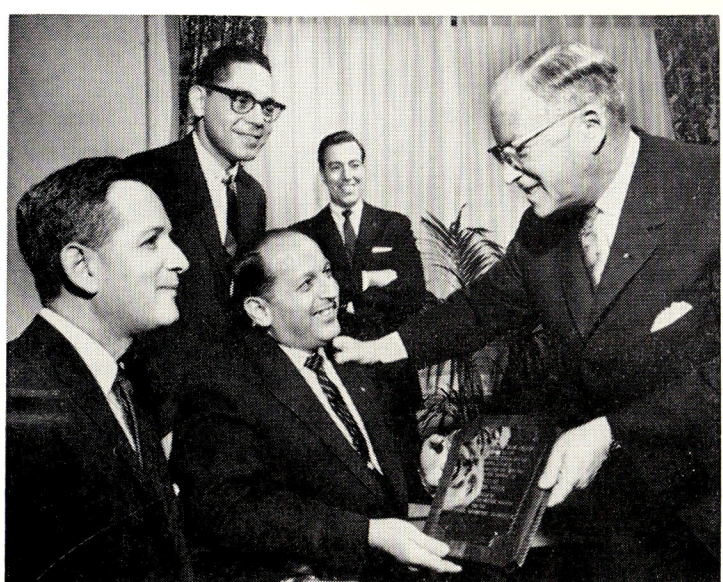

193   Interesting arrangement, high angle photography, and some impression of movement make a good news picture of this group of 116 persons.

194   Even the important but routine presentation picture can be made interesting, as is this one, by use of good composition, good expressions, action, and storytelling quality.
*Photo by Clifford R. Yeich, courtesy Reading (Pa.)* Times

— 155

CHAPTER **19**

# Cutlines Help Pictures Tell Their Stories

FULL SUCCESS with news pictures involves such factors as well-written captions and cutlines, adequate space for photographs, and good integration of illustrations with written materials and headlines.

Most really good news photographs do excellent jobs of telling their stories in picture form alone, but always some details remain to be added in words. Some excellent news pictures are almost without significance until a few words are added to supply some information not pictorially available. How well the captions and cutlines fill in essential detail has much to do with the final effectiveness of the picture. Captions and cutlines usually must be adequate to produce, with the pictures they accompany, brief but satisfyingly complete stories.

Exception to this is the cutline or caption, or both, intended to draw strong attention to the accompanying story and to induce readership of it. In this method, the words that accompany the picture serve as a "teaser" to arouse curiosity about the picture and the accompanying story.

Whether the caption is used traditionally above the picture and the cutlines below, or the caption is used between the picture and the cutlines or as an all-cap. introduction to the cutlines, the words that are integrated with pictures have certain jobs to do.

These six points may serve as a checklist concerning the adequacy of cutlines and captions:

1. For papers that circulate within fairly small communities, identify every recognizable person. In communities so large that the comparative importance of the individual is small, sometimes only the persons important to the story are identified. Your publication's style rules will guide you in how to identify, in addition to names, whether by street address, occupation or some other means.
2. Don't forget to supply orientation whenever it is needed. If there is any chance that viewers might confuse identities, add such information as "left," "from the left" or whatever is needed to make identification foolproof.
3. In general, make cutlines tell as concisely as possible the who, what, when, where, unless some of these points are obvious in the picture.

195   The full emotional value of the emphasis on light doesn't become clear until cutlines explain that the girl is blind.
*Fargo (N. Dak.)* Forum *by Alf T. Olsen*

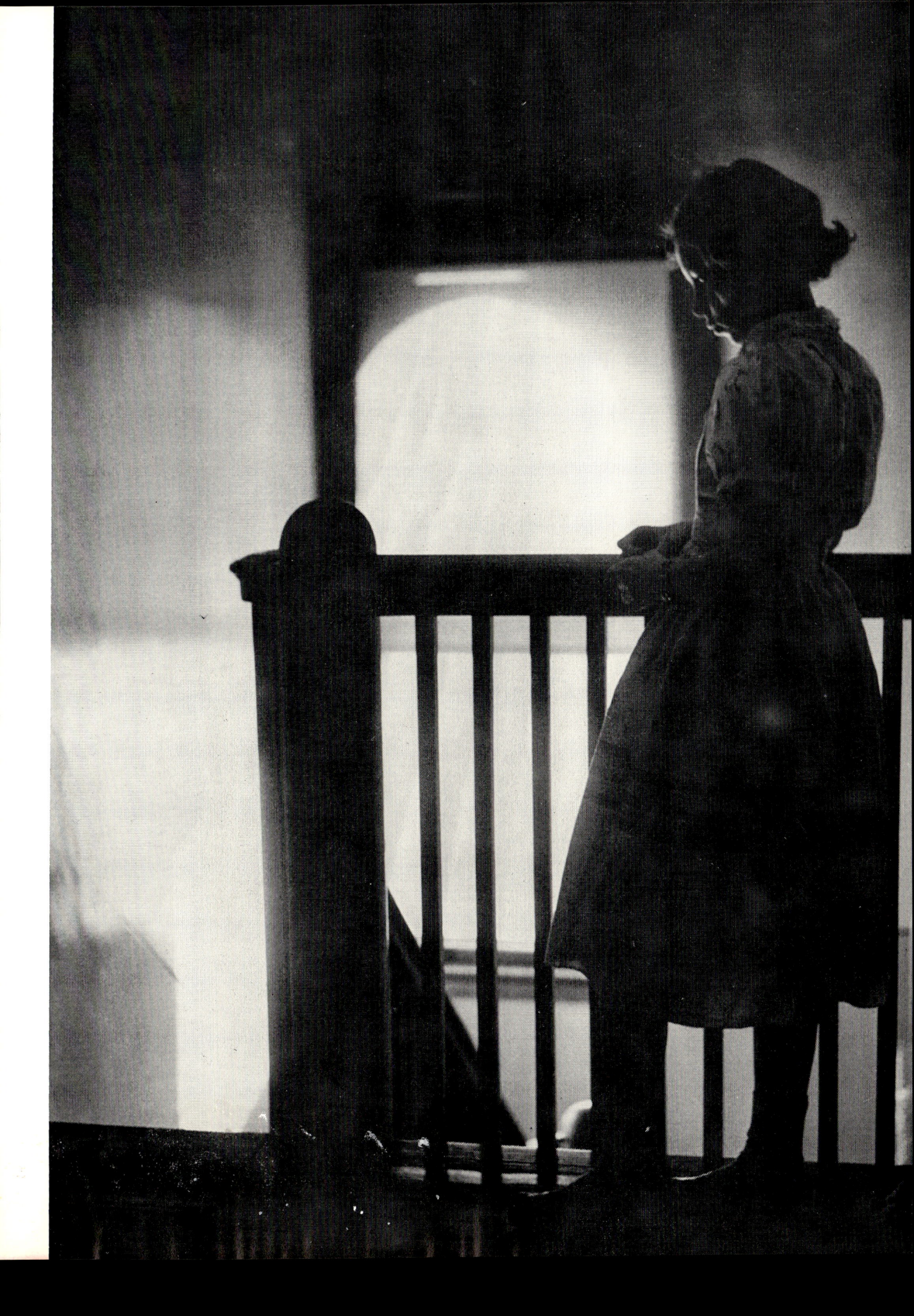

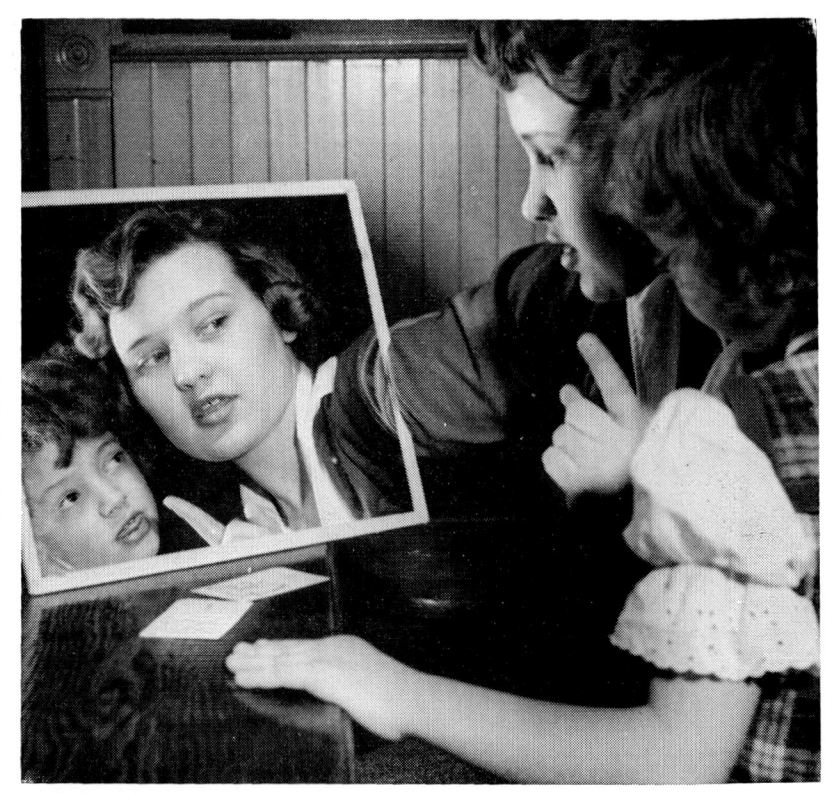

196 Until cutlines make clear that the little girl reflected in the mirror is a mute being taught to speak, a viewer might think the picture just a study in the use of repetition with variation.

4. Be cautious in attempts to be clever or cute. What you think is a smart cutline may seem smart-alecky to a great many readers.
5. Make cutlines contribute to the reader's understanding. Such captions or cutlines as "Rainy Day" or "Firemen Fight Roof Blaze" may be accurate, but they supply the reader with no information he can't obtain by a glance at the picture, if it is doing its job.
6. Don't belabor the obvious. It isn't necessary to write, "Pictured above are . . . .," or to say in cutlines for a basketball picture, "Two players scramble for the ball," when pictures make that evident. Cutlines should supply only essential detail that cannot be drawn from the picture.

Don't belittle the importance of captions and cutlines. Few pictures would be complete without some words. The full effectiveness of most pictures depends on the words used with them.

**Cutlines May Change Attitudes**

For the newsman intent on making his publication as objective as humanly possible, or for the person eager to influence opinion with what he publishes, it is well to remember that captions and cutlines are important in the attitude-changing effect of pictures.

One study showed that captions can greatly modify the judgments of readers regarding the pictures they accompany and may even reverse judgment.[1]

Another piece of research indicates that a photo-caption combination is more effective than a story alone in causing attitude changes. The same study showed that coupling of two persons in a photograph, *without captions,* may also produce an attitude change toward both persons.[2] That finding suggests that what is *not* included in cutlines may be important too.

---

[1] Kerrick, Jean S., "The Influence of Captions on Pictorial Interpretation." *Journalism Quarterly,* Spring, 1955.

[2] Mehling, Reuben, "Attitude Changing Effect of News and Photo Combinations." *Journalism Quarterly,* Spring, 1959.

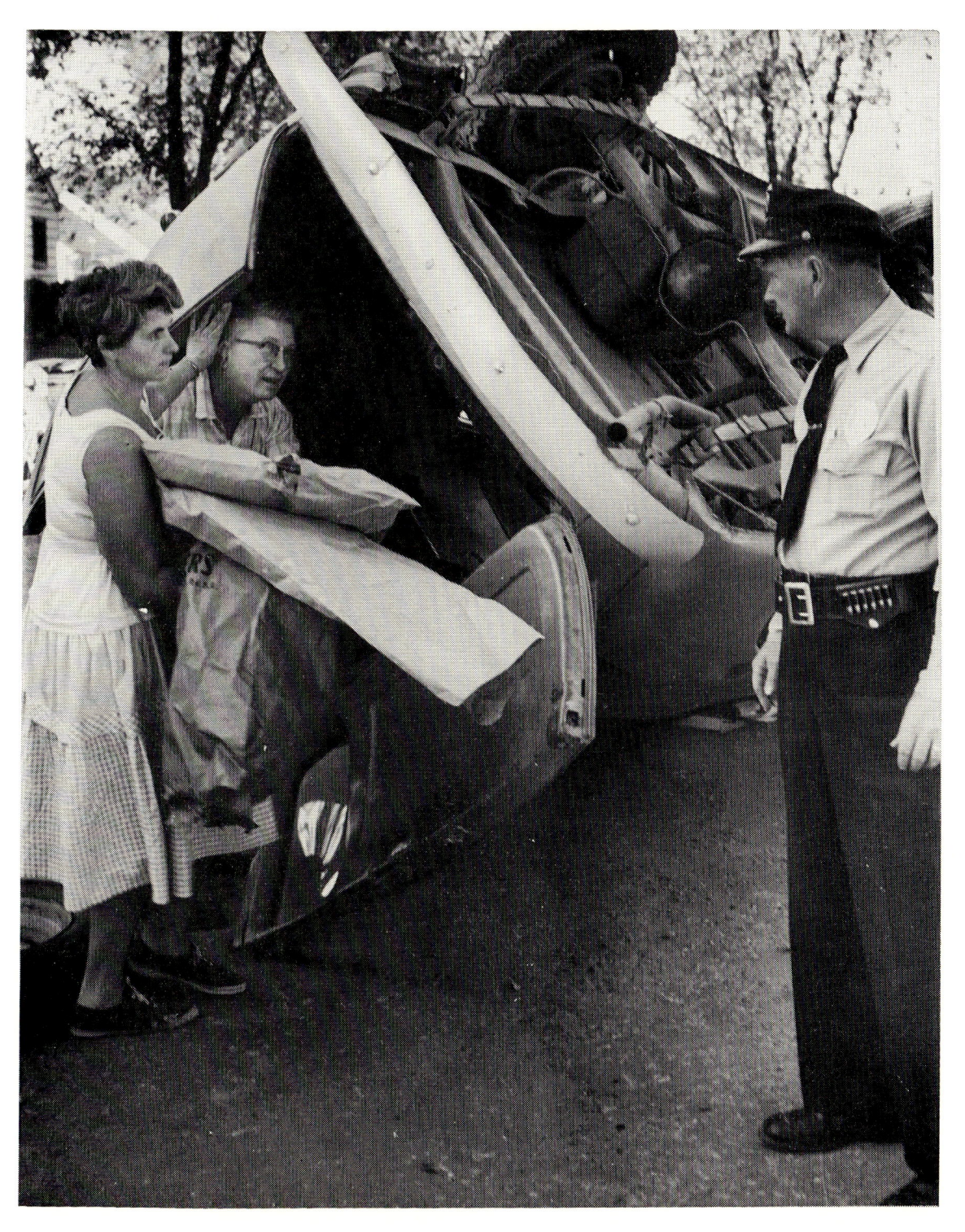

197   An obvious news situation, two rather guilty looking persons taking material from a wrecked car while a policeman looks at them suspiciously, is cleared up quickly by a caption, "But Officer, It's Our Car."

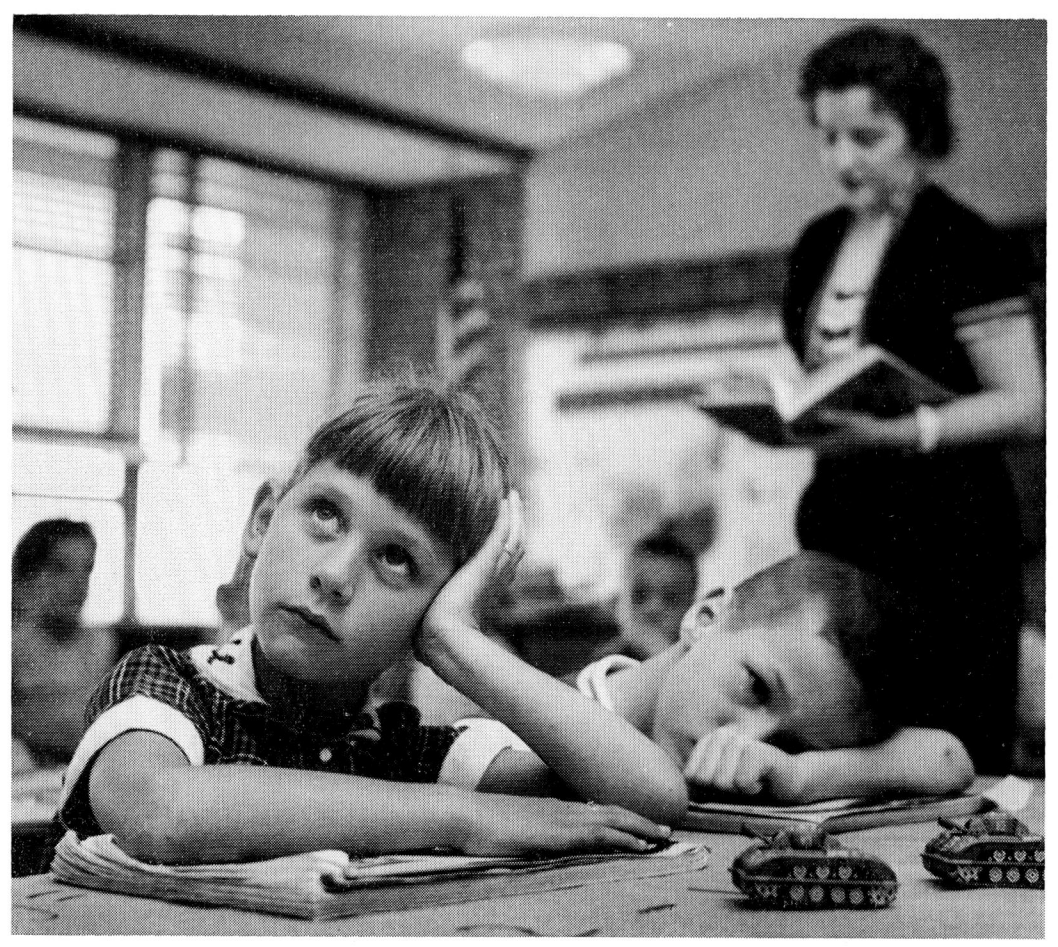

198    Thoughtful planning can eliminate cutline writing problems. In this picture, background and teacher make clear that the photograph was taken to illustrate a school story.

199    But this photograph lacks a revealing background, and cutlines are needed to explain that this is a teacher welcoming a new arrival at school.

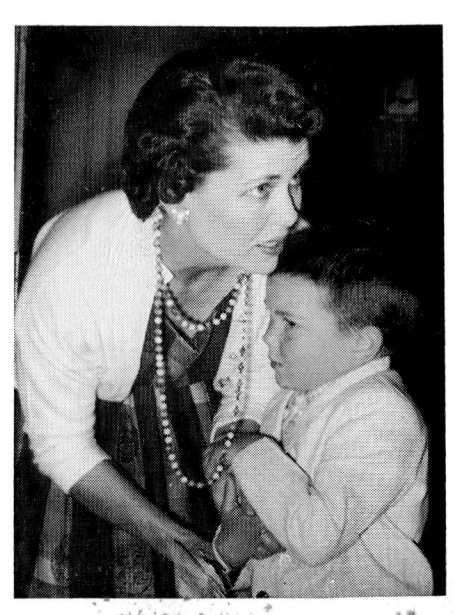

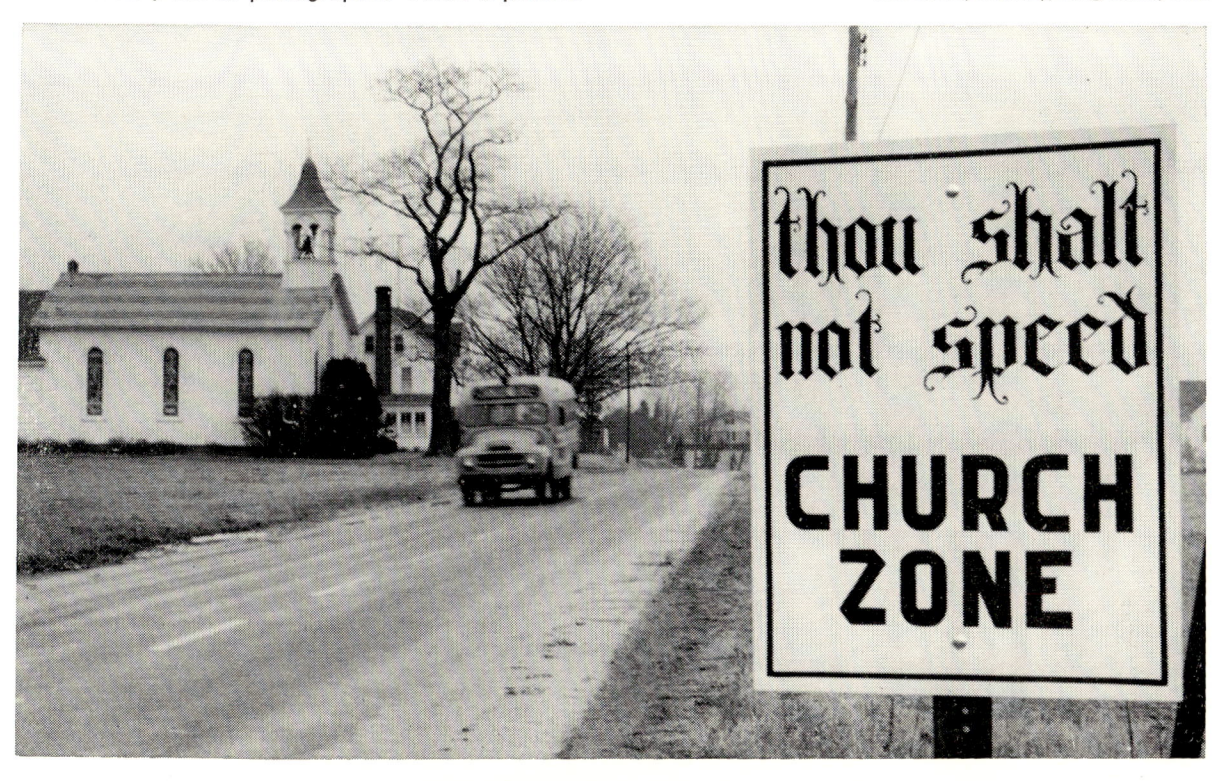

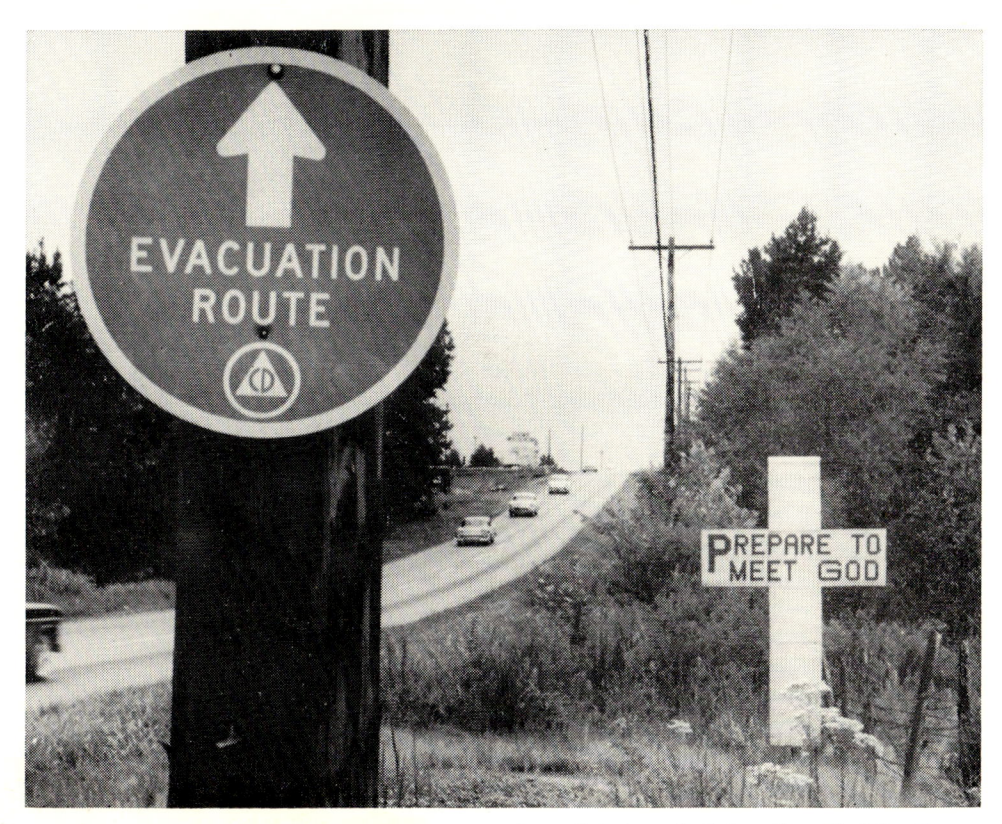

200   Once in awhile most of the words needed to tell a story can be photographed within a picture.

*Max Heine,* Newsday, *Long Island, N.Y.*

*Bruce Roberts, staff photographer,* Charlotte *Observer*

— 161

CHAPTER **20**

# Don't Be Niggardly About Picture Size

WHEN IT IS OBVIOUS that pictures have great readership appeal and that photographs can tell stories vividly and well, why be stingy in giving them enough space to function fully?

Many newspapers have spent much time and effort to find the most legible type faces and use type large enough and with sufficient space around it to provide maximum readability. Yet some of the same papers publish photographs so small that their "legibility" is as reduced as would be the legibility of verbal material printed in 6 point type.

Especially heartbreaking seems the loss of value when an exceptionally good picture is published far too small to achieve its potentials. Such waste of the possibilities of an excellent photograph reflects a lack of good editorial judgment. And every issue of a newspaper should have a few excellent pictures worth playing up. If it doesn't have at least a few good pictures, it needs to start getting them, some way or other. Pictures can contribute much to the popularity and effectiveness of a paper, but the expense and effort of obtaining them will be partly wasted unless they are printed large enough.

That almost all pictures increase in impact as their size increases is too obvious to be argued.[1] But editors do have to weigh the

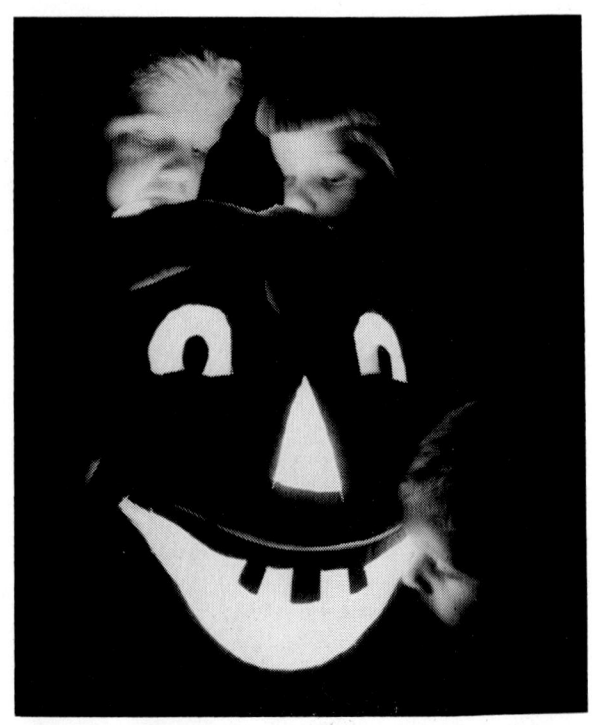

202   Who's afraid of a little Jack-O'-Lantern?
*Dale Westin, Clarion Publications, Naperville, Ill.*

162 —

203   Size helps create effect.

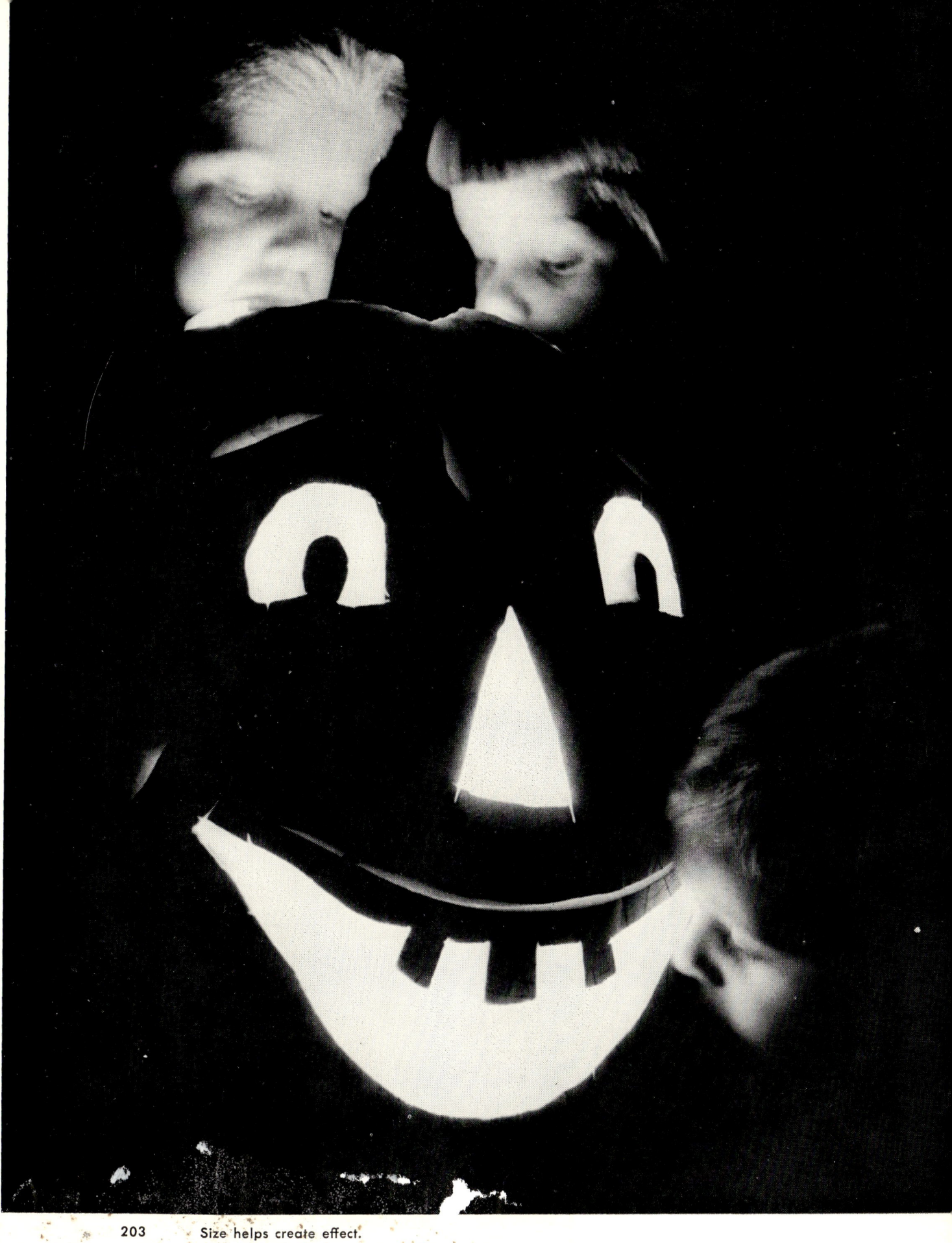

value of increased size for a picture against the demands for space made by other contents of the issue — advertising, stories, other pictures.

No rules can be written to guide editors in making their decisions about size for pictures. Constantly changing are the amounts of space available and the competition of other materials crying for their shares of available space. The size value of any given picture must be determined by weighing its demands against those made by other items against the backgrounds of the day's situation.

Picture enthusiasts who feel that photographs need to be weighted heavily in this constant competition for space offer these arguments for larger news pictures:

1. Good pictures blown up large enough to be effective from a distance should offer a strong appeal to potential readers to buy a paper on the street; or when it is delivered, to pick it up and start looking at it. House organ publishers, although their product is distributed free, are eager to have it picked up and read, and large pictures on the front page or cover should help accomplish this.
2. Effectively large pictures in each section of of a newspaper, such as sports, society, farm, even financial, should influence appreciably more readers to stop at those sections and to seek them.
3. A fairly large picture on every, or almost every inside page should cause readers to pause, then stop to read. After all, most advertising is on inside pages, and unless it is looked at it will not function.
4. Pictures seem an effective way for printed publications to reach a public increasingly used to obtaining information by pictorial or auditory means and apparently more and more unwilling to read. To reach this picture-eager public, pictures kept effectively large would seem essential.

5. It costs money to obtain good photographs. Why waste part of the potential value of such pictures by running them too small?
6. On the day that turns up an exceptionally good picture, spashing that picture big should cause delighted reactions that outweigh criticisms resulting from cutting a few items to make room for the splurge.
7. Some pictures just don't deserve or need large space. This is true when photographs are simple and without interesting detail, when they are short of much potential emotional impact at best and when they are of marginal news value. One column and even half column sizes are big enough for some pictures.

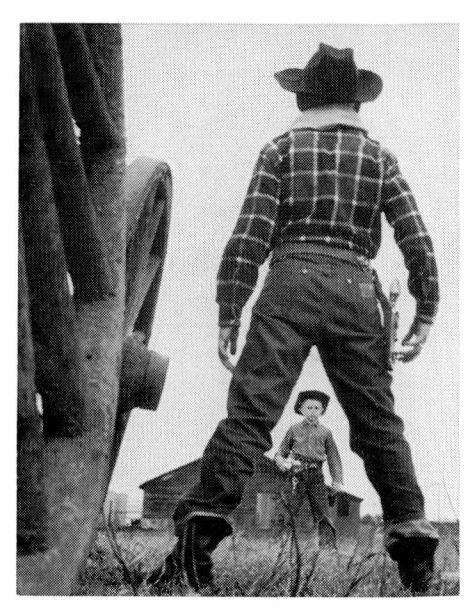

204

205   No matter how tough the gunman, he doesn't look impressive in a small picture. This takeoff on TV westerns makes its point when used larger. Incidentally, this picture was part of a series used on the women's pages showing how Matt Dillon, Jr. got rid of the outlaws on his block.

*Bruce Roberts, staff photographer, Charlotte Observer*

---

[1] Seth Spaulding, in a summary concerning what research has shown about the use of pictorial symbols in educational materials, stated that "The larger the illustration, the more probable that it will attract attenion. However, attention-getting qualities do not increase in mathematical ratio to size." The statement is from his article, "Research on Pictorial Illustrations," in *Audio-Visual Communication Review*, Vol. III, No. 1, Winter, 1955, and was quoted in "Comprehension of Pictorial Symbols: an Experiment in Rural Brazil" by Luiz Fonseca and Bryant Kearl, Bulletin 30, April, 1960, Department of Agricultural Journalism, University of Wisconsin.

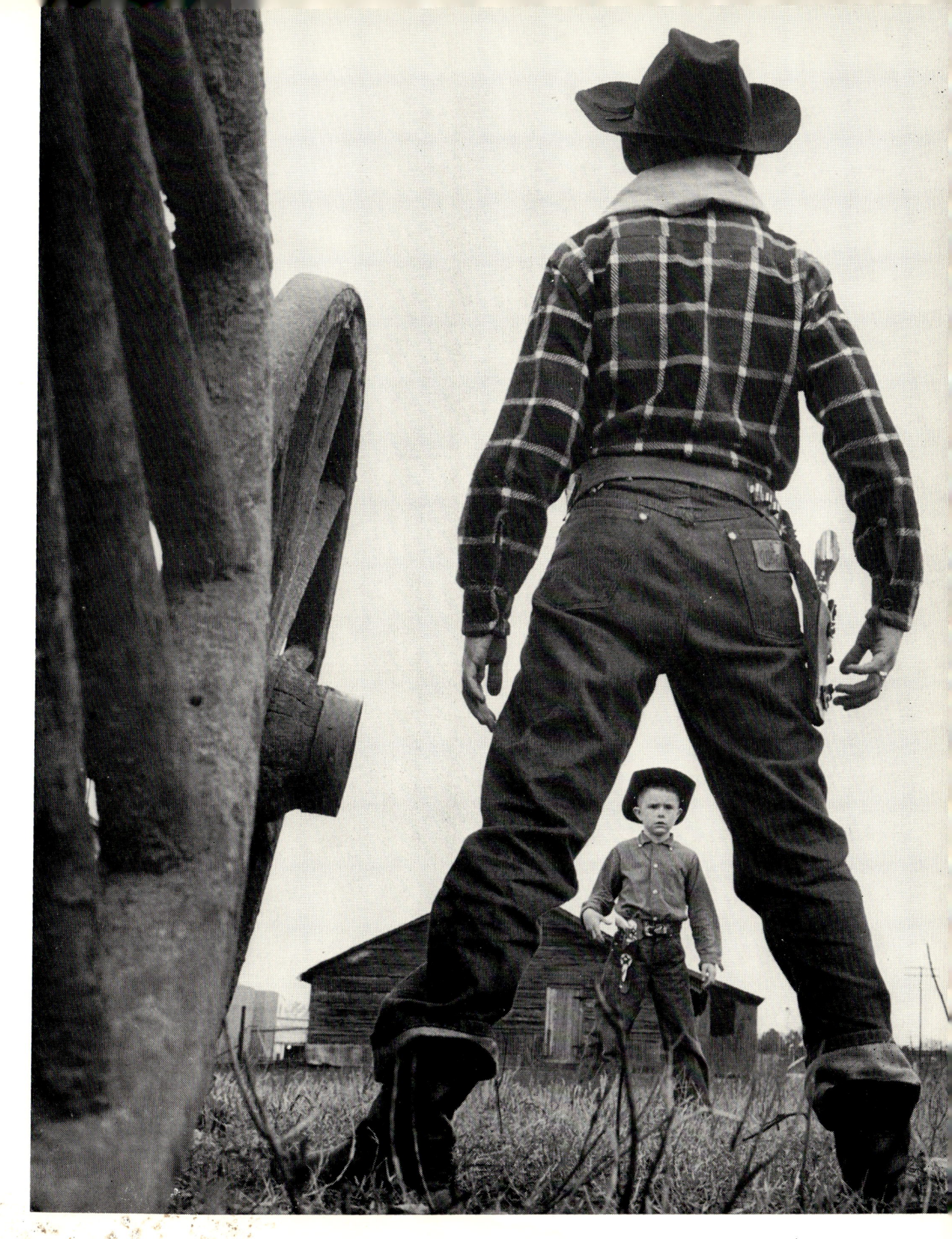

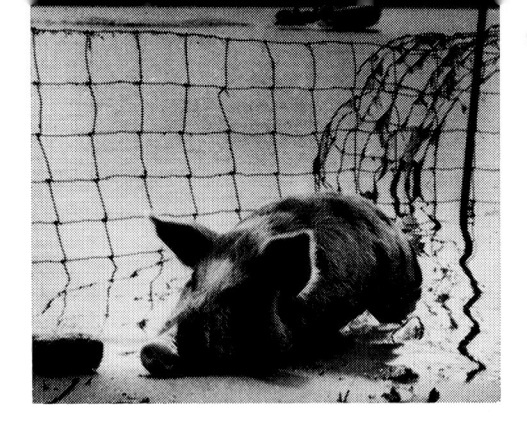

206 A big hog in a big river deserves a big picture. In this case, a compassionate farmer extended his fence into the Mississippi to provide his pigs this watery luxury.
*Davenport (Iowa)* Morning Democrat

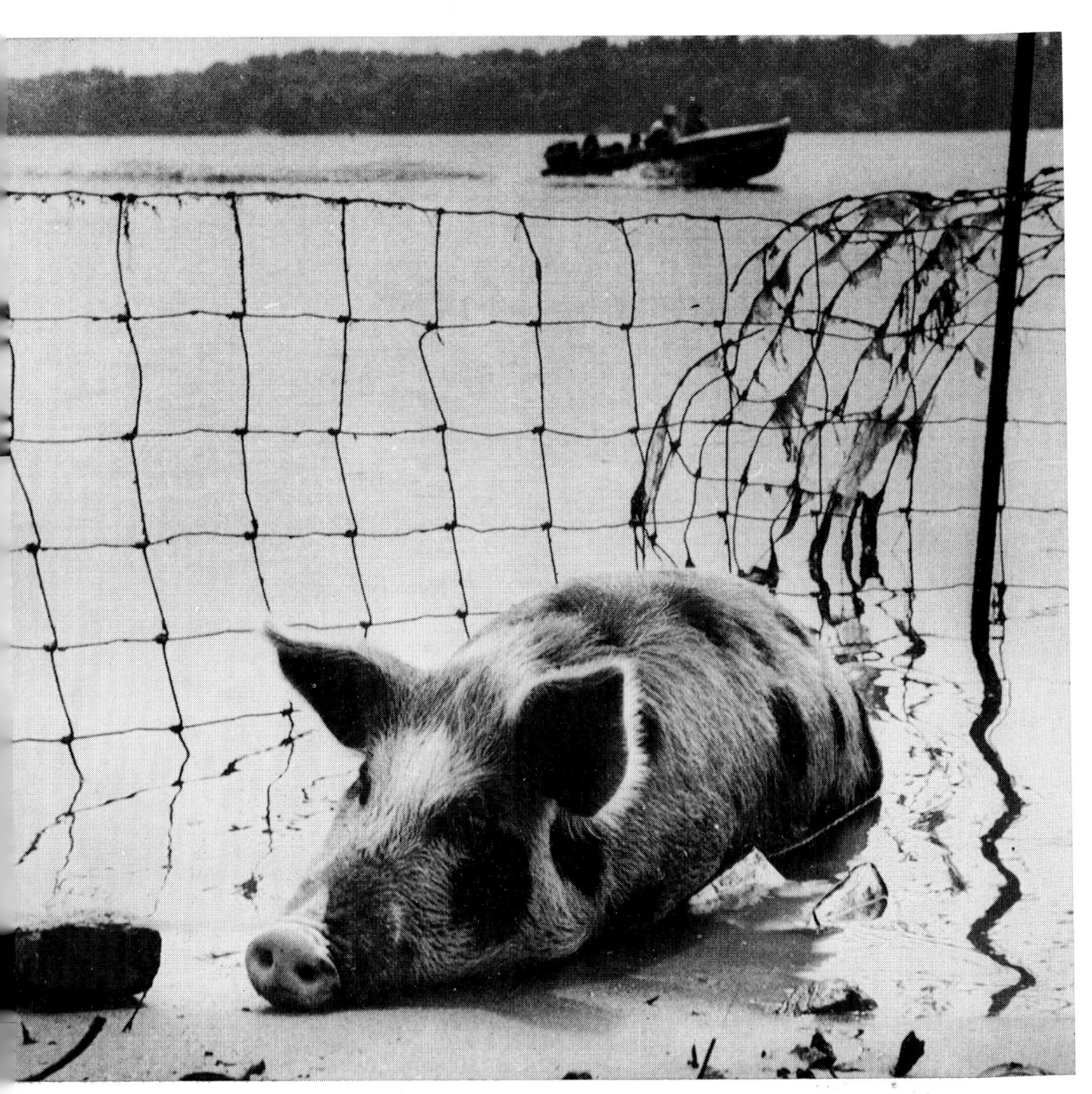

CHAPTER 21

# Retouching Can Save Many Pictures

THE IDEAL NEWS PHOTOGRAPH can be used effectively without retouching. But most pictures, even excellent ones, can be retouched by skilled artists to improve reproduction.

Even when the services of highly trained retouchers are not available, anybody with some knowledge of simple retouching can improve many a picture and save others. Often the picture saved is extremely newsworthy and important and because of time and situation cannot be retaken.

Any photographer with a little practice and a few inexpensive materials can learn to retouch at the newspaper level. Publications with extremely high standards of reproduction will want to turn to professional artists for help.

You can start your retouching activities with only three tools — a fine-pointed brush, some gray poster paint and some India ink. Practice with them for a while on some old prints or discards.

To get rid of distracting backgrounds behind figures, paint the whole background gray. Or cut out the figures and paste them on a suitable background. If tree branches stick out from behind a head, paint out the background. Sometimes only a section of the background needs be painted out, and it can be done to look like a wall panel or some other object.

When dark hair or dark clothing fade into the background, they can be lightened by painting, or the figures can be cut out and pasted against a different background or the background lightened by retouching.

Or you can outline a head with gray paint, then with your thumb feather the line down on the head, creating a kind of highlight. Better practice this one a few times. Its use isn't limited to heads, either.

If you want to darken an area, put a touch of gray paint on a piece of glass or some other hard surface and mix in tiny quantities of India ink to achieve the tone you want.

To lighten gray paint, add some white. Never, never use either pure black or pure white to retouch, because either one will appear to jump right out of the published picture.

If a highlight is weak, you can accentuate it. Never create a highlight, as this will almost certainly damage your picture.

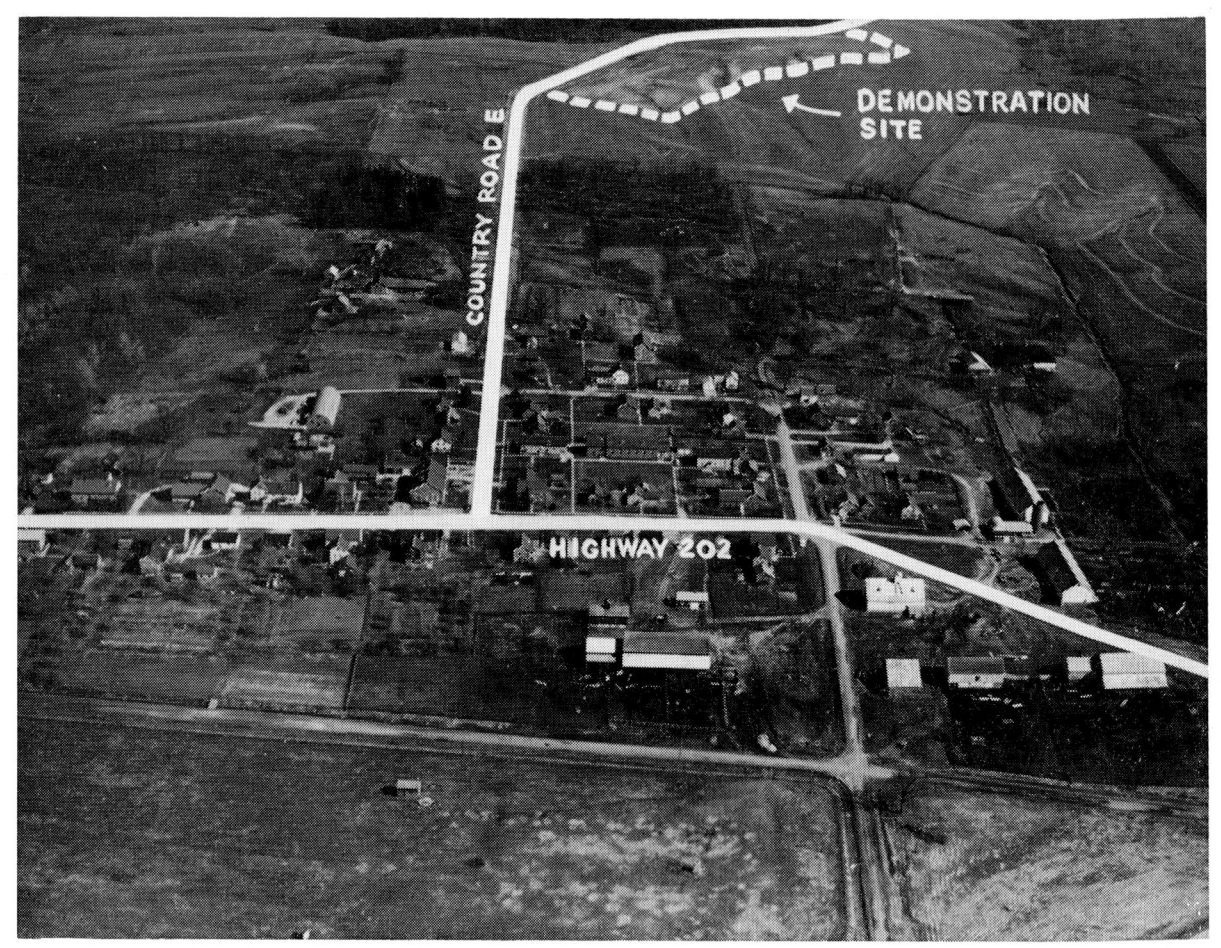

207  A few lines drawn on a photograph often can do the work of many words and in a far superior way.

*Aerial photo by Bob Laker*

Don't retouch more than is absolutely necessary. And above all, be as subtle as possible. Too obvious retouching is offensive, and it destroys the reader's confidence in the authenticity of the picture.[3]

### X Marks Spot Technique Helpful

With India ink and a pen or brush, a little white paint, or even with grease pencil, useful additions to photographs can be made to clarify and increase their story-telling qualities.

Here are some of the possible uses:

X can be superimposed to mark the spot at which the body was found or point out other important locations.

On an aerial photo, such things as the route of the parade, the outlines of the proposed annexation to the city or other information can be indicated.

Arrows drawn on a photograph can indicate direction.

Dotted lines can show the path the automobile careened or other information.

Lines can be superimposed on a picture of a building to show the space the proposed addition will fill.

Just a few simple lines and symbols easily added can increase the value of a photograph enormously.

---

[3] Good advice about retouching is contained in an article, "Retouching Photos Is Easy With Practice," by Edmund C. Arnold in the July 9, 1960, *Publishers' Auxiliary*. Some ideas for this chapter have been drawn from it.

208  Photodiagrams of football plays do a wonderful job of explaining what happened.  *Carl Franks, Cedar Rapids (Iowa) Gazette*

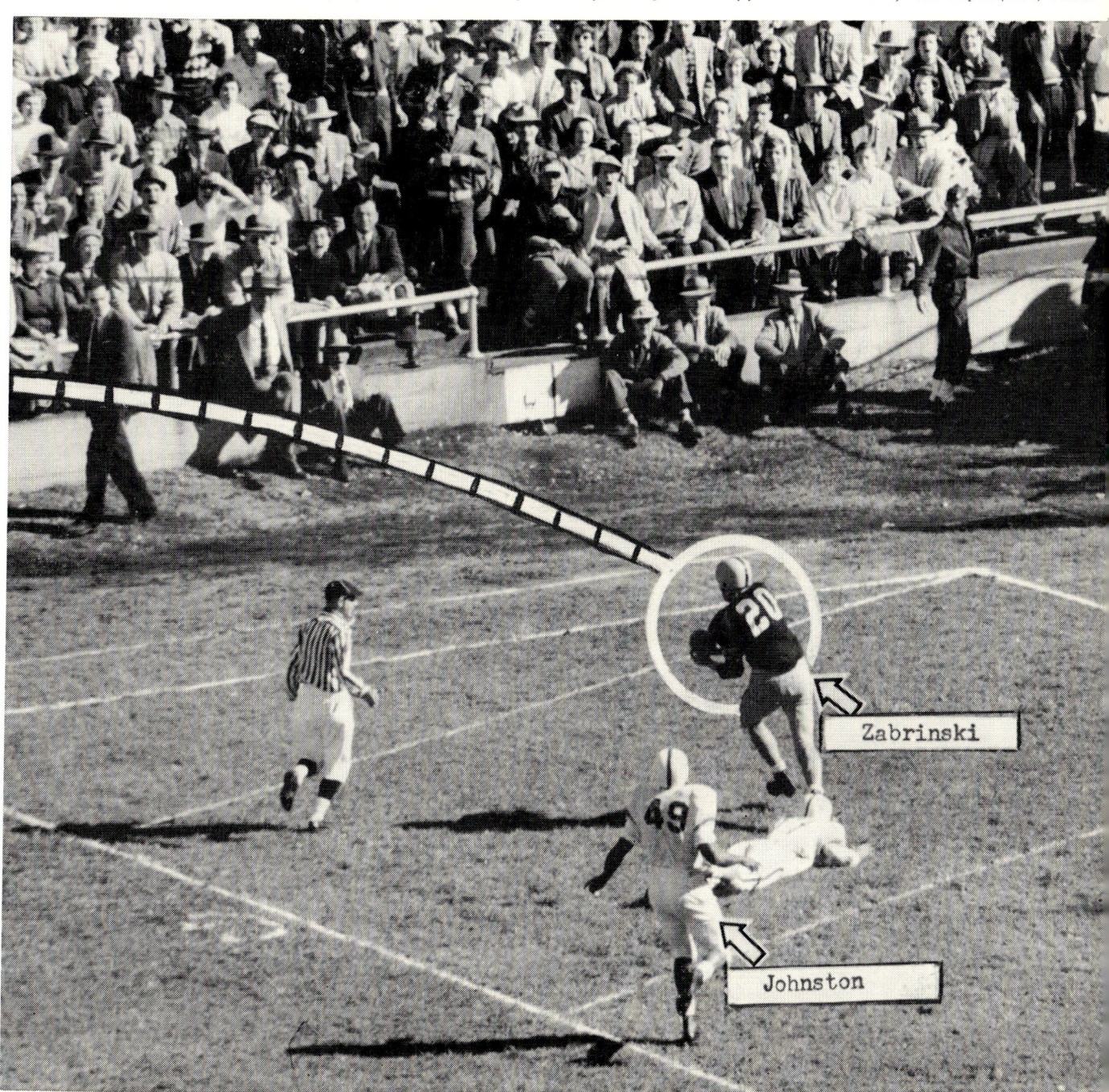

— 169

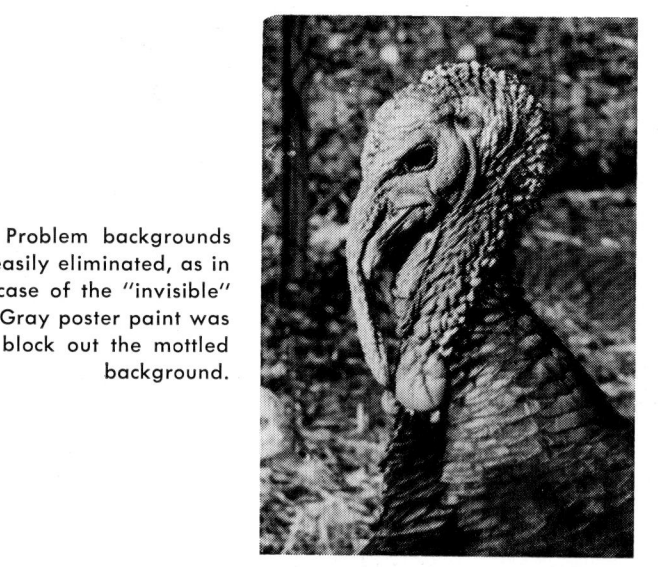

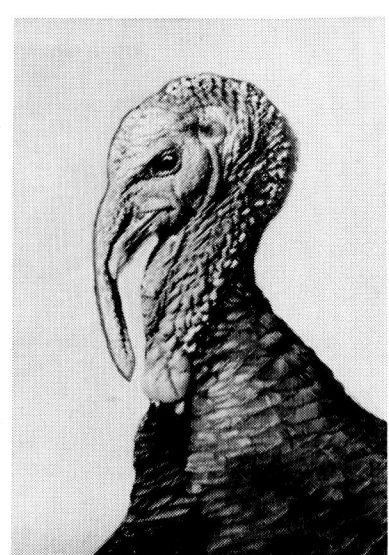

Problem backgrounds can be easily eliminated, as in this case of the "invisible" turkey. Gray poster paint was used to block out the mottled background.

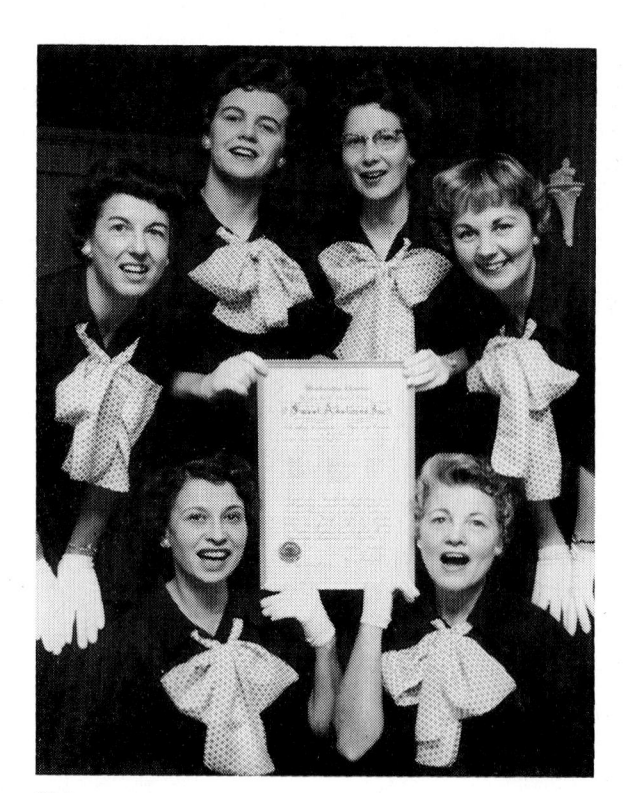

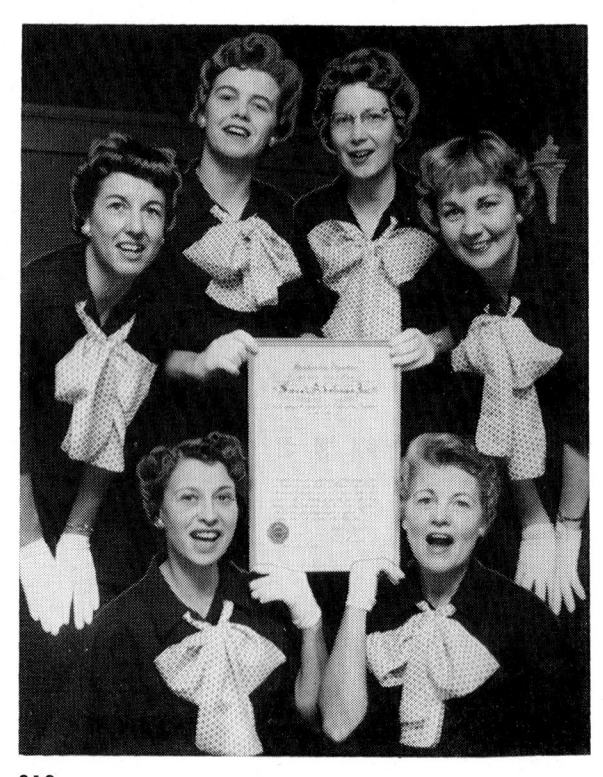

209    210

211    212

When dark hair or clothing fade into the background (Photo 211) they can be lightened by accenting the highlights (Photo 212) or by eliminating the background altogether (Photo 213).

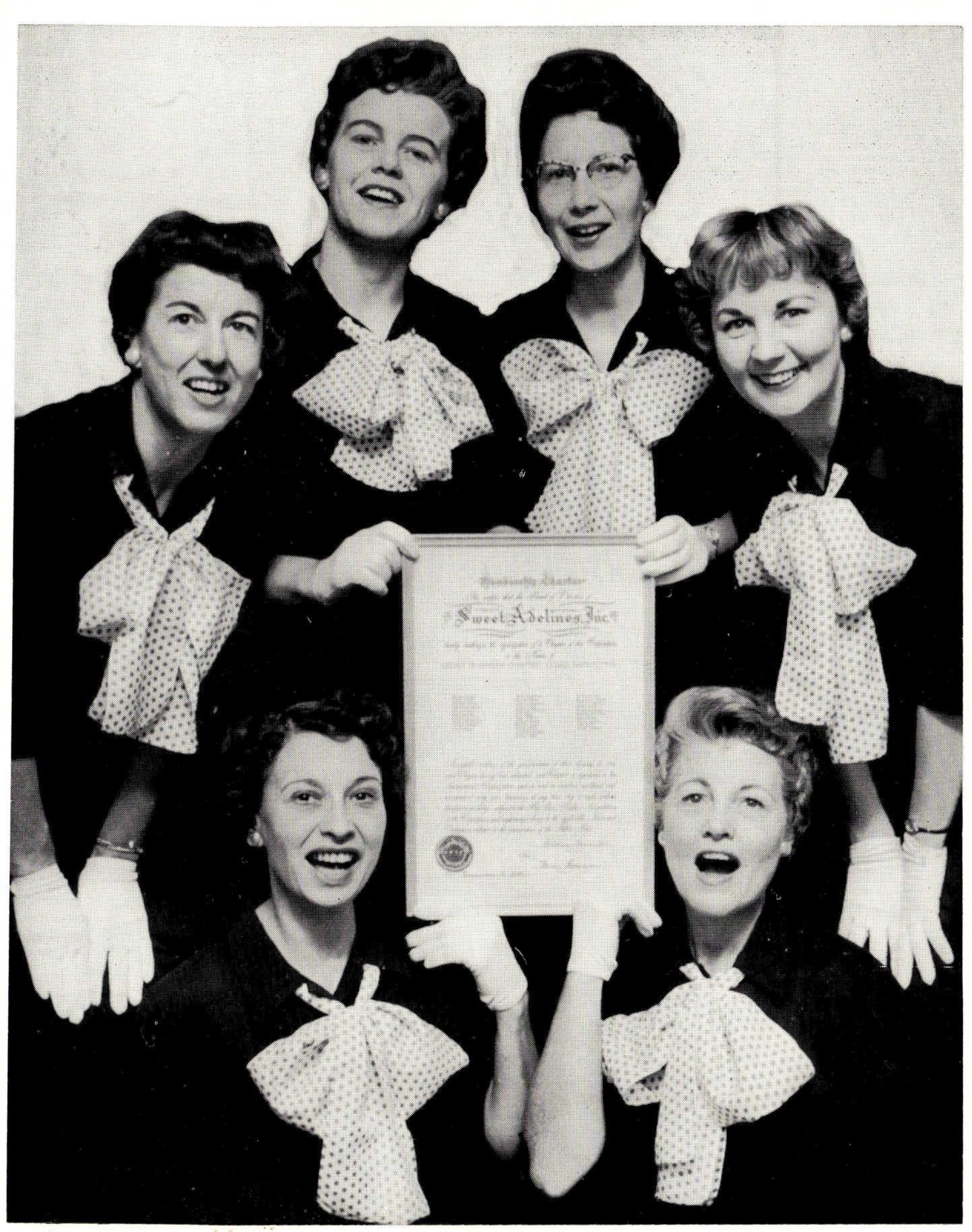

CHAPTER **22**

# Creative Imagination

ADD TOGETHER good, newsworthy subject matter, intelligent pictorial composition and technically good photography and you're bound to have good pictures. But some pictures with all three of these qualities seem better than others rich with the same three essentials. Why?

One answer seems to be imagination. When a photographer sees a subject in a fresh and delightful way, catches in his picture of it little overtones of humor or pathos or whimsey or beauty, his picture is almost sure to be at least a bit exceptional.

Maybe a little of the color of the photographer's personality enhancing his photographs is what makes them imaginative. Maybe it's just that his pictures reflect the warmth and compassion he feels toward the people he portrays. Maybe his picture stands out because he catches some of the delight he feels in the way light falls on objects and the way they group themselves in space. Maybe the joy he takes in telling a story achieves a quality in his photograph just as a similar joy shows itself in the work of a great novelist. Maybe it's just that he feels deeply about the world he photographs.

Whatever the cause, some pictures have this quality of creative imaginativeness. They have the ability to arouse deep, quick emotional responses. Perhaps some people shy away from them to avoid the wear and tear of emotional reaction, but most people seem to enjoy emotions. Probably the imaginative pictures are remembered for more than a few fleeting moments.

**Worth Playing Up**

When a picture rich with this illusive quality presents itself, it's worth playing up in size and placement. Such pictures don't show up often in most papers. A few papers publish exceptionally imaginative pictures often. A few rare publications are consistently filled with them. This quality is worth striving for, for even one or two really imaginative pictures in an issue can lift the feeling toward a newspaper or magazine.

Most of the pictures in this book have some of this quality of imagination. Many of them are loaded with it. Some of the pictures that seem best to illustrate what is meant by creative imagination have been collected in this chapter.

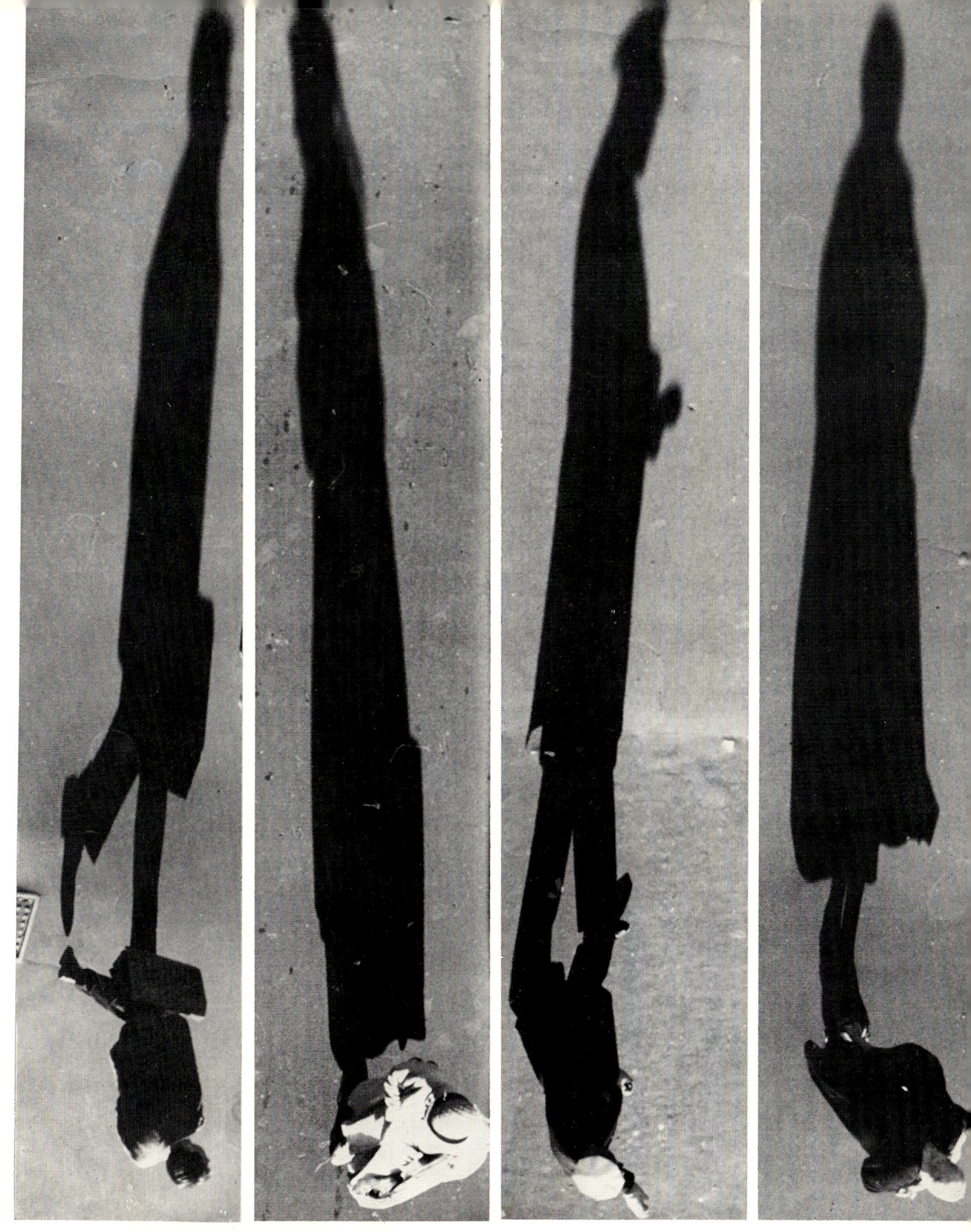

214     Creative imagination discovered this series of shadow caricatures, by Gordon Converse. *Reprinted by permission of* The Christian Science Monitor

215   And creative imagination saw this St. Swithin's Day reflection.
*Harvey Weber,* Newsday, Long Island

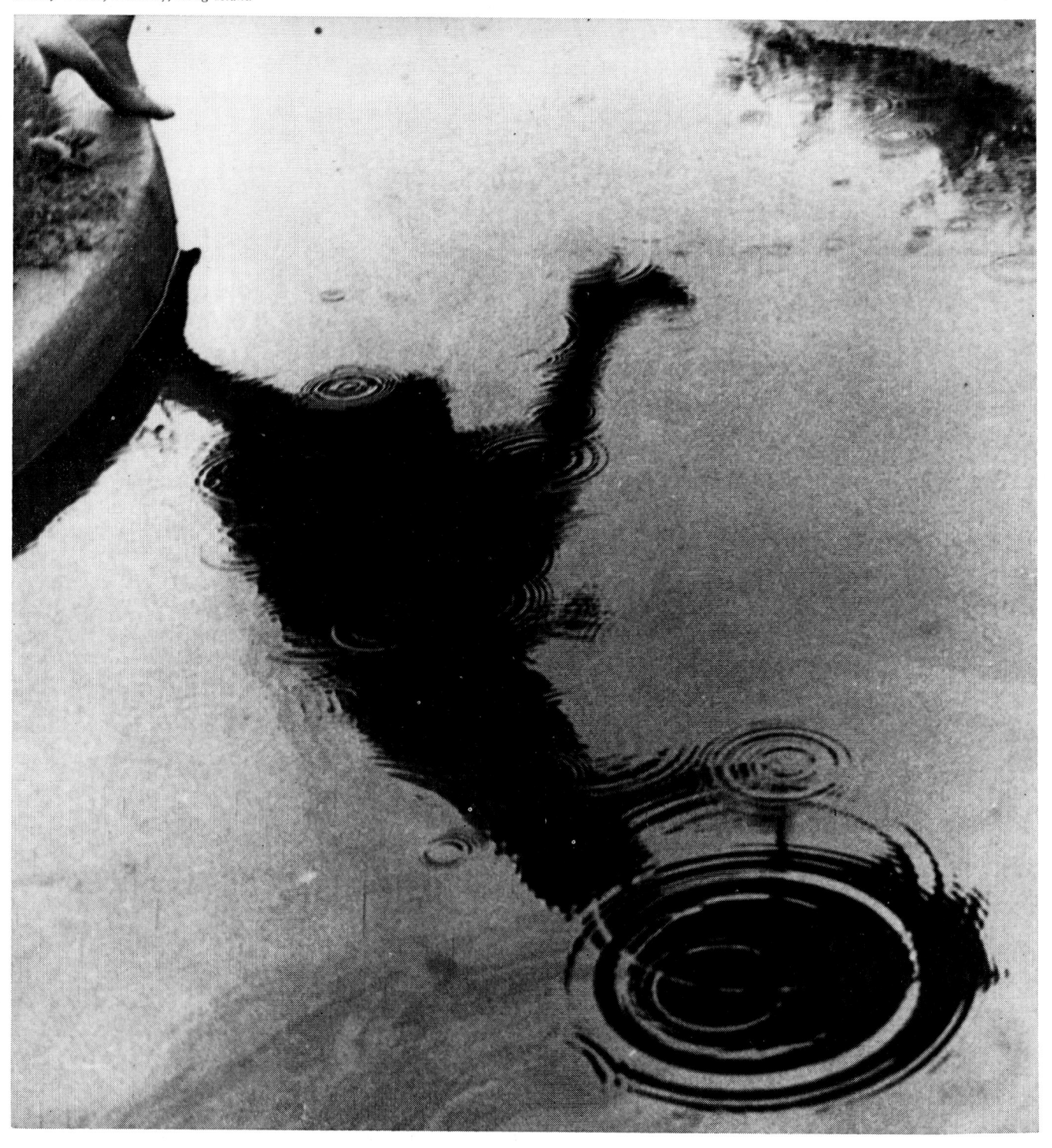

216   Summer fog.
*Rodney Fox*

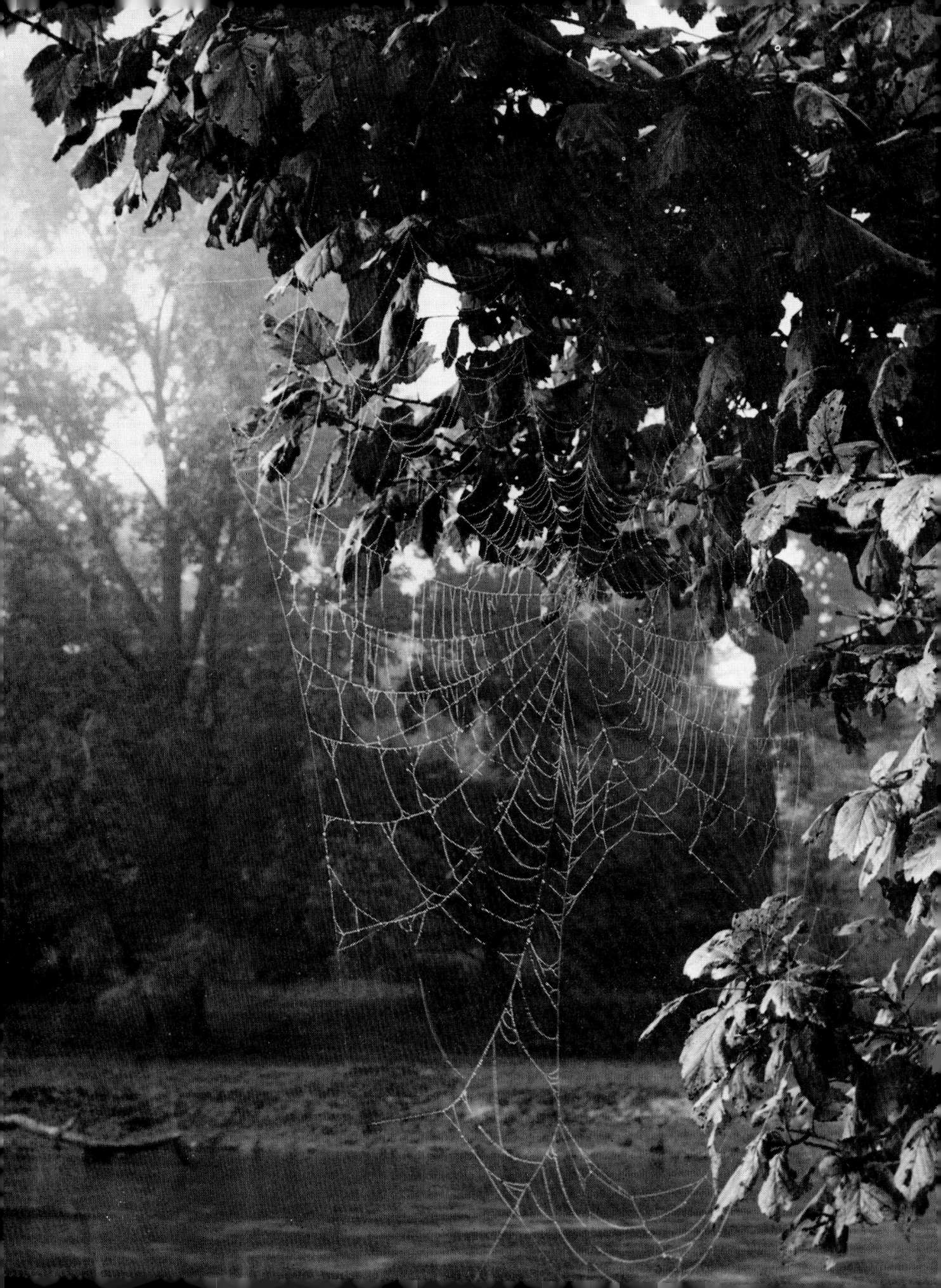

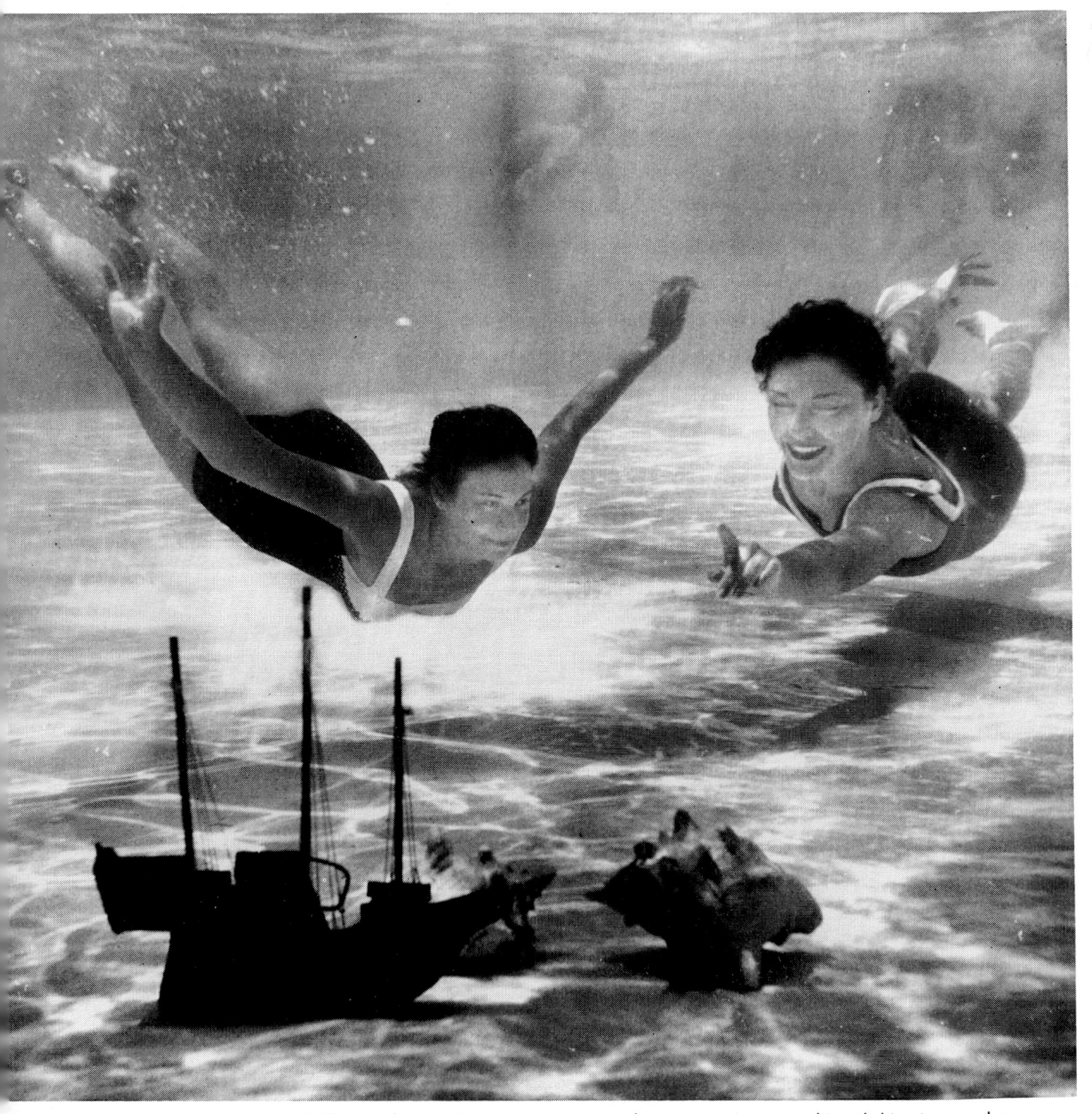

217   Imagination, not expensive underwater equipment, achieved this picture taken by a twin lens reflex on the bottom of a water-proofed wooden box with a glass window on one side.

*Photo by Clifford R. Yeich, courtesy Reading (Pa.) Times*

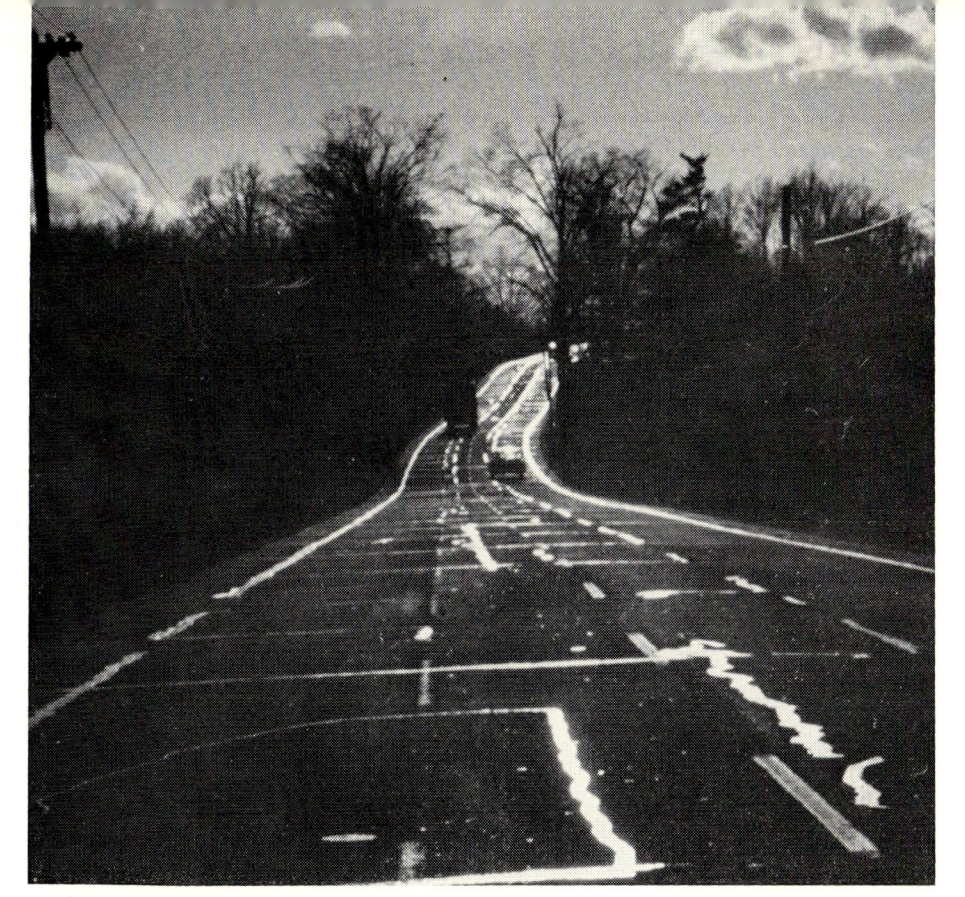

218

*by Larry Mulvehill, Middletown (N.Y.) Daily Record*

A road may be only a road, but to the imaginative photographer a highway can suddenly flame with sunlight or become the setting for comedy.

219

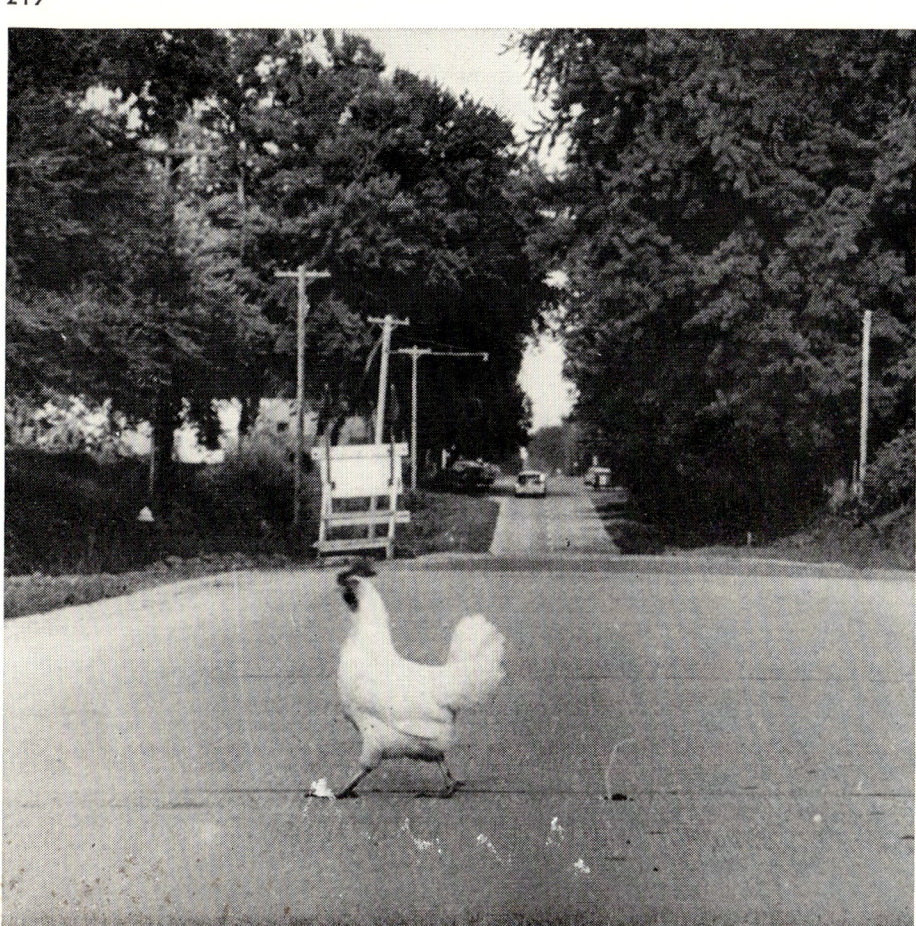

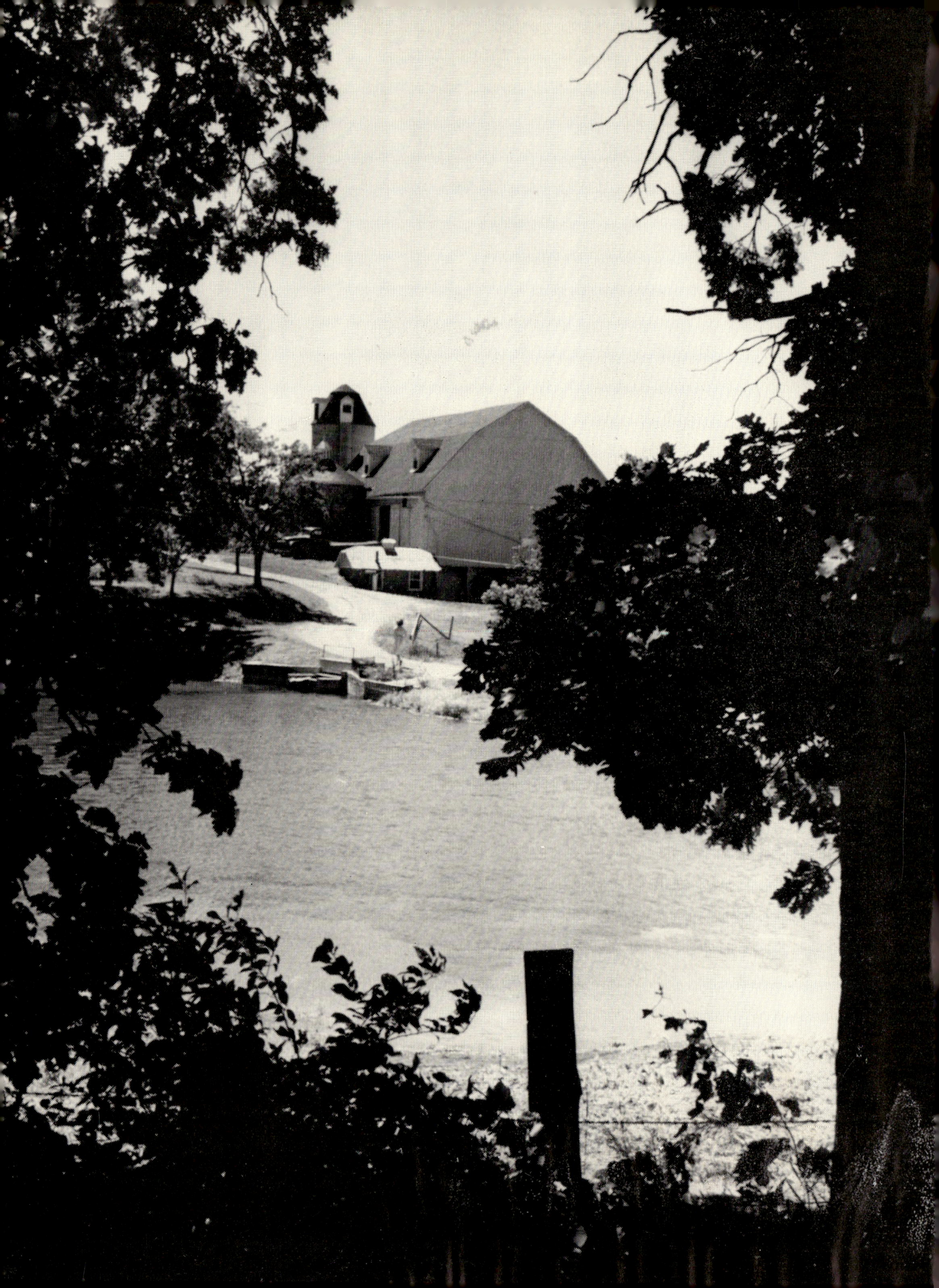

*These magnificent examples of creative photography . . .*

# The Stream

*by* Angus McDougall

*incorporate excellent composition*

*. . . fine camera technique*

*. . . achieve mood*

*. . . and tell a great deal about a country stream.*

*The 19 photographs and map, together with brief cutlines in poetry that made up their original publication, filled eight pages and the front cover of an issue of Harvester World, International Harvester Company publication, which granted permission for reproduction.*

*This picture, used on the cover, served as an introduction and a promise of the things inside.*

— 179

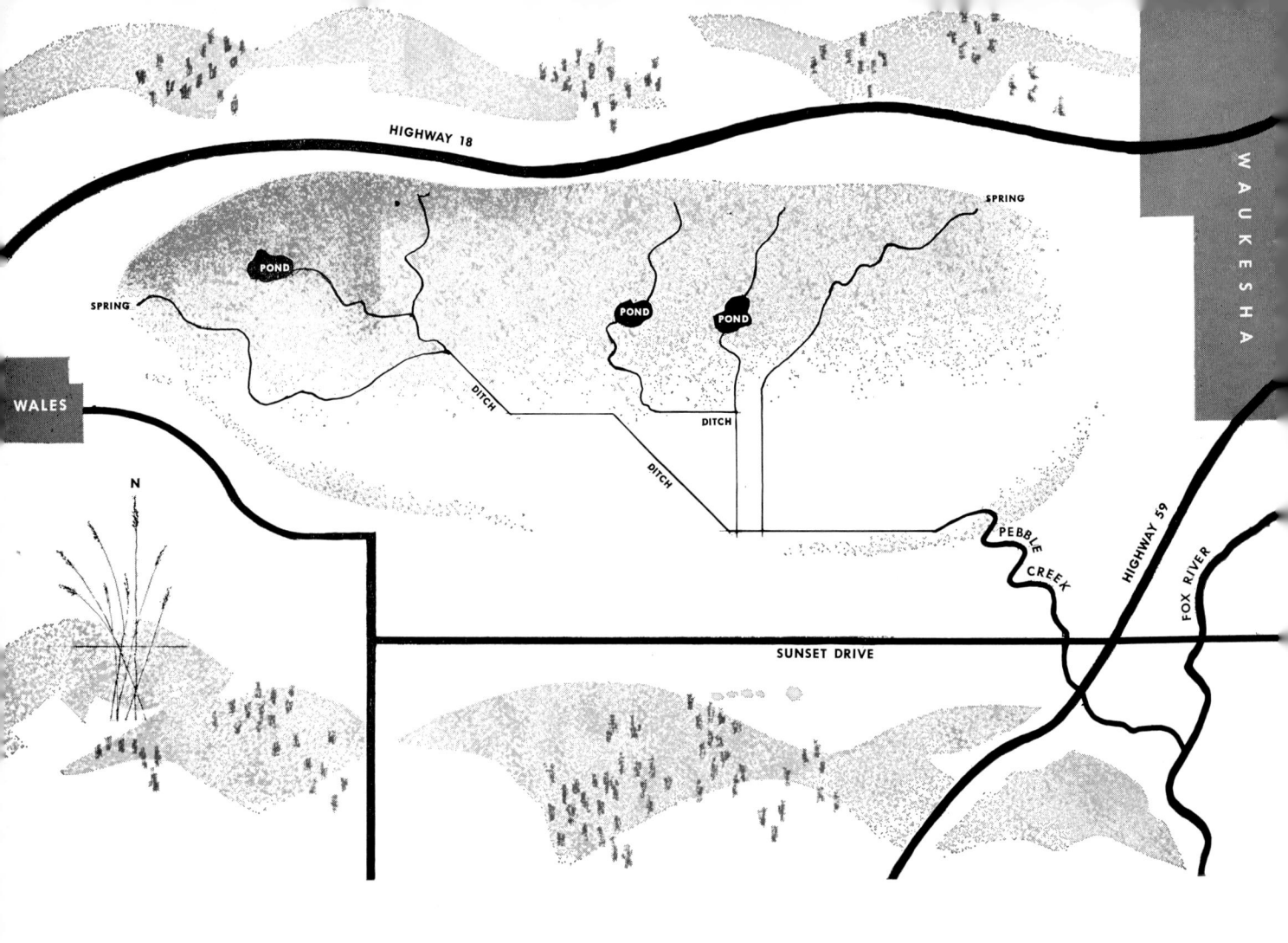

*This map, along with the aerial view, gave an over-all picture ...*

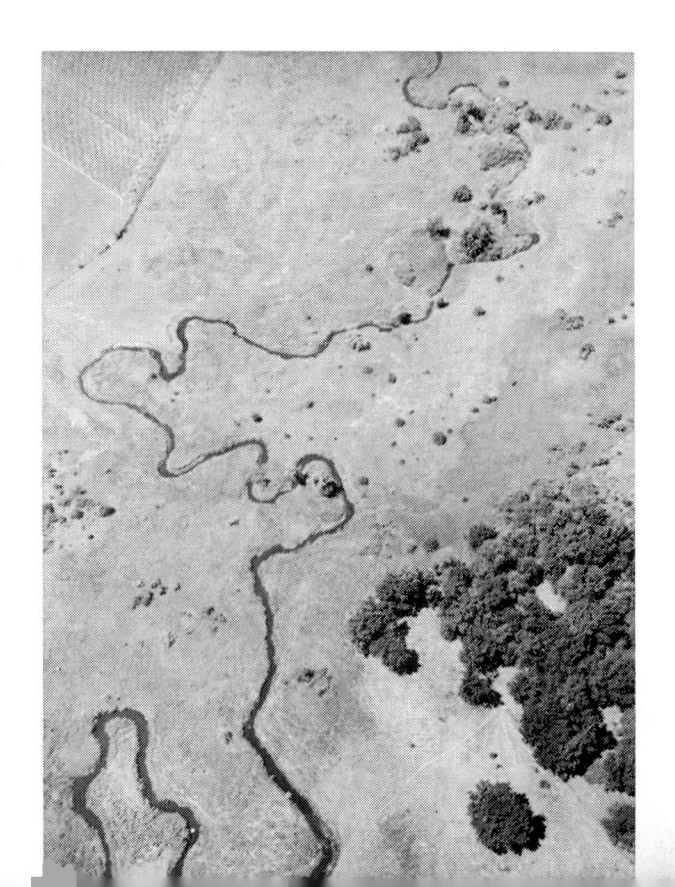

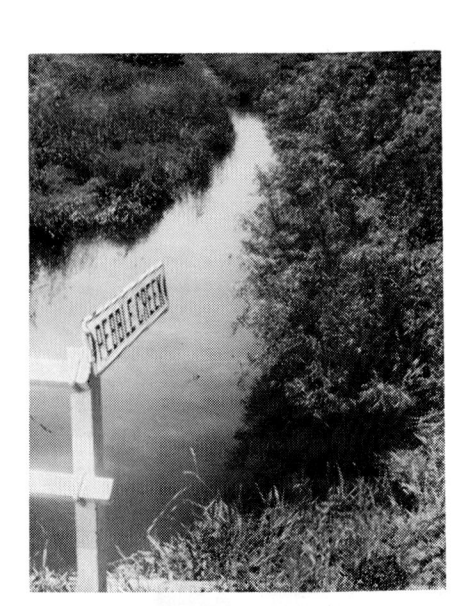

*... of Pebble Creek.*

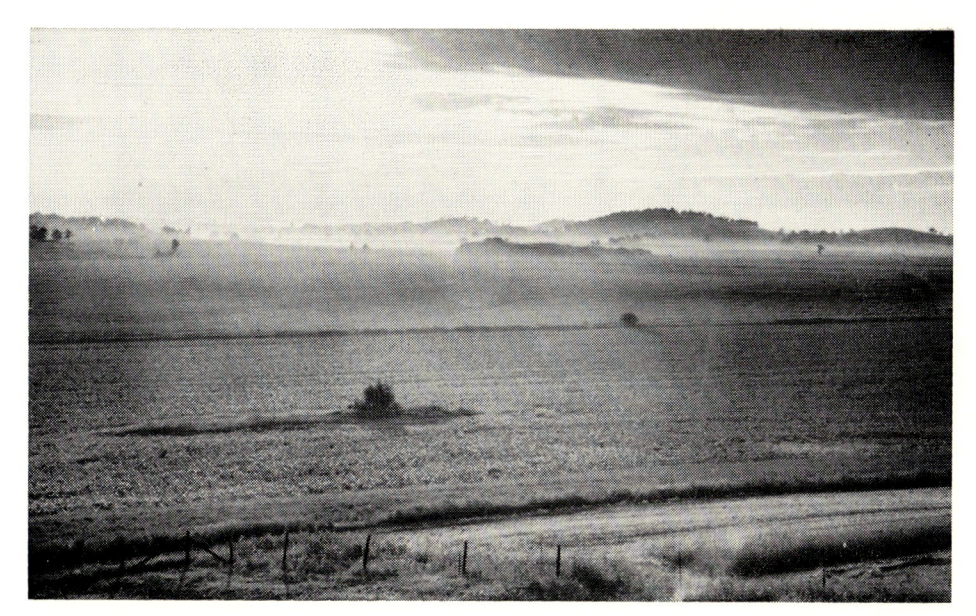

*Here are the hills from which it flows . . .*

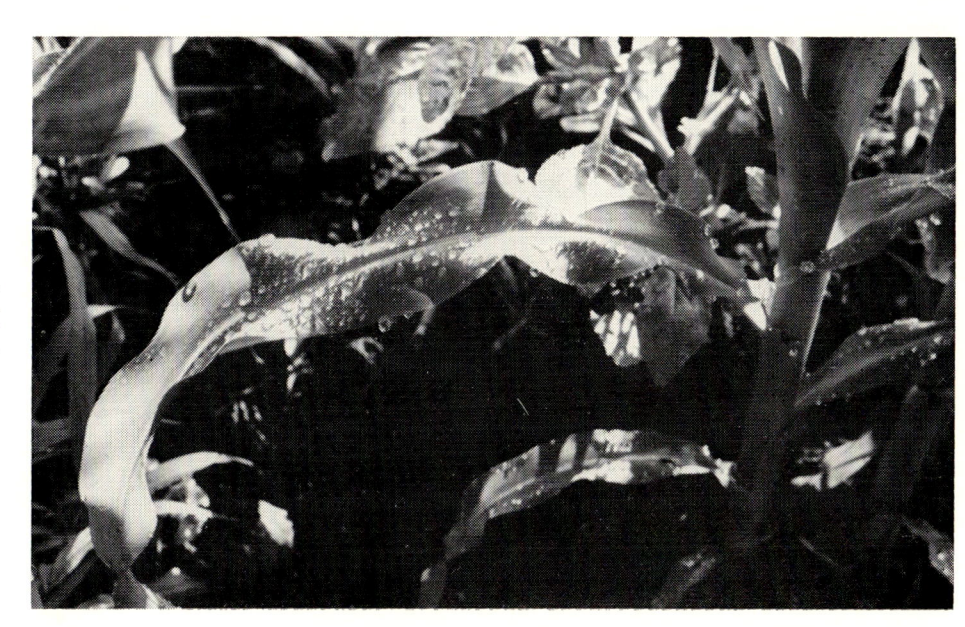

*Past moist corn in fields along its sides . . .*

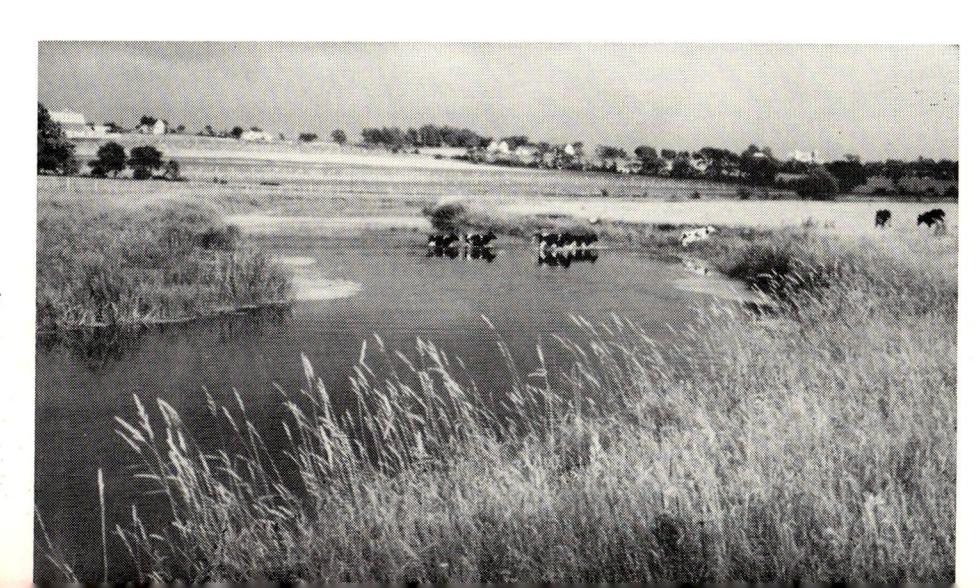

*Until it ends in the river.*

*The clouds bring sustaining rain . . .*

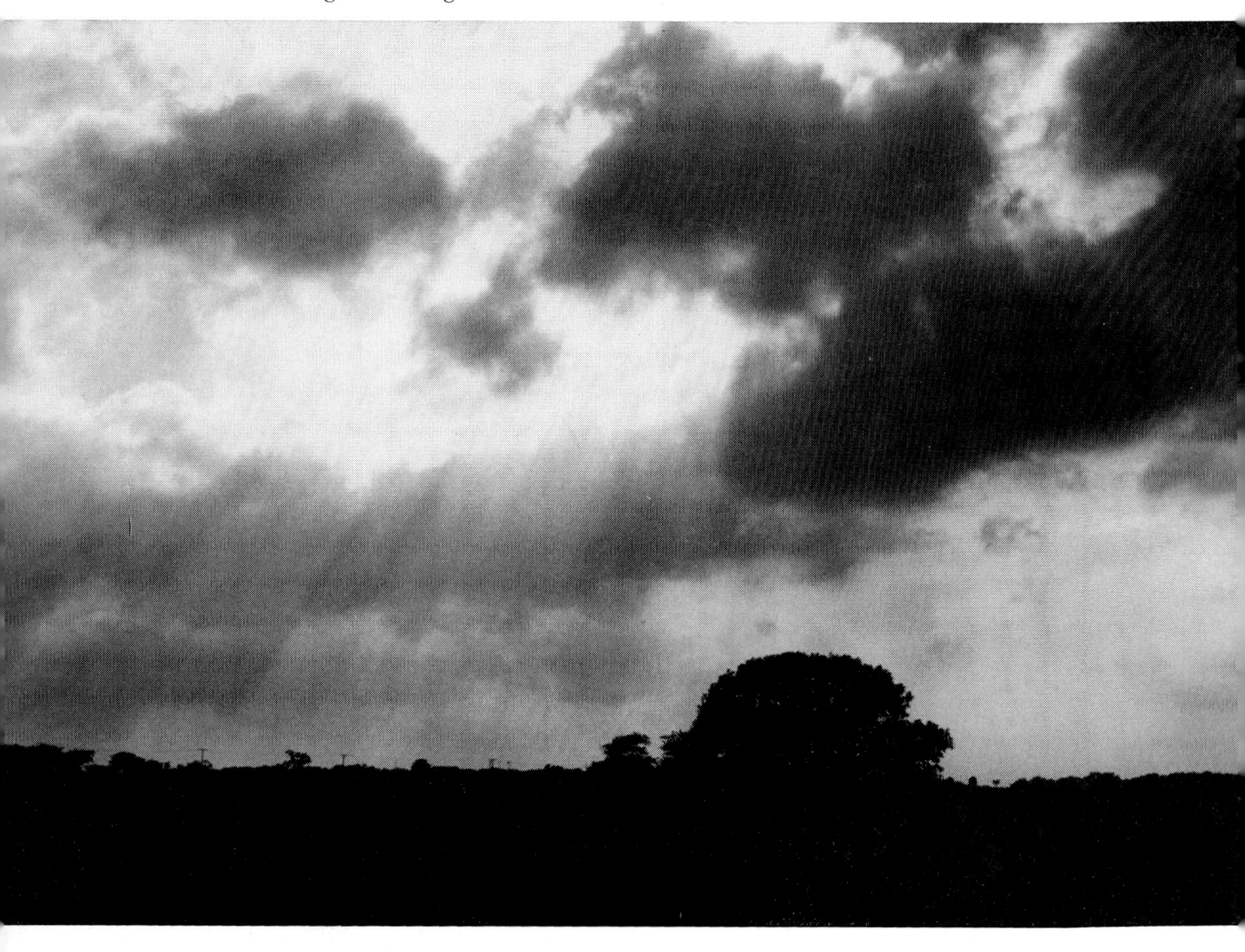

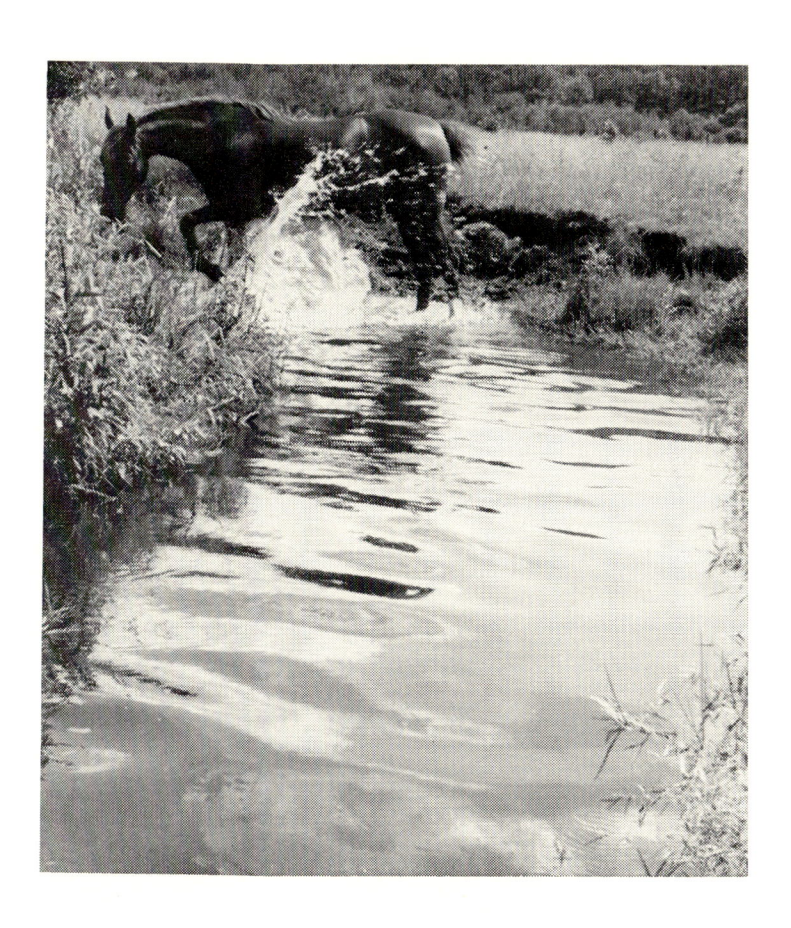

*To keep it full for
mares to splash in.*

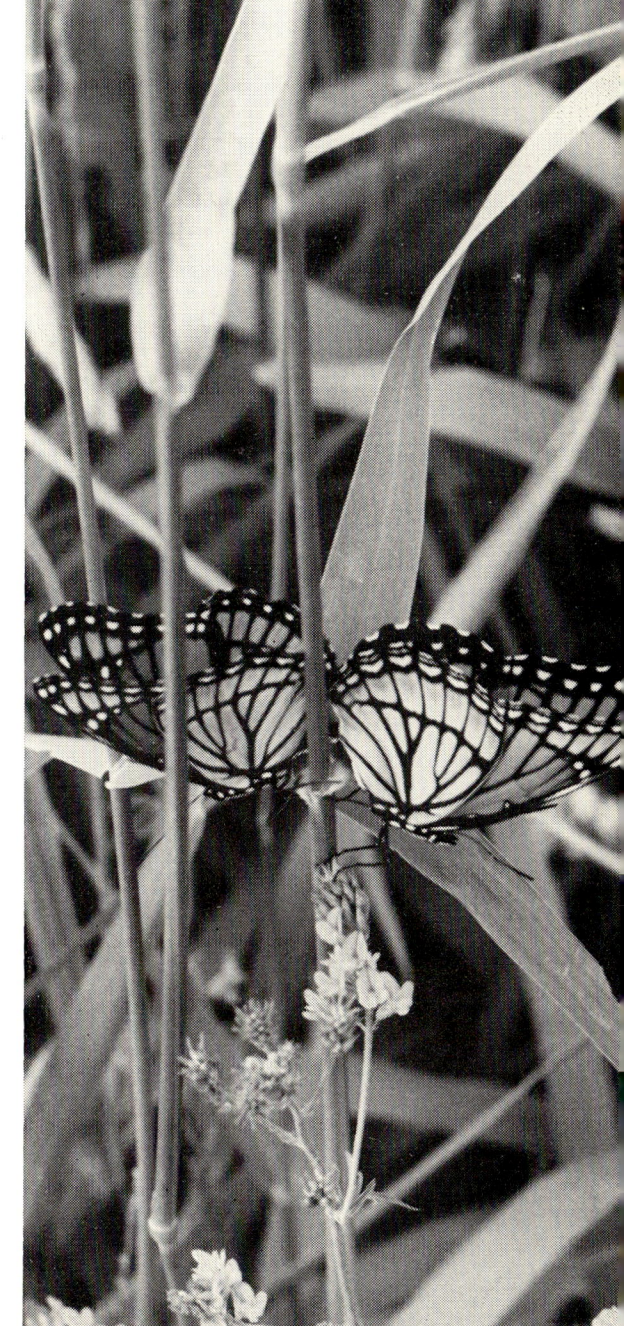

*Beside its course
monarchs mate . . .*

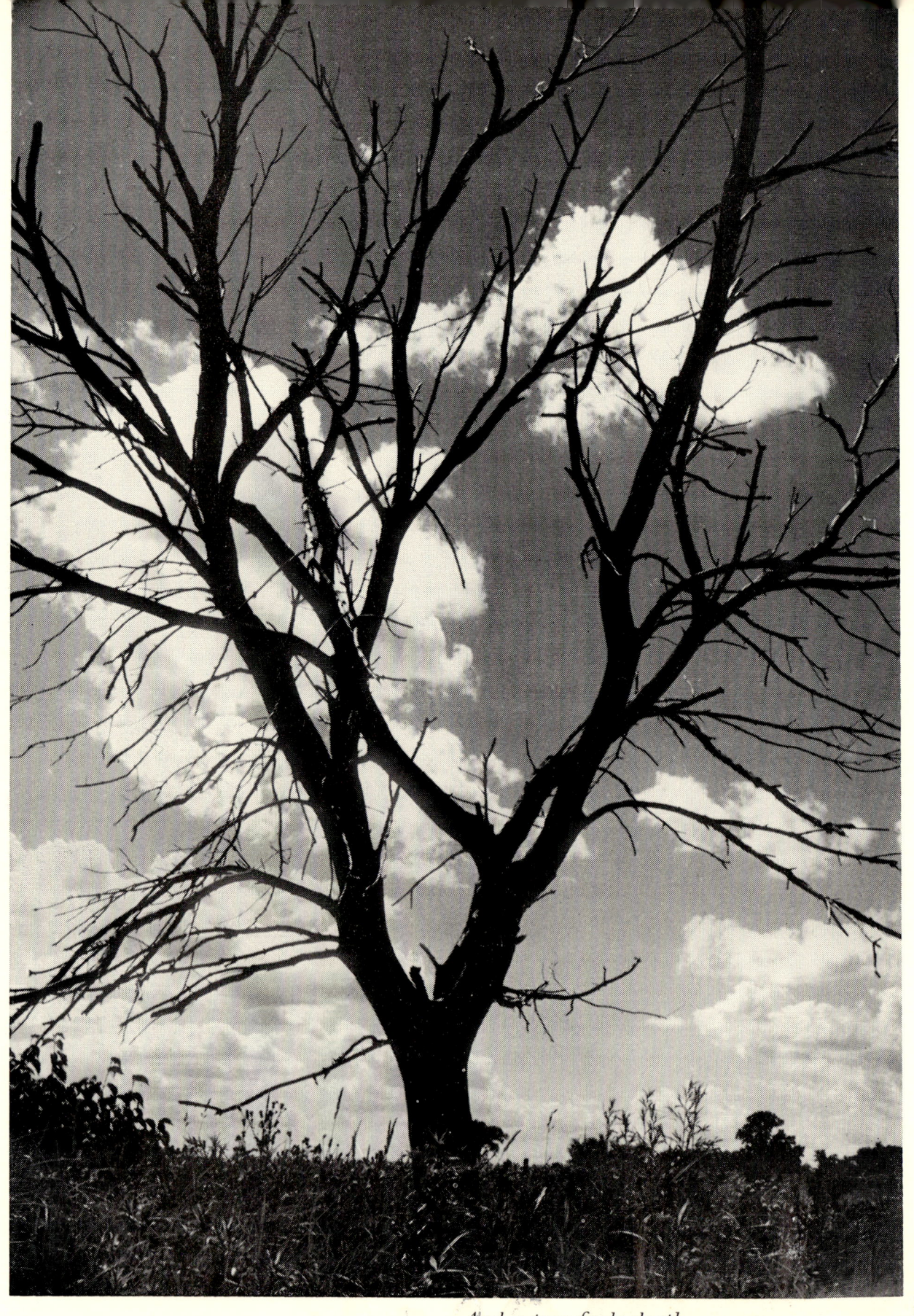

*And a tree finds death.*

*Water striders skate on its surface...*

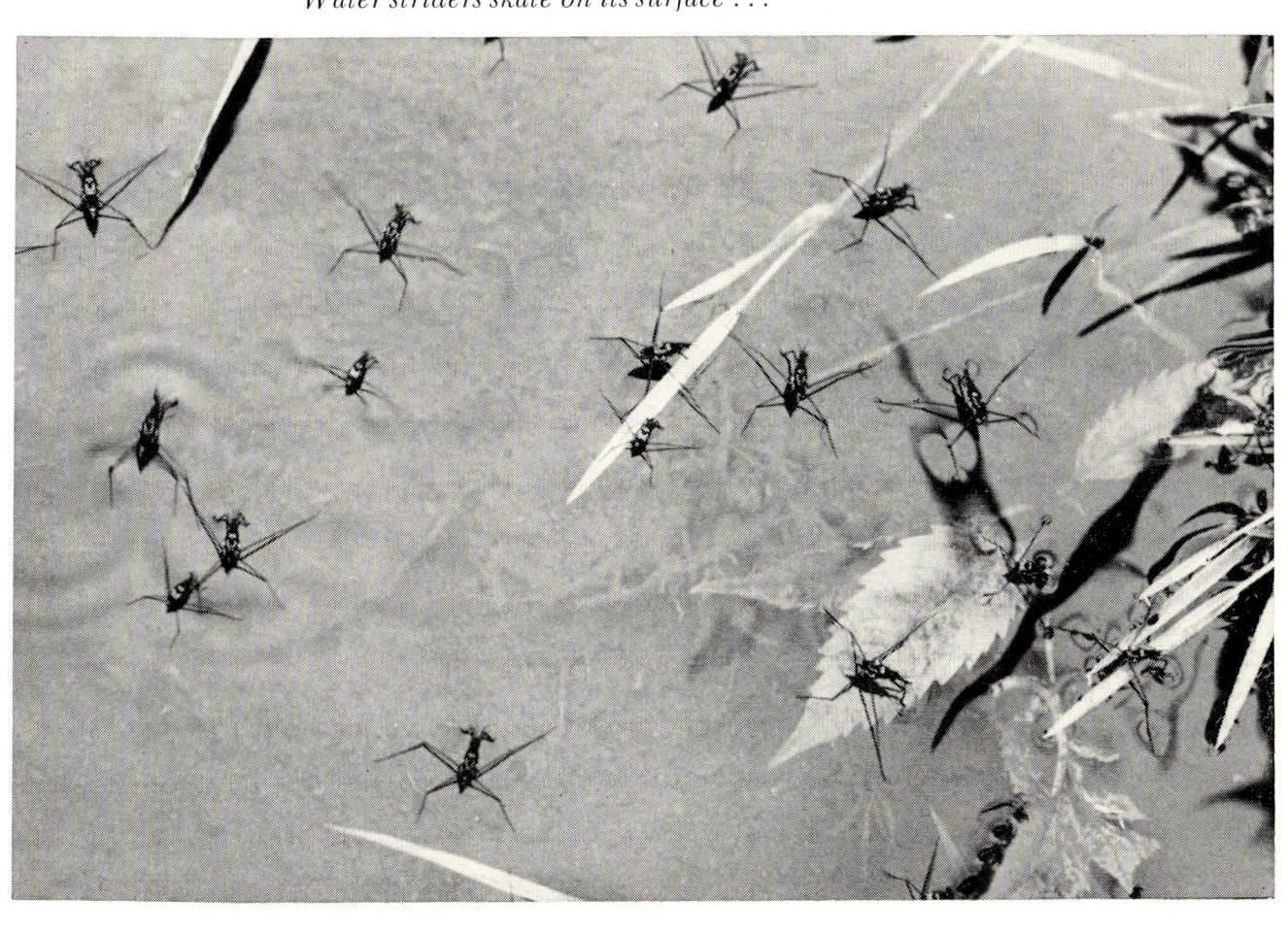

*And seiners seek its minnows.*

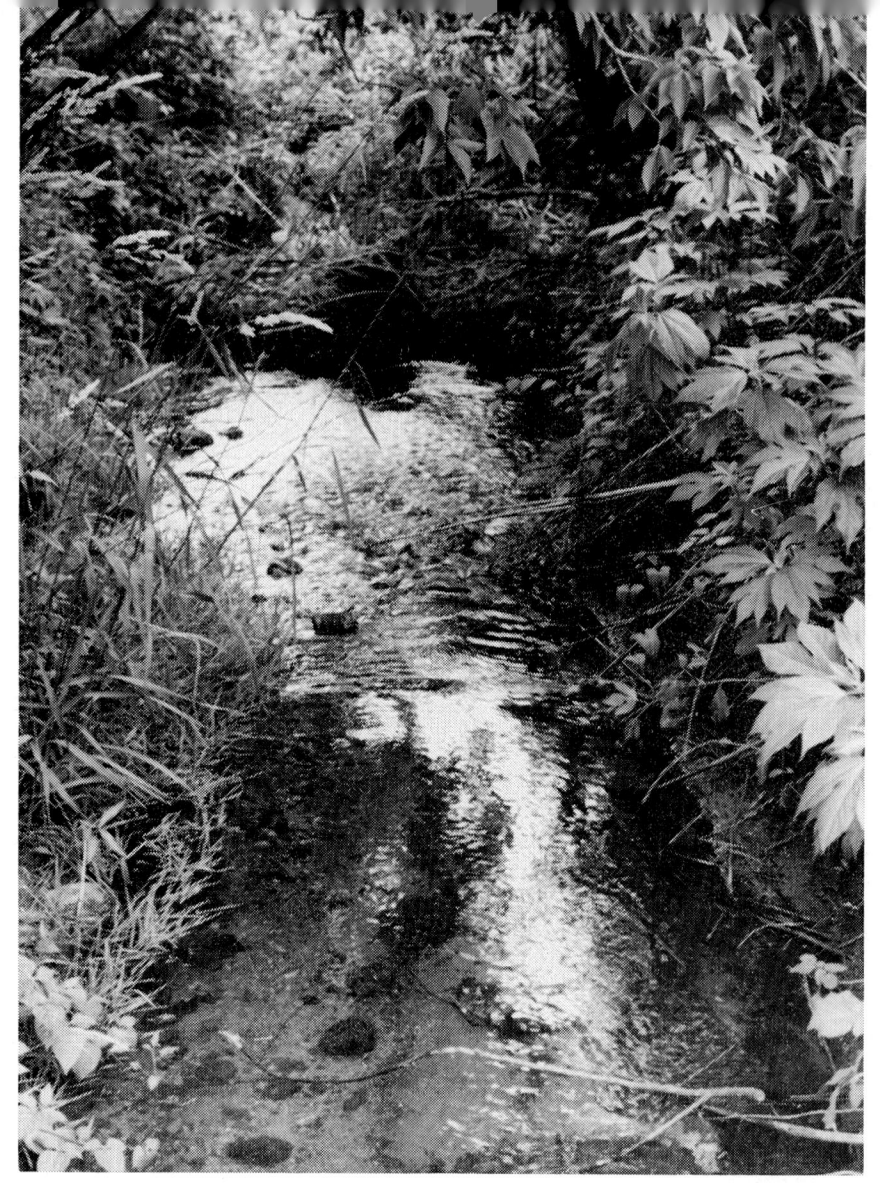

*Light glitters
from its surface . . .*

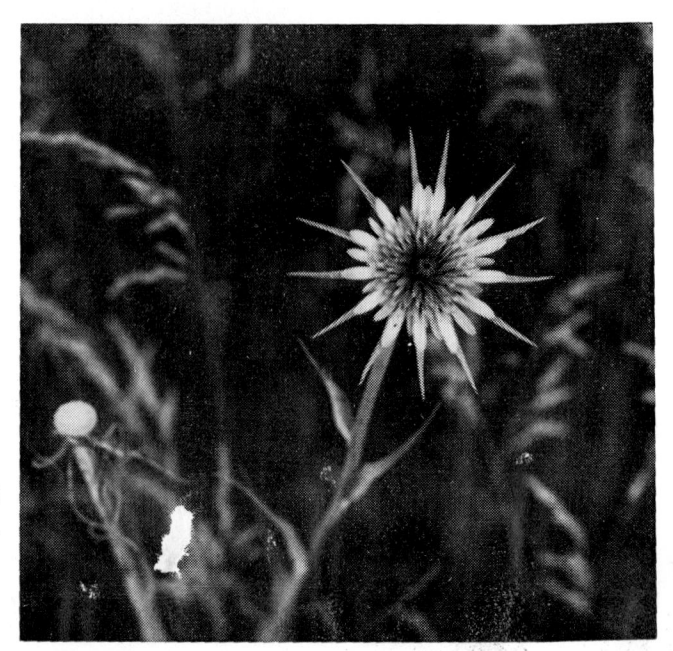

*Wild parsnip
blooms above it . . .*

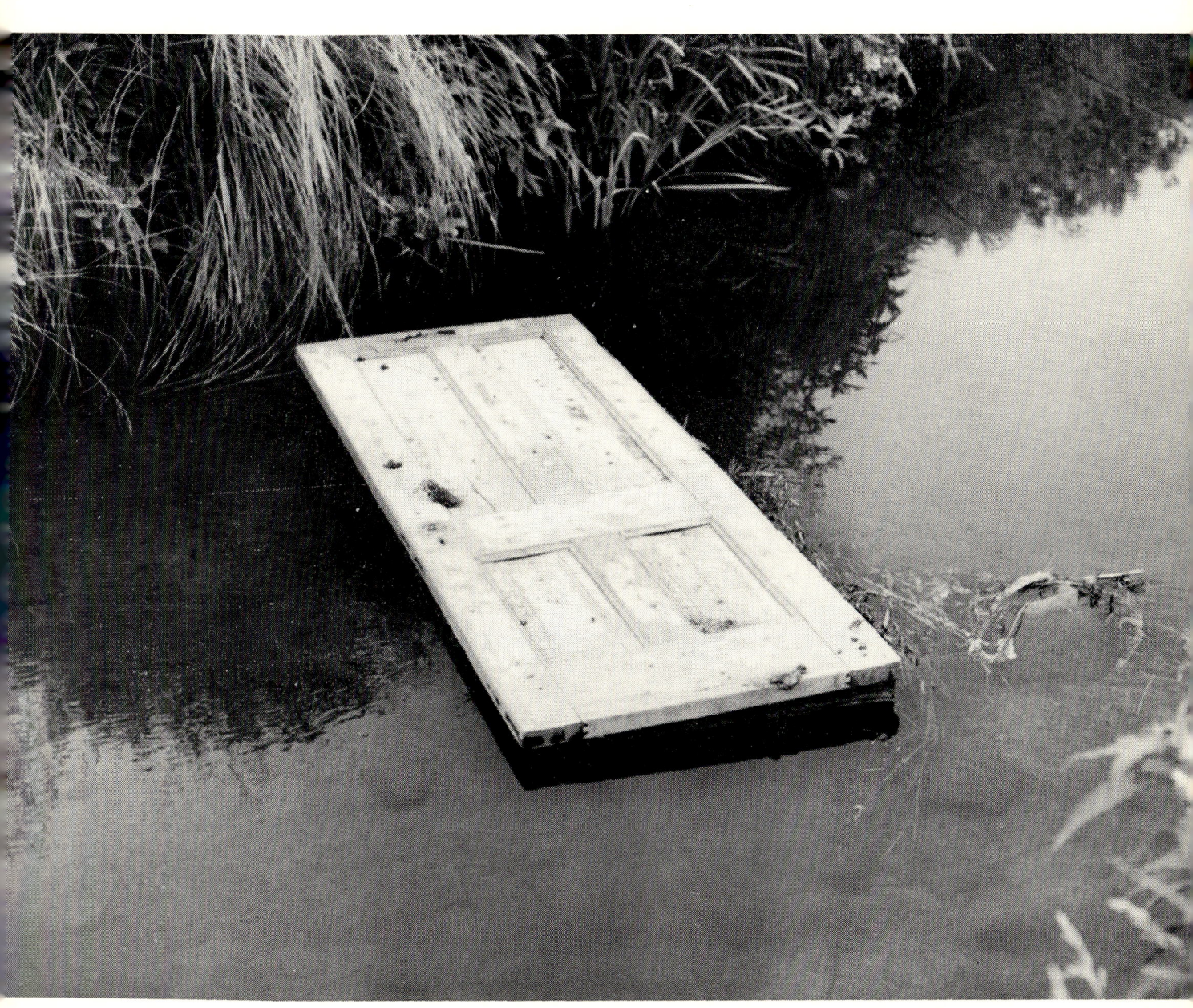

*And a ship abandoned by young sailors floats downstream.*

# Other Books You Might Want To Read

Arnheim, Rudolf, *Art and Visual Perception.* University of California Press, Berkeley, 1957.

A long and somewhat complex book concerning art and research in psychology. Very rewarding for persons interested enough in pictorial composition to read it.

Bethers, Ray, *Photo-Vision.* St. Martin's Press, Inc., New York, 1957.

A simple, imaginative, extremely useful book about pictorial composition. With many pictures and diagrams and few words it does an excellent job of outlining fundamentals.

Deschin, Jacob, *Say It With Your Camera*, Ziff-Davis, New York, 1960.

A book intended for serious amateurs, but it contains many excellent ideas for news photographers.

Evans, Ralph M., *Eye, Film and Camera in Color Photography.* John Wiley & Sons, Inc., New York, 1960.

Mostly about color but strong on photographic esthetics. Not aimed at news photographers, but helpful to determined ones.

Haz, Louise, *Image Arrangement.* The Haz Book Co., Pittsburg, 1956.

A brief, simple and helpful book about photographic composition.

Hicks, Wilson, *Words and Pictures,* Harpers, New York, 1952.

A frequently read book about photojournalism.

Kalish, Stanley E., and Edom, Clifton C., *Picture Editing.* Rinehard & Co., New York, 1951.

This textbook has many excellent pictures and much information concerning news pictures.

Kepes, Gyorgy, *Language of Vision.* Paul Theobald and Company, Chicago, Ill., 1959.

Extraordinarily difficult for persons not familiar with art jargon, but full of creative ideas about photography and art.

Rhode, Robert B., and McCall, Floyd H., *Press Photography,* Macmillan, New York, 1961.

A textbook for photojournalism students.

Rothstein, Arthur, *Photojournalism*: *Pictures for Magazines and Newspapers.* American Photographic Book Publishing Co., New York, 1956.

Beautifully illustrated with the photographs of a master photojournalist.

Sidey, Hugh, and Fox, Rodney, *1,000 Ideas for Better News Pictures.* Iowa State University Press, Ames, 1956.

A simple book intended especially to help editors and photographers on weekly and small daily newspapers but useful for house organ and small magazine editors, too.

# Index

(Boldface page numbers refer to photographs.)

Accidents, 30, 118, 159
Action, 69, 94, 130, 132, 133, 134, 135, 136, 137, 138, 139
    games, rural, 63
    how to photograph, 131
    movement, 86, 94, 101, 131
    in pictures, 131–39
    in portraits, 141
    sequence photos, 39
Advertisers, 53
Advertising, 105
    pictures in, 15
Aerial photography, 32, 44, 102, 180
    photomaps, 168
    photos, 168
    photos, retouching of, 168
Agricultural, Agriculture. see Farms
Albuquerque (N.Mex.) Journal, 26
Ames (Iowa) Daily Tribune, 45
Andre, Paul, photos, 46, 47
Angles, 92, 93
    camera, 73, 105, 133, 147
Animals, 15, 22, 22, 26, 30, 82, 113, 114, 139
    birds, 55
    cats, 22, 82
    cattle, 44, 181
    and children, 1, 15, 22
    deer, 30
    dogs, 15, 21, 22, 61, 62, 66, 99, 130
    farm, 44, 45
    hogs, 45, 166
    horses, ponies, 1, 23, 45, 113, 114, 183
    and man, 23
    poultry, 177
    rodeo, 132
    sheep, 25, 47
    snakes, 18
    swine, 45
    wild, 30, 60, 61
Antiques, 37, 59
Architecture, 14, 85, 86, 87, 90, 93, 104
Arnold, Edmund C., 15
Art, 70, 146, 154
Arts, 71, 72
Attention, 11–16
    reader, 11–16
Auction, 36–38, 46
Aurora borealis, 117
Authenticated News, 101
Automobiles, 66. see also Cars, Transportation
Awards, presentation of, 155. see also Groups

Babies, 48, 88. see also Children, People
Backgrounds. see Composition, Pictures
Backlighting, 112, 113. See also Composition, Pictures
Bacon, Leonard, photo, 110
Balance. see Composition, Pictures
Barnes, Curt, photo, 120, 124
Barns. see Farm, Buildings
Bartley, Bob, photo, 45
Baseball. see Sports
Basketball. see Sports
Beasley, Bob, photo, 25, 43
Beecroft, Dick, 15
Benn, Charles, photo, 102
Bicycling, 12. see also Hobbies, Sports
Birds, 55. see also Animals
Birdwatchers, 55. see also Hobbies
Boats, 13, 57, 103. see also Hobbies

Borer, Del, photo, 136
Breinig, Peter, photo, 94
Bridgeton (N. J.) News, 15
Brinton, Jack, photo, 40
Brownlee, George, photo, 69
Buildings, 14, 25, 32, 33
    churches, 14, 45, 85, 87, 161
    farm, 25, 178
    houses, 32
    schools, 32–33, 68, 157, 160
Burley (Idaho) Herald, 10
Burrows, R. O., Jr., 14
Butterflies, 183. see also Nature

Camera angle, 105. see also Angles
Caricatures, 173. see also Composition
Carlson, Jerry, 47
Cars, 66. see also Automobiles, Transportation
Cats, 22, 82. see also Animals
Cattle, 44, 181. see also Animals
Cedar Rapids (Iowa) Gazette, 39, 46, 47, 52, 63, 73, 132, 147, 169
Charlotte (N. C.) Observer, 12, 22, 23, 27, 82, 83, 84, 113, 132, 144, 145, 164–65
Cheesecake, 65. see also People
Children, 12, 15, 16, 19, 20, 26, 30, 32–33, 50, 51, 54, 73, 81, 85, 88, 96, 117, 132, 133, 134, 135, 137, 138, 146, 147, 152, 157, 160, 162–63, 164–65
    and animals, 15, 22
    Boy Scouts, 93
    group, 149
    at play, 19
Christian Science Monitor, 173
Christmas, 153
Churches. see Buildings, Religious
Circulation, 11, 14
City scenes, 26, 27
Clarion Publications (Napierville, Ill.), 162, 163
Clouds. see Nature, Scenic
Clubs, 54, 144, 154. see also Groups
Colburn, John J., 13, 14
College life, 65, 143, 154
Color photography, 13. see also ROP
    advantages of ROP, 121
    cost of ROP, 129
    Curtis color analyst, 127
    equipment, ROP, 123
    example of ROP, 120, 124, 126, 128
    methodology of ROP, 123
    negative, 121, 123
    newspapers pioneering in ROP, 122
    one-shot, 121
    photos, 25
    printing, ROP, 127
    reflection transmission densitometer, 127
    reversal, 121
    separation print quality, 122
    separation prints, ROP, 127
    separations, three-color (ROP), 125
    transparency, 123
    use of, 102
    value of ROP, 129
Comedy, 23, 27, 69
Committees, 151, 154. see also Groups
Communications media. see Radio, 45
Composition, 10, 15, 87, 112
    backgrounds, 111, 142, 154, 160
    backgrounds in portraits, 143, 146
    backgrounds, retouching of, 167
    backlighting, 112, 113
    balance, 80–87, 82, 83, 84, 85, 87

    balance, formal, 81
    blank space in pictures, 90
    caricatures, 173
    contrast, 29
    cropping, 79, 79, 143
    curves in pictures, 88, 89–98, 95
    depth, 92
    design, 97, 98
    diagonals, 94
    foreground, dramatic use of, 19
    format, 94
    framing, 78, 78, 92, 113, 145, 178
    guide lines in pictures, 94
    high angle, 147
    layout, 32–33, 35–39, 36–37
    lines, 89, 112, 136, 137
    lines, horizontal, 90
    lines, vertical, 90, 91
    lines and shapes in pictures, 89, 97
    low angle, 73, 133
    organization of pictures, 77–79
    pattern, 101, 102, 103, 107
    of portraits, 143
    print quality, 30
    reflection, 99, 100
    repetition, 10, 83, 99–103, 100, 103
    rhythm in pictures, 101, 101, 103
    shades, use of, 102
    shadows, 173
    shapes, 25, 89, 96, 97–98
    silhouettes, 12, 91, 114
    space, use of, 86
    texture in food photography, 109
    texture in foods, 105
    texture in pictures, 105–9
    tone values, 111–18
    variation in pictures, 101
Conductor & Brakeman, 101
Conflict, 20. see also Mood
Construction work, 104. see also Work
Contests, photo, 54, 63
Contrast, 29. see also Composition
Converse, Gordon, photo, 173
Cooperative Consumer, 25, 43
Costumes, 63, 72, 144, 154
Cows. see Animals
Cox, Charles H., photo, 75
Creative imagination, 172–87
Crews, Mildred T., photo, 104, 117
Cropping, 79, 79, 143
Crops, farm, 181
Crowds, 151. see also Groups, People
Curves in pictures. see Composition
Cutlines, 156–61
    necessity for, 157, 158, 159, 160, 161
    not needed, 161

Dancing, 70, 72, 73
Danger, 16
Davenport (Iowa) Morning Democrat, 22, 48, 54, 56, 139, 166
Death, 19, 30
    impending, 16
Delinquency news, 72
Denver (Colo.) Post, 40, 42
Depth, 92. see also Composition, Pictures
Depth reporting, 31–34
Deschin, Jacob, 24
Design, 97, 98. see also Composition
Des Moines (Iowa) Register, 40, 136
Diagonals in pictures, 94. see also Composition, Pictures
Dogs. see Animals
Dougherty, John W., photo, 50
Drama, 18, 29, 30, 45, 118
    pathos, 30

— 189

Dramatics, amateur, 63
Dramatization, 111
 of familiar, 14
Dubuque (Iowa) Telegraph-Herald, 19, 21, 132
Dye, Bill, photo, 100
Eastman Kodak Co., 122, 123, 125
El Crepusculo (Taos, N. Mex.), 104, 117
Elements, photography of, 25. see also Nature, Weather
Emotion, 28, 29, 48, 157. see also Mood
 exuberance, 67
 laughter, 67
 motherhood, 22, 45, 61
 nostalgia, 28
 nostalgic subjects, 13, 14
 pathos, 30
Environment, 24, 25, 26, 27. see also Scenic
Equipment
 farm, 25, 40, 42, 43, 45, 46, 97
 photo, 24, 146, 174
Escape, a symbol of, 14
Essays, picture, 35–39
Expressions. see Mood
Exuberance, 67. see Emotion

Fall, 126. see also Scenic, Seasons
Family, 150. see also Groups
Fargo (N. Dak.) Forum, 16, 157
Farms, 26
 animals, 25, 41, 44, 45, 47, 166
 auction, 46
 buildings, 25, 178
 chores, 26
 crops, 181
 equipment, 25, 40, 42, 43, 45, 46, 97
 field work, 46
 grain, photography of, 117
 harvest, 25, 42, 43, 117
 harvesting, 40
 haying, 43
 how to photos, 46, 47
 land, 181
 landscape, 43, 90, 102
 news, in urban press, 41
 organizations, 47
 photos, 41–47
 ponds, 178
 publicity for, 43
 scene, planting, 46
 scenes, 25, 111, 113
 stock feeding, 47
 topics, most needed, 47
 work, 40, 84
Farmers, 40
Fashion pictures, 53, 53. see also Women's Pages
Father's Day, 50. see also Special Days
Fire, 30, 45, 94, 112, 116, 135
 as light source, 116
Firemen, 45, 94, 112, 116, 135
Fishing, 61, 185. see also Hobbies, Sports
Flowers, 186. see also Nature
Fog, summer, 175
Foods. see also Women's Pages
 pages, 49
 photography, 49, 50, 50
  feature, 51
  texture in, 109
 recipes and menus, 50
 texture in, 105
Football. see Sports
Foreground, dramatic use of, 19. see also Composition, Pictures
Format, 94. see also Composition
Forrest, James, photo, 26
Fox, Rodney, photo, 90, 93, 175
Framing. see Composition
Franks, Carl, photos, 39, 63, 169
Freaks, 57
Frontier Enterprise (Lake Zurich, Ill.), 19

Frost, Robert, 143
Fuchs, Manny, photo, 147
Games, folk, 63
Ganschow, Cliff, photo, 71, 78, 86
Garden features, 56, 57
Georgia, Lowell, photo, 29, 88, 91, 99, 118
Gillespie, Hugh M., photo, 112
Girls. see People
Glickman, Phil, photo, 30
Grain, photography of, 117. see also Farms
Graphs, 47
Green Bay (Wis.) Press-Gazette, 29, 88, 91, 99, 118
Grinnell (Iowa) Herald-Register, 45
Groups, 93, 148–51
 central figure in, 149
 church, 54
 clubs, 54, 144, 154
 committees, 151, 154
 family, 150
 formal arrangement of, 151, 152
 imaginative distribution, 150
 informal arrangement of, 150
 large, 151, 155
 music, 154
 novelty arrangements, 153
 presentation pictures, 155
 religious, 18, 54
 storytelling quality of, 154
 team sports, 152
 triangular arrangement of, 153
 vertical arrangement of, 152
 women, 48
 variety in pictures, 148–55
Guide lines in pictures, 94. see also Composition, Pictures

Halloween, 162–63. see also Special Days
Hartford (Conn.) Courant, 138
Harvest, 25, 42, 43, 117. see also Farms
Harvester World, 44, 178–87
Harvesting, 40. see also Farms
Hatsian, Arman G., photo, 138
Haying, 43. see also Farms
Health, 96
Heine, Max, photo, 161
Herrmann, A. Martin, photo, 15
Historical features, 13, 28
Hobbies, 56–59. see also Leisure-time pictures, Sports
 bicycling, 12
 birdwatching, 55
 boating, 57, 103
 dancing, 72, 73
 dramatics, amateur, 63
 fishing, 61, 185
 gardening, 56, 57
 horseback riding, 137
 music, 71
 sailing, 73, 103
 swimming, 134, 174
 tennis, 138
Hogs, 45, 166. see also Animals
Holidays, 50. see also Seasons
 Christmas, 153
Home, 48. see also Women's Pages
 furnishings, 52, 52
 interior decorating, 52
Home and Highways Magazine, 95, 108, 150
Home economics, 49. see also Foods, Women's Pages
Horseback riding, 137
Horses. see Animals
Houses, 32. see also Buildings
"How to" pictures, 45, 47, 131
Hungry Horse News (Columbia Falls, Mont.), 14, 24, 60, 61, 82, 85
Hunting, 61, 130

Ice, photography of, 97, 98
Imagination. see Creative imagination
Interior decorating, 52. see also Home, Women's Pages
Interior photography, 52
Interviews, 68
Iowa Conservation Comm., 55
Iowa State University, 90, 92, 102
Iowan, The, 1, 13, 25, 90
Isham, Dick, photo, 126

Johnson, Bob, photo, 45

Kerns, Robert, photo, 17, 22, 26, 32, 33, 45, 48, 49, 51, 54, 56, 57, 58, 59, 62, 65, 66, 70, 72, 73, 74, 81, 96, 97, 98, 106, 107, 108, 109, 114, 115, 116, 135, 137, 139, 142, 143, 144, 146, 149, 152, 154, 155, 158, 159, 160, 166, 170, 171, 177
Kingfisher (Okla.) Times and Free Press, 69
Knoxville (Iowa) News-Sentinel, 100
Koenning, Mel, photo, 150
Kraus, Richard, photo, 57

Laker, Bob, photo, 168
Lakes, 110. see also Nature, Scenic
Landscapes. see Nature, Scenic
Laughter, 67. see also Emotion, Mood
Lawrence (Kans.) Journal-World, 110
Layout. see Composition, Pictures
Leisure-time pictures, 55–63. see also Hobbies, Sports
 bicycling, 12
 birdwatching, 55
 boating, 57, 103
 dancing, 72, 73
 dramatics, amateur, 63
 fishing, 61, 185
 gardening, 56, 57
 horseback riding, 137
 music, 71
 sailing, 73, 103
 swimming, 134, 174
 tennis, 138
 vacation photos, 60, 61, 73
Liffring, Joan, photo, 1
Light, 104, 110, 111, 112, 112, 117, 118, 186
 dramatic use of, 115, 157
 emphasis on, 157
 magic of, 111–18
 source of, 115, 117
Lighting, 26, 29, 70, 71, 83, 84, 105, 146
Lindquist, Nils, photos, 36–38
Lines in pictures. see Composition
Lipton, Thomas J., Inc., 50
Local news, pictorial coverage of, 31
Logging, 82
Los Angeles (Calif.) Examiner, 30
Louisville (Ky.) Courier-Journal, 18, 59

McDougall, Angus, photo, 178, 180–87
McIvor, John, photo, 52
Machines, 128
Magazines, picture, 11
Malden (Mass.) Press, 53, 152
Maps, 47, 180
 retouching of, 168
Marriage, 48. see also Women's Pages
Mason City (Iowa) Globe-Gazette, 103, 117, 138
Mathias, Dave, photo, 40, 42
Merryman, Tom, photo, 14, 132
Middletown (N. Y.) Daily Record, 111, 147, 177
Midwest, 25. see also Scenic
Miller, Thomas V., Jr., photo, 18, 59
Milwaukee (Wis.) Journal, 49
Minneapolis (Minn.) Star, 30

Minutes magazine, 36–38
Models, 53. *see also* Women's Pages
Montgomery County (Md.) Sentinel, 112
Mood, 25, 59, 83, 84, 90, 93, 113. *see also* Emotion
    conflict, 20
    expressions, 36–37, 138, 139, 141, 146
    laughter, 67
    nostalgia, 28
    nostalgic subjects, 13, 14
    restlessness, 91
    struggle, 93
    tranquility, 13, 14, 19, 24, 25, 87, 90
Motherhood, 22, 45, 61. *see also* Emotion
Mountains, 24. *see also* Nature, Scenic
Movement. *see* Action
Movies, 11
Mulvehill, Larry, photo, 111, 177
Music, 71, 154. *see also* Hobbies
Musser, Elwin, photo, 103, 117, 138

Nationwide Insurance, 36–38
Nationwide World, 140
Nature, 24, 30. *see also* Environment, Scenic, Seasons, Weather
    aurora borealis, 117
    butterflies, 183
    clouds, 90, 111, 182
    elements, photography of, 25
    flowers, 186
    ice, photography of, 97, 98
    lakes, 110
    landscapes, 14, 24, 25, 86, 110, 126, 178, 182
    landscapes, farm, 40, 43, 90, 102
    landscapes, photography, 24
    mountains, 24, 60
    photography of, 25
    picturesque, 10, 83, 84
    rain, 26, 27, 144, 176
    river scenes, 13
    sky, 25, 91
    snow, 26, 62
    spider web, 175
    spring, 55
    storms, 25, 26
    streams, 180, 181, 183, 185, 186, 187
    studies, 180–87
    summer, 12, 57
    summer fog, 175
    trees, 184
    tornado, 16
    water, 19, 24, 59, 69, 73, 100, 103, 110, 174, 176, 178
    winter, 26, 62, 78, 82, 97, 98
    woodland, 58
New York (N.Y.) Times, 24
News
    photography, material for, 17
    pictures, 30
    quality, 30
Newsday, 57, 69, 133, 154, 161, 176
Newspapers
    city, 17
    small town, 17
    special sections, 60
Night pictures, 26
Nostalgic subjects, 13, 14, 28. *see also* Emotion, Mood
Novelty, 27, 69, 99, 164–65, 174
    arrangement of groups, 153
    shots, 57

Oconto County (Wis.) Times-Herald, 100, 151, 152
Older persons. *see* People
Olsen, Alf T., photo, 16, 157
Organized picture, 77–79
Outdoor photography. *see* Environment, Nature, Scenic, Seasons, Weather

Pageants, 153, 154
Painterly photos, 10, 13, 59, 83, 106

Parades, 66
Parties, costume, 72
Party photography, 52
Pathos, 30. *see also* Emotion, Drama
Pattern in pictures. *see* Composition
People, 17, 18
    crowds, 17, 18, 36
    faces, 108, 109
    girls, 18, 53, 65, 67, 68, 69, 174
    older, 20, 53, 109, 113, 140, 145
    pedestrians, 27
    personalities, 20, 53, 108, 138, 140, 142, 143, 145, 146
    personality, 124
    students, 158, 160
    as subjects, 17
    teachers, 158, 160
    women, 144, 154
    young, subjects to interest, 67–71
Pets. *see* Animals
Photo coverage, improvement of, 11, 13
Photodiagrams, 169
    maps, 168
    sports, 169
Photos
    aerial, 168
    aerial photos, retouching of, 168
    cost of, 15
    photomaps, 168
    quality of, 18
Picture
    essay, 35–39
    size, 162–66, 166
    story, 31, 32–33, 34, 35–39, 36–38, 51
Picture balance. *see also* Composition
    asymmetrical, 80
    formal, 80
    isolation, 85
    problems of, 86
    shapes in, 85
Pictures. *see also* Composition
    action in, 131–39
    backgrounds, 111, 142, 154, 160
    backgrounds in portraits, 143, 146
    backgrounds, retouching of, 167
    backlighting, 112, 113
    balance, 80–87, 82, 83, 84, 85, 87
    balance, formal, 81
    blank space in, 90
    contrast, 29
    cropping of, 79, 79, 143
    curves in, 88, 89–98, 95
    depth, 92
    design, 97, 98
    diagonals in, 94
    as escape, 28
    foreground, dramatic use of, 19
    format, 94
    framing of, 78, 78, 92, 113, 145, 178
    in government, 45
    guide lines in, 94
    information, 11
    layout, 32–33, 35–39, 36–37
    lines in, 89, 112, 136, 137
    lines, horizontal, 90
    lines, vertical, 90, 91
    lines and shapes in, 97
    night, 26
    organization of, 77–79
    pattern in, 101, 102, 103, 107
    presentation, 155
    print quality of, 30
    in publications, 11
    reflection in, 99, 100
    repetition in, 10, 83, 99–103, 100, 103
    rhythm in, 101, 101, 103
    shades, use of, 102
    shadows, 173
    shapes in, 25, 89, 96, 97–98
    silhouettes in, 12, 91, 114
    space, use of, 86
    texture in, 105–9

    tone values in, 111–18
    variation in, 101
Picturesque, 10, 83, 84. *see also* Scenic
Pittsburgh (Pa.) Press, 15
Police, 144, 159
Portraits, 140–47
    action in, 141
    backgrounds in, 143, 146
    composition of, 143
    lighting in, 146
Poultry, 177. *see also* Animals
Power, 16
Prayer, 19, 81, 115. *see also* Religious
Prestige, 11
Print quality, 30. *see also* Composition
Properties, 144, 144, 145, 146
Publications, pictures in, 11. *see also* Pictures

Quality. *see* Composition, Pictures
Queens, 147
Quinn, Johnnie, photo, 61

Radio, 45
Rain. *see* Nature, Weather
Readers, young, 64–74
Readership, 11, 64
Reading (Pa.) Times, 52, 153, 155, 174
Recreation, 55, 57, 58, 61, 63. *see also* Hobbies, Leisure-time pictures, Sports
Reflections, 99, 100, 176
Relaxation, 23
Religious subjects, 14, 19, 29, 45, 81, 85, 87
    churches, 14, 45, 85, 87, 161
    groups, 18, 54
    prayer, 19, 81, 115
Repetition in pictures. *see* Composition
Restlessness, 91. *see also* Mood
Retouching, 167–71, 170, 171
    aerial photos, 168
    backgrounds, 167
    maps, 168
Rhythm in pictures. *see* Composition
Richmond (Va.) Times-Dispatch, 13
Riding, horseback, 58, 114. *see also* Hobbies, Leisure-time pictures, Sports
River scenes, 13. *see also* Nature, Scenic
Roadman's Magazine, 101
Roads, 126, 161, 177. *see also* Transportation
Roberts, Bruce, photo, 12, 22, 23, 27, 82, 83, 84, 113, 132, 144, 145, 164–65
Rochester (N.Y.) Times-Union, 120, 124, 126, 128
Rockwell City (Iowa) Advocate, 117
Rodeo, 132. *see also* Animals, Sports
ROP, 121–29. *see also* Color Photography
    advantages of, 121
    cost of, 129
    Curtis color analyst, 127
    equipment for, 123
    example of, 120, 124, 126, 128
    methodology, 123
    newspapers pioneering in, 122
    printing, 127
    reflection transmission densitometer, 127
    separation prints, 127
    three-color separations, 125
    value of, 129
Ruder, Mel H., 14, 17
    photo, 24, 60, 61, 82, 85
Rural. *see also* Farms
    church, 45
    games, 63
    news, 41, 45
    scene, 14, 25, 43, 44, 90

Sailing. *see* Sports
San Antonio (Tex.) Light, 130

— 191

San Francisco (Calif.) Chronicle, 94
Safranek, Frank, photo, 19
Scenic. see also Environment, Nature, Seasons, Weather
   aurora borealis, 117
   clouds, 90, 111, 182
   environment, 24, 25, 26
   fall, 126
   flowers, 186
   ice, photography of, 97, 98
   lakes, 110
   landscapes, 14, 24, 25, 110, 126, 178, 182
   landscapes, farm, 40, 43, 90, 102
   Midwest, 25
   mountains, 24, 60
   photography of, 25
   picturesque, 10, 83, 84
   river scenes, 13
   rural, 14, 25, 43, 44, 90, 111, 113
   sky, 25, 91
   snow, 26, 62
   spider web, 175
   spring, 55
   streams, 180, 181, 183, 185, 186, 187
   summer, 12
   trees, 184
   water, 24, 59, 73, 100, 103, 110, 174, 178
   winter, 26, 62, 78, 82, 97, 98
   woodland, 58
Schools, 32–33, 68, 157, 158, 160. see also Buildings, Children
Schwartz, Karl F., 117
Seaman, William, photo, 30
Seasons, 26. see also Scenic
   Christmas, 153
   fall, 126
   spring, 55
   summer, 12, 57, 88
   winter, 26, 62, 78, 82, 97, 98
Separation print quality, 122. see also Color Photography, ROP
Sequence photos, 39. see also Action, Sports
Sex, 20
Shades, Shadows, Shapes. see Composition, Pictures
Sheep, 25, 47. see also Animals, Farm
Shellman, Fritz, photo, 100, 151, 152
Signs, photography of, 161
Silhouettes. see Composition
Sky, 25, 91. see also Nature, Scenic
Smoke, 112
Snakes, 18. see also Animals
Snow, 26, 62. see also Nature, Scenic
Social events, 52. see also Women's Pages
Society pictures, 48, 49. see also Women's Pages
Space, use of, 86. see also Composition
Spaulding, Seth, 164
Special days, 50, 163, 176. see also Holidays
Spider web, 175. see also Nature, Scenic
Sports, 12, 20, 39, 71
   baseball, 39, 120
   basketball, 124, 132, 152
   bicycling, 12
   fishing, 185
   football, 67, 100, 122
   high school girls, 69
   horseback riding, 137
   hunting (season), 61
   minor, 59
   novelty shots, 152
   photodiagrams of, 169
   rodeo, 132
   sailing, 73, 103
   sequence photos of, 39
   spectators, 67
   stadium, 86
   swimming, 134, 174
   symbols of, 65
   team photograph, 152
   tennis, 138
   track and field, 136
   water, 69
Spring, 55. see also Nature, Scenic, Seasons
Stability, 93, 94
Stage photography, 63, 70. see also Theatre
Statistics, 43, 44
Stierman, Dale, photo, 21, 132
Still life, 83
Storms, 16, 25, 26. see also Nature
Story telling quality, 12
Streams. see Nature, Scenic
Street scene, 26
Structures, 100
Struggle, 93
Students, 158, 160. see also People
Subject matter, 17–30
Summer, 12, 57, 88. see also Nature, Scenic, Seasons
Survival, 18, 19, 30, 45
Sussman, Marvin, photo, 154
Swimming. see Hobbies, Leisure-time pictures, Sports
Swine, 45. see also Animals, Farm Animals
Symbolism, 28, 29

Teachers, 158, 160. see also People
Technique, photo, 11
Television, 11, 64
Tennis, 138. see also Sports
Texture, 25, 83, 104, 105, 105–9, 106, 108. see also Composition, Pictures
   fabrics, 109
   in food photography, 109
   in foods, 105
   metal, 107
   in pictures, 105–9
   plastic, 108
   skin, 108
   wood, 106
Theatre, 70
   costume photos, 63
   stage photography, 63, 70
Tone values, 111–18. see also Composition, Pictures
Tornado, 16. see also Nature, Weather
Traffic, 26. see also Transportation
   pedestrians, 27
Tranquility. see Mood
Transportation, 95
   cars, 66
   cars, antique, 59
   traveling, 95
Trees, 184. see also Nature, Scenic

Underwater photography, 174
Uniforms, 144, 144, 154

Vacation. see also Leisure-time pictures
   photos, 60, 61
   summer, 73
Ville Platte (La.) Gazette, 61
Vogel, Bert, photo, 13, 25
Ward, L. W., photo, 18, 68, 73, 146, 147
Water. see Nature, Scenic
Weather, 16, 25, 26, 27, 41, 182. see also Nature
   elements, photography of, 97, 98
   fog, 175
   rain, 26, 27, 144, 176
   storms, 25, 26
   tornado, 16
Weber, Harvey, photo, 69, 133, 176
Weddings, 49
Weir, Bob, photo, 53, 152
Westin, Dale, photo, 162, 163
Wild animals. see also Animals
Wildlife, 30, 60, 61. see also Animals
   birds, 55
   snakes, 18
Windmills, 111
Women, 144, 154. see also People
   bridal photo, 49
Women's Pages, 48–54
   bridal photo, 49
   charity, in support of, 54
   clubs, 54
   fashion pictures, 53, 53
   foods pages, 49
   foods photography, 49, 50, 50, 65
   feature, 51
   texture in, 109
   foods, texture in, 105
   groups, church, 54
   groups, women, 48
   home, 48
   home furnishings, 52, 52
   interior decorating, 52
   marriage, 48
   models, 53
   pictures, 48–54
   recipes and menus, 50
   social events, 52
   society pictures, 48, 49
   weddings, 49
Woodland, 58, see also Nature, Scenic
Woody, Bob, photo, 10
Work, 10, 26, 40, 42, 43, 57, 79, 104, 138
   construction, 104
   farm, 84
   logging, 82
   railroad, 101
Workers, 10

Yeich, Clifford R., photo, 52, 63, 153, 155, 174
Young people, subjects to interest, 67–71. see also People
Young readers, 64–74
Youth, 12, 18, 61, 64–74, 69, 70, 72, 74, 100, 146, 154
   college, 68, 92

Gaashart Bros.
Book Bindery
West Spfld., Mass.